Praise for
Breasts: The Owner's Manual

"I love this book! In *Breasts: The Owner's Manual*, Dr. Kristi Funk's evidence-based advice will have you kicking breast cancer—and all of life's major killers—to the curb."

> —MICHAEL GREGER, MD, FACLM
> Founder, Nutritionfacts.org
> *New York Times* Bestselling Author

"Dr. Funk writes *Breasts: The Owner's Manual* just like she talks: with conviction, passion, and a laser focus on *you*."

> —DR. MEHMET OZ
> Host, *The Dr. Oz Show*
> Professor of Surgery, New York Presbyterian Columbia University
> Director, Integrative Medicine Center,
> Columbia University Medical Center
> *New York Times* Bestselling Author

"*Breasts: The Owner's Manual* is an empowering guide to the latest life-saving information. It has everything you need for protecting and improving your health, tackling medical questions, planning health-supporting meals, and breaking through the myths that could hold you back, all in an easy-to-read format."

> —NEAL D. BARNARD, MD, FACC
> Adjunct Associate Professor of Medicine,
> George Washington University School of Medicine
> President, Physicians Committee for Responsible Medicine
> *New York Times* Bestselling Author

"Dr. Funk has written an incredibly detailed and carefully documented book on the very complex topics of breast health and breast cancer. She lays out a clear plan for breast health, cancer prevention, and, in reality, a *lifestyle* that we all could use to improve our health. Presented in an easily approachable manner, *Breasts: The Owner's Manual* does not spare the science (in fact, it really ladles it on), but Dr. Funk makes the science readable in a conversational style that both calms and empowers the reader (exactly how I imagine she talks with her patients!). As she writes in the introduction, 'Knowledge is power, and power replaces fear with confidence and joy, which motivates you to implement changes'—words that all patients (and all of us) can take to heart, making positive changes and taking control of our futures!"

— PETER D. BEITSCH, MD, FACS
Director, Dallas Breast Center
Past President, American Society of Breast Surgeons

"Dr. Funk uses scientific facts, complex theories, and clinical experience to artfully compose and communicate pearls of advice that are actionable and sensible. *Breasts: The Owner's Manual* will become an indispensable and valued guide for women looking to optimize health and minimize breast illness."

— DEBU TRIPATHY, MD
Professor and Chair, Department of Breast Medical Oncology, University of Texas MD Anderson Cancer Center
Editor-in-Chief, *CURE Magazine*

"In *Breasts: The Owner's Manual,* I can hear Dr. Funk's straight-talking, witty voice as she debunks breast myths, simplifies complex choices, and inspires you to become your healthiest self. An important read for anyone looking to take charge of their health."

— TRAVIS STORK, MD
Host, *The Doctors*
Emergency Medicine Physician

"*Breasts: The Owner's Manual* not only provides a clear path to breast health, but a road that leads straight to your healthiest self. As someone who has faced breast cancer, I suggest you follow it."

—ROBIN ROBERTS
Coanchor, *Good Morning America*

"Dr. Kristi Funk distills the complex topic of cancer causation and promotion down to practical, actionable advice and cutting-edge nutritional science. *Breasts: The Owner's Manual* will become a cherished, life-saving manual shared among all generations of women throughout the world, for both breast health and breast illness. There's simply no guide like it—and it's so compelling to read!"

—CAROLYN "BO" ALDIGÉ
President and Founder, Prevent Cancer Foundation

"*Breasts: The Owner's Manual* is highly readable, informative, and practical. Dr. Funk is a trustworthy and knowledgeable source of information. If you're searching for the comprehensive book on breast health, look no further."

—MIKE DOW, PSYD
Psychotherapist
New York Times Bestselling Author

"I believe that *Breasts: The Owner's Manual* will change and save lives and serve as a gateway for many women to enter into a total health transformation: physical, mental, and spiritual. It is a comprehensive how-to, go-to book addressing the lifestyle issues of anyone with breasts. Somehow Dr. Funk has been able to neatly dissect, define, and package this explosive information. You now hold in your hands knowledge of revolutionary proportions. The light of this manual chases away the darkness that can be associated with breast health. Now sit back and enjoy the ride."

—BEVERLY "BAM" CRAWFORD, DD
Chancellor, Bible Enrichment Fellowship International Church

"We all have (or had) breasts, but who has ever told us how to care for them? What should you eat, not eat, do, not do—and what about all those risk factors over which you have no control? There are so many mixed messages about screening and even about what to do after you've been diagnosed. In *Breasts: The Owner's Manual*, Dr. Funk helps you sift through all the confusion as though you're having coffee with a dear friend—a friend who just happens to know a lot about breast health and illness! So grab a cup and turn the page."

—LISA LING
TV Journalist
Producer and Host of *This Is Life with Lisa Ling*

BREASTS

THE OWNER'S MANUAL

EVERY WOMAN'S GUIDE
TO REDUCING CANCER RISK,
MAKING TREATMENT CHOICES,
AND OPTIMIZING OUTCOMES

DR. KRISTI FUNK

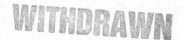

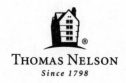

THOMAS NELSON
Since 1798

Published in Nashville, Tennessee, by W Publishing, an imprint of Thomas Nelson.

Thomas Nelson titles may be purchased in bulk for educational, business, fund-raising, or sales promotional use. For information, please e-mail SpecialMarkets@ ThomasNelson.com.

Any Internet addresses, phone numbers, or company or product information printed in this book are offered as a resource and are not intended in any way to be or to imply an endorsement by Thomas Nelson, nor does Thomas Nelson vouch for the existence, content, or services of these sites, phone numbers, companies, or products beyond the life of this book.

This book is not intended to provide therapy, counseling, or clinical advice or treatment, or to take the place of clinical advice and treatment from your personal physician. Readers are advised to consult their own qualified health-care physicians regarding medical issues. Neither the publisher nor the author takes any responsibility for any possible consequence from any treatment, action, or application of information in this book to the reader.

Scripture quotation is taken from the King James Version (KJV). Public domain.

ISBN 978-0-7852-1882-1 (e-book)

ISBN 978-0-7852-1872-2 (HC)

Library of Congress Cataloging-in-Publication Data

Names: Funk, Kristi, author.
Title: Breasts : the owner's manual : every woman's guide to reducing cancer risk, making treatment choices, and optimizing outcomes / Kristi Funk, MD.
Description: Nashville, Tennessee : W Publishing, [2018]
Identifiers: LCCN 2018000692| ISBN 9780785218722 (hardback) | ISBN 9780785218821 (e-book)
Subjects: LCSH: Breast--Care and hygiene. | Breast--Cancer--Prevention. | Breast--Cancer--Risk factors. | Breast--Cancer--Treatment.
Classification: LCC RG492 .F86 2018 | DDC 616.99/449--dc23
LC record available at https://lccn.loc.gov/2018000692

Printed in the United States of America
18 19 20 21 22 LSC 10 9 8 7 6 5 4 3 2 1

To the women and girls
all over this wonderful world
who have—or had—breasts.

Contents

PART 1:
Breast Health Basics

PART 2:
Reducing Cancer Risk

PART 3:
Learn Your Personal Risk Factors
and Control What You Can

PART 4:

Making Medical Choices and Living with Risk

Foreword

I'm embarrassed to say that when I first walked into my appointment with Dr. Kristi Funk, I wanted to turn around and leave. I thought, *There's no way this young woman whose beauty rivals Jessica Simpson's can be the doctor I've heard so much about from my gynecologist and my internist as being someone who is widely known for her dedication and expertise to breast surgery.* Boy, was I wrong! And furthermore, that appointment was one of the big blessings to come from my cancer experience. Not only was she then—and remains now—one of the finest breast surgeons a woman could have, but she also has been an inspiration and a friend to me ever since I walked into her office.

It was February 2006, and I was due to have my yearly mammogram. This one seemed to be more of a nuisance than ones in the past, because my engagement had just fallen apart five days before and I really didn't want to be bothered with something I knew would be a waste of time. I was healthy and extremely fit, having spent the better part of the previous three years riding my bicycle up the sides of mountains—and I had no family history of breast cancer. I licked my wounds and went ahead and got it over with.

A few days after my mammogram, my gynecologist called me and suggested that I have two biopsies just to answer any questions that had shown up on the film, rather than waiting the recommended six months to view the areas again. She advised me to see Kristi Funk, who performed surgery a few days later.

I went through the painful process of a wire-localized open surgical biopsy and went home to resume the business of getting on with life. Four days later, I went in for my postoperative appointment with Dr. Funk. I will never forget the look on Kristi's face when she told me that, although the odds of my having invasive cancer had been extremely minimal, mine *was* invasive, and I would need additional treatments. It was a blow of the first degree to someone who, until that point, had had complete and total control over every aspect of her life, or so I thought. And it seemed a blow to Kristi as well.

Now that I know Dr. Funk as I do, I believe each time she has had to deliver the outcome of a cancer screening that renders a malignant diagnosis, it has felt like a blow to her.

I got through my treatment uneventfully and went about rebuilding my life, personally and physically. Cancer was a game changer in the best and hardest of ways. I had to learn to put myself first, and I had to challenge what it means in a woman's life to always nurture others but never to allow anyone to nurture her. I had to learn to say no and to be okay with not everyone liking or respecting me. I had to learn how symbolic breasts truly are and to accept that reality.

Accepting these truths seemed to be the lesson in the cancer experience for me—and from what I have heard from the countless women I have met in the most random of places who come up to me and share their cancer experiences, there is a lesson in it for everyone. Additionally, cancer changed my behavior; I had to learn about self-care and quality of living through nutrition and alleviating stress.

After some time passed, Kristi and her husband, Andy, and I met about their dream of opening a place that offered a "one-stop shop" where breast cancer screening, diagnosis, and treatment happened seamlessly and comfortably under one roof. I was all in. Their dream would eventually become Pink Lotus, including the free care they provide to underserved women via the Pink Lotus Foundation. The Pink Lotus Breast Center would offer the first contrast-enhanced digital mammograms in North America, combining Western medicine with complementary and alternative medicine, nutrition, psychology, physical therapy, genetics, and innovative technologies—and offering women holistic, whole-body view of health and wellness.

Over the years, I have learned so much about how to live a healthier life through diet and exercise and meditation. I wince every time I hear from someone I know or someone who is distantly connected that they've been diagnosed with breast cancer or cancer in general. The 1 out of 8 statistic seems to hold on, but we are learning more about prevention, and until there is a cure . . . well, early detection is a great help, but prevention is the greatest hope for us all.

Over a decade later, I remain grateful to Kristi for continuing to be driven to learn more about how to outsmart this insidious disease. Whether you live with or without breasts, there is so much to know and so many things one can do. Navigating it all can become confusing, especially with all the contradictory advice out there. Dr. Funk's book is a gift to women everywhere looking for answers to breast issues and to health in general. Kristi shares what she learns in the hopes that eventually she will be out of a job as a breast cancer surgeon!

—Sheryl Crow

Author's Note

My mom was thirty-six years old and had five children under the age of fourteen (I was two) in December 1971. She was in peak fitness as a competitive A-level tennis player who swam daily when she suffered a stroke and inexplicably fell into a coma that lasted three weeks. The UCLA doctors told my father on multiple occasions not to leave for home that night, for she would surely die by morning. A priest administered the sacrament of last rites, which I believe made heaven take notice: *Oh heck no, we aren't ready for that ornery MaryAnn; give her another fifty-plus.* So she woke up! (If you ever meet me—and I hope you do—ask me *how* she woke up.) My mom remained in rehab for a year before returning home, relearning how to speak and how to walk, since she would never move her right side again (hemiparesis). All of my parents' "friends" disappeared and my dad downsized the house, but his love for her never diminished; in fact, it grew. To this day, in their late eighties, he defends her fiercely and assists her tenderly. How could you not cherish a warrior who stared down death and won—without speaking a word?

That's where I come from, and that's what I offer you. I possess the dogged determination and tenacity of my mother, mixed with the empathy and compassion of my father. So when you fling excuses and hopelessness at me, I will whack you with a reality check. And when you come to me scared and broken, I will hug you until you're whole again.

After my relationship with God, I only really care about two things in this life: loving family and killing cancer. You picked up this book. You're family now, so let's get going.

Introduction

From the age of four, I wanted to be an actress. (Ha! You thought I was going to say I always wanted to be a doctor, didn't you?) I performed in every school play, beginning with *Sleeping Beauty* in the second grade and continuing all the way through college, when I starred as Oedipus in an all-female production. Yet Hollywood was never my endgame. I actually pictured myself helping children heal from illness, using drama and imaginative play to explore the feelings and fears brought on by sickness.

Cut to my sophomore year as a psychology major at Stanford University, when I experienced an epiphany that would both change my course and guide it to this day. In the midst of studying for a neuropsychology final, painstakingly trying to memorize which neurotransmitters in the brain led to which functions of the body, I experienced an unmistakable and repetitive "interrupting thought" that made my own neurotransmitters buzz. It came from God.

You're going to be a doctor, it said. Whoa.

Okay, that was interesting. *Incorrect*, but interesting. You see, my female role models married young, and all I wanted was to raise a family and work as a drama therapist. I traveled to Africa a week later on a summer missionary trip that had been planned for months. When I saw firsthand the health challenges that millions of men, women, and children face, my life's purpose snapped into shape—and not in the form of theater or therapy. I felt newly inspired to care for people in the one way that matters most to them—by helping them maintain the very vessel that carries them around all day: their bodies. Disease robs far too many people of joy, replacing hope with chronic illness and death. It isn't right. As I sat cross-legged in a dung hut, balancing potatoes on my head to make the tribal kids laugh, I decided to do something with my life to try to stop the killer of joy: I heeded God's voice and resolved to become a doctor.

I went to medical school, did my residency in general surgery, and then completed a surgical breast fellowship at Cedars-Sinai Medical Center. I stayed on to become the director of patient education at their breast center, where I gave a number of community and physician lectures. Most women don't want to hear about cancer unless they have it and need to make some decisions, so rather than bore them to tears with medical jargon, I challenged my audiences by discussing attention-grabbing studies that would incite them to alter their behavior. I delved into risk reduction and discovered all sorts of lifestyle game changers. I loved the work, and patients responded like crazy. I couldn't wait to get to the office to spend all day examining and educating women, operating with curative intent, and becoming creative when a diagnosis or cosmetic issue became challenging. Everything I did back then and continue to do today—helping women boost their health, reduce their breast cancer risk, make sense of a diagnosis, or find their way after treatment—inspired the book you're reading now.

A MULTILAYERED PROBLEM

Whether perky or droopy, full or flat, for two organs perched front and center on half the population's chests, it is pretty crazy that breast health remains rather mysterious to many breast owners. Most women don't know much about their breasts, what their purposes are, and how to keep them healthy so *the rest* of their bodies can thrive. Everyone knows that breasts can grow cancer, which is the number-one killer of women ages twenty to fifty-nine, yet there's never been a solid and informed conversation about how to reduce our risk factors for this disease and why certain precautions might help.

Any breast health conversation needs to focus on two problems: numbers and knowledge. First and foremost, breast cancer is a pandemic concern, and the numbers sure prove it. In the United States alone, 1 in 8 women will be diagnosed with breast cancer at some point in their lives. Every year, we identify 1.7 million new breast cancer cases worldwide, with over 300,000 in the US. Interestingly, incidence rates vary fourfold across the globe, ranging from 27 per 100,000 in Middle Africa and Eastern Asia, to 93 in the US, to 112 in Belgium, and it's not the weather that accounts for these global disparities. If this freaks you out, you're not alone.

Based on my experience as a board-certified breast cancer surgeon who has helped tens of thousands of women navigate breast health issues, I know *for a fact* that we have the power to reduce our breast cancer risk in achievable and dramatic ways. Enter our second big problem with breast cancer awareness: erroneous public perception. Most women believe that family history and genetics determine who gets breast cancer, but for most people, they don't. Inherited mutations, like BRCA, only cause 5 to 10 percent of breast cancer; in fact, 87 percent of women diagnosed with breast cancer *do not have a single first-degree relative* with breast cancer.[1]

I'll give you a minute to pick your jaw up off the floor.

For the last thirty years, the medical community has not corrected the false notions held by the majority of breast cancer survivors who attribute their breast cancer *entirely* to family history, environmental factors, stress, or fate—all factors predominantly *not* under their direct control.[2] Yet research tells us that if, before reaching menopause, women embrace a lifestyle that prioritizes exercise, not smoking, not drinking alcohol, and a diet shifted away from meat and dairy toward whole food, plant-based eating, their odds of getting breast cancer are slashed in half. And for older women, risk drops by 80 percent.[3]

That's right. You have the opportunity to impact the way you behave toward your breasts and how your breasts respond to that behavior. Rigorous science and firsthand experience in the trenches back up everything I know to be true about breast cancer risk reduction and care. The women I treat are exactly like you. They share your concerns about any new mammogram finding, pain, lump, itch, or discharge. They want to know if there's anything new under the sun that they can do to ward off this disease. Most of the patients who heed my diet, lifestyle, and medical advice come away from our conversations feeling empowered and relieved, gaining clarity over "the right thing to do." Depending on the changes they make, women might also notice that their fibrocystic lumps and pain disappear, their obesity or diabetes improves, or they find themselves cancer-free year after year.

I must mention here that having an *unhealthy* lifestyle doesn't guarantee a future breast cancer diagnosis; similarly, we can never know with certainty that lifestyle choices caused the cancer you might have already had. Moreover, even women following an ideal lifestyle get breast cancer (although not as frequently, as we shall repeatedly see), and boy, are they upset. "I did everything right!"

That being said, the changes I'm about to suggest in this book don't just serve your breasts well. Oh no, ladies. They also yield lower cholesterol, better triglycerides, perfect blood pressure, fewer heart attacks, a leaner body, less diabetes, painless joints, more energy, better sleep, a happier mood, an improved sex life, a sharper mind, less dementia, smoother skin, regular bowel movements, cleaner lungs, less cancer in every single organ in your body, a healthier planet, and a longer life. If you practice what I teach, you will radically reduce, if not completely prevent, many of the illnesses that ultimately lead to chronic and life-threatening diseases. You'll feel a boost of happiness and satisfaction. You'll implement your goals with ease—and never look back.

A PIONEERING APPROACH TO BREAST HEALTH

Since I founded the Pink Lotus Breast Center in Los Angeles in 2007 alongside my husband, Andy Funk, our mission has been to fuse state-of-the-art breast cancer screening, diagnosis, and treatment with preventive strategies and holistic, compassionate care. We're out to save lives in a way that eliminates fear, instills confidence, and provides hope in a moment of panic. Pink Lotus aims to transform the delivery of breast health care in America and to help as many women as possible, regardless of their income or status in life. We see thousands of patients every year, with a wide range of concerns, and do our best to accept most insurances, including Medicare. For low-income uninsured or underinsured women, the Pink Lotus Foundation provides 100 percent free breast cancer screenings, diagnoses, treatment, and support to those who otherwise might not be able to receive any care at all.

I am incredibly grateful that occassionally working with prominent celebrity voices affords me the unique opportunity to get my message about breast health and risk reduction into the world. Three days after I removed Sheryl's breast cancer, she arrived in my office with a paper in hand and revealed, "I want to go public about this. Can you please fact-check this press release?" And Angelina Jolie's *New York Times* op-ed, "My Medical Choice," led to a permanent increase in BRCA testing documented around the world.[4] I consider it an honor and duty to continue the conversations they started.

While I'm best known as a surgeon, my ultimate mission as a physician is to get to people *before* they need to go under the knife. I do everything I can to teach others about breast health—I appear on television, contribute to our *Pink Lotus Power Up* blog, give lectures, publish articles, perform research, and sponsor campaigns. I want to empower you with facts and arm you with strategies to help you understand your breasts, reduce your cancer risk, and open your eyes to life-changing interventions and treatments if you are diagnosed with the disease.

HOW TO USE THIS BOOK

Educating yourself on breast health simply requires a commitment to living your best life. We should never die from something we can largely control. Can we control breast cancer? Admittedly, a percentage of breast cancer occurs in women who seem to have mastered all the things that promise to maintain health and wellness throughout life. Until that elusive cure or prevention vaccine shows up, our best efforts will occasionally be thwarted by uncontrollable mutations and unrecognized causes. Nevertheless, you do have significant power over this disease—let's use it. A solid 50 percent—and perhaps as much or more than 80 percent—of all breast cancer could be eliminated from planet Earth if women understood that daily choices like food, drink, exercise, weight, toxic exposures, and mind-set create the environment inside the very cells of our breasts, which either stay healthy or turn malignant.[5] Every single day, we make countless choices that bring us closer to cancer or move us farther away. The easiest cancer to cure is the one you never get.

Here's what you can expect as you move through all these pages. I suggest reading the entire book to best comprehend all the important information it contains, but I certainly understand if you want to jump directly to the sections that apply to you and your interests. To that end, let me give you a little direction so you can navigate straight to the topics that intrigue you most.

In the first half of the book, I focus on boosting your breast savvy and teaching about lifestyle choices that reduce your breast cancer risk. In part 1, you'll learn how to care for your breasts and never again mind the myths surrounding breast cancer's causes. I have spent much of the last two decades researching the connection between lifestyle and cancer, and many of the things you've heard cause breast cancer are false. In part 2, we'll discuss what else you can do besides showing up for your yearly mammogram and hoping that you don't find a lump in the following 364 days. I'll help you reduce your cancer risk based on food and lifestyle changes, particularly those that keep estrogen in check, since estrogen fuels 80 percent of all breast cancers. The healthiest meals are plant-based, low fat, and high fiber: an abundance of fresh fruits and vegetables (preferably organic), 100 percent whole grains like brown rice and oats, nonanimal proteins such as lentils, beans, and soy, with a cup of green tea on the side. I will also talk about choices like supplements, exercise habits, weight control, and hormones that can impact risk.

In the second half of the book, I'll explore uncontrollable risk factors for breast cancer, plus outline your medical choices if you're at elevated risk for, newly diagnosed with, living with, or navigating life after breast cancer. In part 3 specifically, I'll detail the operations and medications that mitigate risk. I field a lot of questions from patients about genetics and BRCA mutations in particular, and will share the latest research on mutations and what they mean for you. The key with uncontrollable risks is to understand them and then to use them to inform controllable choices. And if you do have elevated risk, this doesn't mean there is a one-size-fits-all protocol. Some patients choose prophylactic surgery. Others don't want to go anywhere near the knife but take preventive medications. Still others decide to improve lifestyle factors combined with an aggressive screening regimen. If you're struggling with medical choices, in part 4 I'll help you find a path that leaves you feeling confident and comfortable with your decisions. I will review surgical options, explain the differences between lumpectomy and mastectomy, endocrine and immunotherapy, radiation and chemotherapy, and address specific questions I repeatedly hear at my center.

It turns out acronyms abound in medicine, and in the interest of keeping you easily moving through our time together in this book, I use a number of them. To that end, please reference the appendix, a handy-dandy table that puts all those acronyms into a tidy little list.

So let's get started! I firmly believe that knowledge is power, and power replaces fear with confidence and joy, which motivates you to implement changes—changes that I know could save your life, and in turn, make the lives of all those whom you love, and who love you in return, all the more joyful too.

PART 1

BREAST HEALTH BASICS

CHAPTER 1

Breast Care ABCs

Take it from someone who's around breasts all day, every day, and has been known to dream of them at night—women can have very emotional associations with their breasts. It takes a strong sense of self, which I hope we all strive to achieve, to say, "I am not my breasts," because breasts connect in undeniable ways to femininity, sexuality, body image, and womanhood. Our feelings about our breasts run the gamut from pride in their shape and size, to awe over their milk-producing and life-affirming function, to trepidation and dread that someday they may give us cancer. To this last point, despite our fears, there have been few solid guidelines on how to improve your breast health, lower your risk of getting cancer, optimize your outcomes if you're faced with a diagnosis, and make informed medical choices after treatment—until now.

I'd like to start off here with a few basics about breast health: the parts and functions of your breasts, surprising facts about the "girls," and how to take good care of them so you live a long, vibrant life. Understanding the breasts you're caring for will ultimately go a long way to reducing their cancer risk. While you can't control all your risk factors—some, like being a woman and getting older, are nonnegotiable—you can influence and reduce more than you may know by recognizing the factors that *are* under your control and then adjusting your life choices accordingly.

BREASTS 101

When it comes to your chest's general anatomy, breasts remind me of a funky Jell-O fruit salad. Imagine one of your breasts as many bunches of grapes that you're holding by the top of the largest stems (at the nipple). As you picture these bunches, see all the tiny connecting stems as the tubes that carry milk out of the nipple during lactation (they exist whether you ever get pregnant or not). The stems all connect to grapes, which represent the milk-producing lobules of your breast. The entire breast has fifteen to twenty lobes (grape bunches), and all the stems coalesce toward the nipple, with eight to twelve milk ducts opening on your nipple's surface.

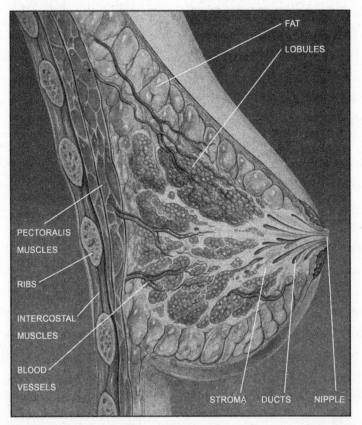

Patrick J. Lynch, medical illustrator; C. Carl Jaffe, MD, cardiologist. https://commons .wikimedia.org/wiki/File:Breast_anatomy_normal.jpg.

Now, push that entire bunch of grapes and stems, which together comprise what we call *glandular tissue,* into a mold of Jell-O that's shaped like your breast and sits on top of your chest wall muscles. (By the way, imagine if Tupperware *actually* made breast molds. They'd make a killing at "bye-bye breast" parties—or as one of my patients called hers, "Ta-ta, ta-tas!") The Jell-O represents the supportive structures that surround the breast gland, composed of stroma (a kind of connective tissue), adipose tissue (fat), ligaments, lymphatics, and blood vessels. The lobules and ducts, or grapes and stems, are usually what become cancerous (milk ducts alone are responsible for 75 percent of all breast cancers), but the Jell-O rarely does. For example, a Mayo Clinic review of all breast cancers in women over fifty-nine years old showed that a stromal-based breast cancer, called primary breast sarcoma, accounted for only 0.0006 percent of breast malignancies.[1]

Breasts range in size from absent, as seen in a rare disease called Poland Syndrome, to ones that swing down to your knees. Cups go from AAA to L—with the average American cup size being a D; Russia, Sweden, Norway, and Finland have cup sizes larger than D; Australia, France, Italy, the UK, Canada, and South America average a C; in Africa and Asia, women are A/B. Few women have a perfect match. In most, the left breast is up to 20 percent larger than the right (sudden one-sided changes in size are not normal, so if that happens, see your doctor). Your breast size and "perkiness" mostly come from a genetic patchwork of markers handed down from both of your parents to you, plus nutrition and the influence of estrogen, progesterone, insulin, and growth factors during your early years, puberty, pregnancy, lactation, and menopause. Fatness, exercise, aging, skin quality, and hormone use also influence size and shape. Since your breasts contain a genetically predetermined amount of fat, your breasts expand when you do. And contrary to what you may have heard, there's no direct connection between the size of your breasts and your risk of getting breast cancer.

Your actual breast takes up more space on your body than you probably realize—a point to keep in mind when you do your breast exam every month, as I'll discuss next. The girls aren't limited to the two fleshy mounds nestled into your bra. Each breast technically goes all the way up to your collarbone (the *clavicle* superiorly), centrally to your breastbone (the *sternum* medially), down to the curve you associate with being the bottom of your breast (the *inframammary fold* inferiorly), and off to the side of your chest wall (the anterior border of the *latissimus dorsi muscle* laterally). Another bit of breast tissue extends like the point of a teardrop toward the armpit, called the *axillary tail*, located just beneath the hair-bearing part of your axilla. Sometimes this tissue actually extends into the armpit itself, which is called *axillary accessory breast tissue*. When rather pronounced, it bulges out, covered by skin. Depending on whether this happens on one or both sides, you might feel as though you have three or four breasts. An axillary accessory nipple could even connect that breast tissue to your skin, and yes, this means you could actually breastfeed from your triple nipple one day.

All breasts are lumpy, not just cancerous ones. Who in the world ever referred to breasts as melons? Did that person ever feel a breast before? Melons are uniformly firm, round, and very smooth—and they don't budge when you poke them. The natural terrain of the breast is more like a mountain range with peaks and valleys covered in a blanket of snow (fat) and then wrapped in skin. When you run your fingers across that skin, the snow feels soft until you push deep enough to feel a mountain peak, and with a valley on both sides, that peak sure feels like a lump. The only way to trust that that's a mountain and not a malignant intruder is to either see a doctor, or to know that it's been there forever and it's just your normal anatomy. All breasts have lumps, breasts *are* lumps, and they feel lumpy. The denser your tissue, the lumpier you feel. Genetics determine breast density, as do the estrogen levels in your body.

Lastly, there's the surface of the breast. Arteries and veins circulate blood flow to nourish the breast skin, and in lighter-skinned ladies, sometimes we can see the veins rather clearly; also, conditions that increase blood flow will dilate those veins, making them more apparent—especially after exercise, or during pregnancy, or in certain cancers. Nipples can be dark or light, smooth or textured, pointing out, level, or inward, and range in size from flat to a pencil eraser or sugar cubes—it's all normal. The colored skin around the nipple base is called the *areola*, and its diameter varies from dimes to saucers, generally 1.5 inches to 4 inches (4–10 centimeters). Some people have additional nipples, called supernumerary nipples, located along two vertical "milk line" arcs from the armpits to the normal nipples to the left and right groin. Occurring in 1 per 8,000 people, these either look like flat moles or have a raised bump.[2] Celebs with extra nipples include Mark Wahlberg (three) and Harry Styles (four), so no shame there.

If you zoom in on the areola, there's so much more to see. All women have hairs that grow at the areolar edge coming from hair follicles. We have fifty million follicles on our skin, so sometimes a few unwelcome strays grow right there. They usually show up in response to hormone changes: puberty, pregnancy, menstruation, menopause, or birth control pills. You can safely tweeze them out or get electrolysis. Tweezing sometimes leads to ingrown hairs, which then cause tiny raised pimples and white sebum to collect. Makes you wonder why you thought tweezing would make the area *more* attractive. Areolar bumps called Montgomery glands are tiny sebaceous glands whose function is to lubricate the nipple (per textbooks), but since that seems like a fairly useless function and doesn't even make sense anatomically since they are not *on* the nipple, I just tell people they are normal and benign and won't go away no matter how much you squeeze them. You can also get tiny blackheads at the edge of the areola; just wash the area and occasionally exfoliate as you would do to your face at night. If you notice an itchy, scaly, flaky rash on your nipple or areola, call your doctor.

MORE NIPPLE FUN FACTS!

- Some people are born without nipples, which is called *athelia*. There are about seven thousand diagnosed cases worldwide.
- Nipple stimulation and genital stimulation affect the same part of the brain. One-third of women can reach orgasm solely through having their nips caressed.

- If you use a magnifying glass to examine the areola, you will find hairs growing on the areolar border of all adult living human beings.
- When supernumerary nipples occur outside the milk line, they're called *ectopic*, and can be as far from your chest as the sole of your foot.
- Why do men have nipples? Because we all start out as girls! Nipples show up in utero before sex organs do. And then they just stick around (and out).

GET HANDSY IN THE NAME OF HEALTH

Healthy breasts require regular at-home breast exams, but don't let them stress you out. The goal here is to get a lay of the land and learn what all your lumps feel like. This way, if you develop something new or different, you'll be the first to find it. Next to risk reduction, early detection ranks second as our best defense against cancer. I suggest starting a self-exam routine in your teens and doing one every month. Teenagers virtually never get breast cancer, but it helps them later to be familiar with their breasts now. Whatever your age, time exams to one week after your period since that's when they're the least lumpy, tender, and confusing. If you don't menstruate anymore, make the first day of every month your exam day. The whole exam should take three minutes, and it may just be the most reassuring part of your day. If anything seems out of the ordinary, trust your intuition and see your doctor. Ready?

1. First, give your breasts a good stare. Disrobe from the waist up, stand in front of a mirror, and then scrutinize the breasts peering back at you. Visually scan them for shape, size, or contour changes, plus skin alterations like thickening, redness, dimpling, retraction, and bulging out. Your nipples should be pointing the way they always point—straight ahead, left, right, naturally inverted, or headed south checking for spare change on the floor.

2. Next, check to see if your breast tissue dimples or bulges out while watching your breasts in the mirror in two different positions. In the first posture, put your hands on your hips and push in so that you're flexing your chest muscles. Any funny dents or bumps? In the second pose, raise both hands overhead like you're getting arrested. All clear?

3. Exam time! Either reclining on your bed or standing in the shower—whatever is comfortable for you—put a little lotion or shower gel on your fingers to help them glide across the breast tissue. Pick one of the following four patterns to trace over your breast tissue: (1) up and down the length of the breast vertically, (2) left to right across the breast like words on a page, (3) concentrically in circles like a target sign, or (4) radially like spokes on a wheel. Whatever pattern you choose, the results will be the same—just be sure to use the same technique every month so your fingers develop an unconscious memory of the tissue.

4. Start with your left breast, and raise that left arm behind your head to flatten the tissue as much as you can (I know—some breasts are way too floppy to flatten). Use the fat pads of the three middle fingers on your right hand to do the exam. You're feeling for a new lump or thickening. Start in your armpit, then transition to the upper outer part of your breast and make tiny circles gliding across the breast until you've evaluated the entire breast in whatever pattern you chose from number 3 above. Don't ever lift your fingers off your breast skin as you do this. Repeat the entire exam three times—first with a light touch, then medium, then deeper still.

5. Gently squeeze your nipple a few seconds. At some point in your life, you will probably elicit discharge from your nipples due to tiny amounts of fluid always present in the breast ducts. It's normal to have discharge when you squeeze or stimulate the nipples, but fluid should never come out by itself without touching the nipple

(e.g., staining your bra cup or PJs). If you squeeze out bloody or clear-like-water fluid, or if discharge is spontaneous, see your doctor. I don't care about *non*spontaneous discharge that's any color other than bloody or clear like water.

6. Repeat on your right breast. You're done for the month!

7. Visit easybreastexam.com to watch a demonstration video.

WHAT TO LOOK FOR DURING A BREAST SELF-EXAM (BSE)

In 2017 an image from Worldwide Breast Cancer depicting bright, cheerful lemons in an egg carton went viral with the caption "What Breast Cancer Can Look & Feel Like."

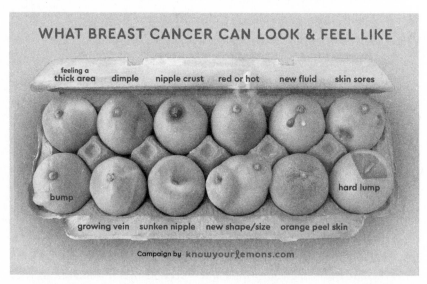

Worldwide Breast Cancer, "What Breast Cancer Can Look & Feel Like," © Worldwide Breast Cancer, 2017. Used by permission. Knowyourlemons.org.

So smart. I love this! Certain signs of breast cancer are seen and not felt, so they should be *seen*. It's said a picture is worth a thousand words. And looking at lemons, well . . . they don't make you squirm or feel embarrassed, and it's hard not to associate these yellow balls of fruit with sunshine and lemonade.

Here's the list of signs shown in the picture:

- a thick area
- a dimple
- nipple with crusting, itching, pain, rash, cracks, peeling, flaking, scaly, or bleeding skin
- redness or heat
- new fluid from the nipple (especially bloody/brown or clear like water)
- skin sores (that are not typical skin conditions)
- a bump
- a growing vein
- a sunken nipple that is pointing in a new direction, getting flatter, or inverting (retracting inward)
- a change in size or shape (especially one side only)
- skin that looks like an orange peel (larger pores, orange/red discoloration)
- a hard lump deeper inside the breast

Also worth noting:

- swelling or lumps where lymph nodes are located: armpit, around the collarbone, in your neck
- pain or tenderness in one spot, constant, not changing with your periods

Any one of these findings is a good enough reason to check in with your doctor. No one will think you're paranoid, and most times we discover a noncancerous reason behind the signs. So if your breast reminds you of one of those lemons in the egg carton, get it checked out. On the other hand, don't fret that finding breast cancer is all up to you. That's why you get breast imaging and annual breast exams with your doctor.

BREAST HEALTH BY THE DECADE

Though you can improve your breast health at any age, you'll want to keep a certain level of vigilance in mind based on where you are in life. Let's take a look at my recommendations for optimal breast health, based on the decades in life. The median age for breast cancer in the United States is sixty-two years old, so half of women are diagnosed at or after sixty-two, and half before sixty-two; so if you're at, over, or under sixty-two, I want you to pay attention.

As a teenager, you're in a sweet spot for breast health. With a lifetime of conscientious habits ahead, I don't want you to worry about your breasts as they develop. Learn to do a breast self-exam (BSE) and do it every month, one week after your period starts, because the younger you learn to recognize lumps and bumps, the more familiar you will be with any changes that occur in the future. My unforgettable friend Mary Ann Wasil began the Get In Touch foundation to help young girls demystify and understand their breasts by teaching them the potentially lifesaving skill of breast self-exam. Check out their site, getintouchfoundation.org, to learn creative ways to spread knowledge and skill regarding BSE.

If you have a family history of breast cancer prior to age fifty, your mother or father (whoever is blood-related to the person with cancer) should schedule a genetic counseling and risk assessment visit for her/himself, the result of which will further inform you about your own risks. Know, though, that breast cancer as a teen is a reportable phenomenon, with chances being less than one in a million.

Women in their twenties and thirties need to take breast health more seriously than they did when they were younger. If this is you, do your BSE once a month, one week after your period starts or the first day of every month if you do not have a period. Visit the gynecologist for an in-office manual exam, called a clinical breast exam (CBE), every three years, plus schedule a genetic counseling and risk assessment visit if it's appropriate due to family cancers. Women under the age of forty with breast cancer have more aggressive tumors, so it's crucial to stay aware.

A decade or two later, in your forties, continue doing a BSE once a month, but start seeing your gynecologist *annually* for a CBE for the rest of your life. You'll also need to add a mammogram once a year, and if your breasts are dense, get an ultrasound too. And from here on out, that's the deal, ladies, whether you're in your fifties, seventies, or nineties.

If you're considered *high risk*, we layer a little extra on top of all this advice. Various factors determine what makes a woman high risk, with the most outstanding being whether any marker lesions have been identified in your own breast tissue, and how many of your relatives have had breast cancer, especially under age fifty. If this sounds like you, take our anonymous, free genetics quiz at pinklotus.com/genequiz. Talk to your doctor about more frequent testing beginning ten years prior to the age of your youngest relative with cancer, and be sure to inquire about CBE twice a year, annual mammograms, and possibly ultrasound and/or breast MRI. You might also want to discuss the benefits of risk-reducing medications and operations. More on this in part 3.

WHAT IT MEANS TO LOWER YOUR RISK FACTORS

We're going to spend a lot of time discussing risk factors for breast cancer in this book, so I want to be sure you understand what I'm talking about straight away. Simply put, a risk factor is anything that increases your chance of getting a disease, but does not definitely cause the disease. We don't understand all of what causes breast cancer, so it's impossible to eliminate every last variable and declare, "There, I prevented it!" with the same assurance that you could cry, "Five in a row. Bingo!" In that way, prevention doesn't exist, but risk reduction does—and you, my friend, are in the driver's seat.

Think of it this way: driving fast doesn't automatically mean you will have a car accident, but it certainly increases the odds. Car accidents are caused by the collision of a vehicle with something else, and driving fast is just one risk factor for collisions. Deciding to drive fast backwards while also texting on a dark road in the rain combines multiple risk factors for a collision, but the actual cause would still be the undeniable imprint of that tree trunk smashed into your car trunk.

So how do you avoid colliding with breast cancer? Know your breasts, understand what they're about, and take good care of them. This last point includes making the strategic and rather simple dietary and lifestyle improvements I outline in this book. After all, as I mentioned in my intro, researchers find that among women who, prior to menopause, (1) exercise, (2) don't drink alcohol, (3) don't smoke, and (4) shift their diet away from meat and dairy toward whole food, plant-based eating slash their odds of getting breast cancer in half. And postmenopausal women's odds are sliced by 80 percent. In the medical world, this represents an incredible triumph when you consider that women endure chemotherapy for a mere 10 percent average improvement in survival over those skipping chemo.

How has all this powerful information eluded you so far? It's hardly your fault. Evidence-based advice on breast health, particularly when it comes to cancer prevention, is publicly doled out in drips and drabs—a magazine article here, a brief morning show segment there. And when we do hear a tip, it's often in isolation and gets lost in the shuffle of everyday life. So you might find out that consuming cinnamon improves breast health, but who, with so many spinning plates, remembers to make this part of her daily diet—and without guidance, who actually knows how? Our daily habits are set in stone or bring us comfort, so it's hard to make changes to an established routine. But I will show you how.

I also need to point a manicured finger at our flawed educational system. During my four years of undergrad, four years of med school, five years of general surgery training, and my surgical breast fellowship, nutrition was a fleeting mention in the form of the Krebs cycle in the middle of one lecture—and for many of us physicians, that was twenty to forty years ago. Most doctors do not explore the science of eating or the impact of lifestyle choices to the degree that knowledge affects *their own behavior*, let alone yours. I know this is true because when I shared some of this book's content with my cancer patients, countless times I heard, "Wow, I had no idea. You know, I asked my doctors what I should do and eat now that treatment has ended, and they just told me, 'You did everything you were supposed to do. You're fine; don't worry about it. Live your life.'" Not so, my friend. You're not done yet.

Even when doctors do recognize the nutrition–illness connection, part of the reason they don't tell you much is a reimbursement issue. Just as insurance companies don't pay for your gym membership, weight-loss program, or stress management course, they don't reimburse us doctors to spend time detailing preventive strategies. Doctors already need to stay up-to-date on what you expect from them, like screening guidelines and the best treatments for all the diseases they handle, which leaves no time for researching and dispensing extra freebies like, "Hey, did you know that three cups of green tea a day cuts breast cancer risk in half?" (By the way, did you?)

So when you put all that together, the question isn't how did you *not* know this—but how could you have possibly known at all? Nobody's taught you to connect food and lifestyle to breast health the same way you might relate it to, say, the strength of your heart or brain. Which is funny, because your breasts coexist with the same body as these vital organs. The good news is that food science matters now more than ever, as the global health outlook becomes increasingly dismal. Both patients and doctors are becoming more interested in how nutrition and lifestyle affect risk reduction, causation, and reversal of disease processes.

Of course, my central concern right now is your breasts (well, and your heart, since the number-one killer of women is heart disease; lucky you, my advice helps both problems). Up to 90 percent of the risk factors that determine optimal breast health lie entirely in your hands—so *you* are in control of you. Not your doctors, genes, or fate. You are with your breasts all day long, every single day. If you spent that much time with anything or anyone—a child, a spouse, a pet, even a car—you'd make sure they were in good shape.

Why treat your breasts any differently?

TRUE, THAT'S FALSE

In coming chapters, we'll discuss how to keep your breasts and body as healthy as they can be, but first let's set the record straight on what does *not* cause breast cancer. Myths abound out there that puzzle my patients and the public, and they don't hold up in studies. (Quoting studies is a theme you'll find throughout this book because the pervasiveness of myths is such a peeve of mine.) If you're aiming for optimal breast health, there's no room for bogus claims.

CHAPTER 2

Debunking Breast
Cancer Myths

In this book, we'll talk at length about how to eat, drink, exercise, and behave in ways that optimize breast health and reduce your risk of cancer—all supported by credible, exciting research. But for as much useful information that's out there, way too many myths persist that confuse and distract us from what we need to know. I can't tell you how often patients come to me paralyzed with fear because they've read or heard that something they've done in the past—or currently do—will ruin their health. Genetic myths, hormone-related myths, dietary myths, environmental myths: I could play volleyball all day with all the false ideas flying around—set up, smash, repeat.

I know, I shouldn't be carrying my cell phone in my shirt pocket . . .

My nutritionist said to eat grass-fed beef. That reduces cancer, right?

Did my IVF drugs give me this breast lump?

Oh, ladies. Let's let go of the anxiety and misinformation you've unwittingly come to trust and start implementing the meaningful changes that science shows will help you live a longer and more vibrant life. It's time to debunk the most common breast myths that have kept your armpits smelling and your cell phone ten feet from your wireless bra.

THE TRUTH ABOUT GENES, GENDER, AND DESTINY

As I've mentioned, genetics play a less important role than you probably think. Consider this fact: the identical twin sister of a woman with breast cancer has only a 20 percent chance of getting breast cancer one day—which, by the way, is the same risk as anyone with an affected sister.[1] Since these twins share the exact same DNA, if genetics called all the cancer shots, risk should approach 100 percent—but it doesn't, because genes aren't the be-all end-all many people think they are.

Patient after patient tells me that there isn't any breast cancer in her family, so she's not really at risk. Yet 87 percent of women diagnosed with breast cancer do not have a *single* first-degree relative with breast cancer. In fact, only 5 to 10 percent of breast cancers currently prove to be hereditary, meaning that they occur because abnormal gene mutations pass from parent to child.

Of course, a vitally important part of assessing your risk includes genetic screening and family history, and I encourage every woman to use the free test on our website to see whether further testing would be warranted (pinklotus.com/genequiz). But if we can only blame our parents' DNA 10 percent of the time, then factors outside of inherited genetics cause breast cancer 90 percent of the time. A major goal of this book is to teach you how to proactively make daily choices that reduce nongenetic cancer risk. Why passively await a breast cancer diagnosis when you can get actively involved in deterring it?

Patients also think their mother's family history of breast cancer matters much more than their father's. Clearly, you are 50 percent your father's DNA. You inherit genes from both sides—your maternal *and* paternal family histories count equally. Even doctors get this wrong. So when assessing familial risk, don't just pay attention to your maternal lineage. Look at first-, second-, and third-degree relatives on both sides: parents, siblings, and your own children; grandparents, aunts/uncles, nieces/nephews, your own grandchildren; great-grandparents, great-aunts/great-uncles, first cousins, grandnieces/grandnephews, and your own great-grandchildren. When reviewing your father's side, look for breast and ovarian cancers hiding in the women of more distant generations. Especially when the family tree lacks ladies, pay attention to mutation-associated cancers that show up more frequently in men than breast cancer, such as early-onset colon, prostate, and pancreatic cancers.

And speaking of the guys, most think they can't get breast cancer, but since they actually do have breast tissue, they're susceptible too. Male breast cancer accounts for approximately 0.8 percent of all breast cancer cases, about 2,470 men annually.[2] In American men, the lifetime risk of breast cancer approaches 1.3 in 100,000.[3] Interestingly, stage for stage, men survive cancer at the same rates as women; however, due to a lack of awareness that male breast cancer is even a possibility, their diagnoses usually come at later stages, increasing overall mortality rates.

Another erroneous myth about breast cancer relates to age—that it only happens to older people. While certainly less common among premenopausal than postmenopausal women, breast cancer does not discriminate when it comes to age. In the United States, 19.7 percent of all breast cancers and 11 percent of all breast cancer deaths occurred in women under fifty years old (specifically, 48,080 invasive breast cancer diagnoses, 14,050 *in situ* cancer diagnoses, and 4,470 breast cancer deaths befall women under fifty years old).[4] In fact, the median age of breast cancer in the US is sixty-two years old, which means that exactly 50 percent of breast cancers are diagnosed under age sixty-two, and 50 percent are diagnosed at or over age sixty-two. No matter what your age, cancer cells shrink at the sight of healthy living, so we can employ the anticancer strategies in this book during all decades of life.

Finally, the misunderstood stat that all women have a 1 in 8 chance of getting breast cancer is one of the most commonly quoted statistics out there. While it's correct, truth be told, you don't walk around every day of your life with 1 in 8 odds of getting breast cancer! If that were true, you'd probably have cancer by next month. Breast cancer risk increases as you get older. A woman's chance of being diagnosed with breast cancer during her twenties is 1 in 1,567 (not 1 in 8); her thirties, 1 in 220; forties, 1 in 68; fifties, 1 in 43; sixties, 1 in 29; seventies, 1 in 25; finally reaching the oft-quoted 1 in 8 as a *cumulative* lifetime risk once she hits eighty.[5] You know those pictures with a lineup of eight "woman" icons like the ones you see on a public restroom door? They sport a caption that reads, "One in eight women will develop breast cancer in her lifetime." Really, the icons should not be youthful triangles. We need a few canes and wheelchairs in there to more accurately reflect risk as it pertains to age.

FACT: YOUR DIET MATTERS—A LOT

Frankly, one of the most dangerous falsehoods circulating out there states that your diet doesn't impact breast health, which is completely bananas and wrong. What you put into your body influences estrogen levels, inflammation, blood vessel formation, cellular function, and destructive free radicals, to name a few cancer-related processes. What's more, the core genetic mutation within a cancer cell cross-talks with hundreds of other genes, turning them on or off to suit the cancer's survival instincts. Cancer growth isn't the handiwork of a single gene; it's the product of a network of genes. A human study in men with prostate cancer proved that by using *only diet and healthy lifestyle* interventions, the cross-talking chatter got turned down in 453 bad genes, and turned up in forty-eight good ones.[6] Oh yes, nutrition matters, you can bet your life on it. I've devoted the next two chapters to foods that work to enhance breast health or flat-out destroy it, but a few phony food rules come up so often that I'd like to take a moment to slam them down.

First up, wake up to coffee. A lot of the women I meet believe that coffee causes breast cancer, but absolutely no link exists between your sacred cup of joe and breast cancer.[7] In fact, mounting evidence suggests that coffee might actually have a preventive effect.[8] That being said, the caffeine in coffee isn't always a plus for your breasts, as it can increase breast pain and breast cysts, particularly in young women with fibrocystic breast changes—but that's not cancer. So if your breasts don't hurt, it doesn't hurt your breasts to love a latte.

And speaking of lattes, the idea that dairy causes breast cancer is unproven. Evidence from more than forty case-control studies and twelve cohort studies does not support an association between dairy product consumption and breast cancer risk.[9] It sounds intuitive to say that the presence of hormones, growth factors, fat, antibiotics, and chemical contaminants often found in dairy would lead to a proliferation of cancer cells, especially hormonally sensitive breast cancer cells, but the evidence contradicts our intuition. That being said, dairy *is* a major source of saturated fat, so you must be mindful of how fat influences your risk, which we discuss in chapter 4.

At first blush, the evidence seems to point toward the fact that no causative link exists between the consumption of red meat, white meat, total meat, or fish and breast cancer.[10] Hit the brakes and screech to a skidding stop! Ladies, it took my writing this book to live inside the hundred-plus confusing and contradictory breast/meat studies and really figure it out. Meat is *so toxic* to your breasts that even the *slightest* consumption of it nullifies a measurable difference between "high" and "low" meat consumers. Only when you compare *zero/zippo* meat consumption to *any* meat consumption might you arrive at the truth. Minimize meat. See you in chapter 4 to understand why.

Finally, I hear from a lot of my most nutrition-savvy patients that acidic foods alter the body's pH balance to the extent that it could cause breast cancer. But here's the thing: your body tightly regulates your blood pH to be 7.35 to 7.45 no matter what you eat, and even minor changes to this range would cause severe symptoms and life-threatening illness. According to the American Institute for Cancer Research, this myth clashes with everything science teaches about the chemistry of the human body. There isn't much wiggle room, since a pH outside of 6.8 to 7.8 equals certain death. And don't be fooled by test kits said to rate your body's acidity through urine. If you check the pH of your urine, and it's not a perfect 7.35, that's because your body constantly fine tunes excess acid or base to maintain proper *blood* pH balance, and it does so by excreting the excess in your urine.

That said, it's true that cancer cells flourish in acidic microenvironments.[11] However, it's the cancer *itself* that creates the acid it bathes in, so consuming low pH foods doesn't provide a happy place for cancer; cancer doesn't even need you for that.[12] Besides, stomach juices are pure acid at pH 1.5 to 3.5. Your alkaline water slides down the esophagus and splashes right into an acidic bath; it will not change your body's pH, and it will not neutralize a cancer cell's acidic little world. I will say that the foods (nuts and veggies) you would consume in a (futile) effort to change your pH to more alkaline actually pack a massive punch to cancer cells via high antioxidant levels, DNA–damage control, and immune system support, but it's not from making you alkaline.

BOGUS LIFESTYLE BELIEFS

We'll dive into the lifestyle changes that matter most in chapter 5, but I'd like to first clear the decks on certain popular myths so you don't think I'm skipping these.

Let's talk bras. They don't start or stimulate breast cancer, thankfully, because we need their unwavering *support*. Underwire bras, tight bras, sleeping in a bra, or wearing a bra more than twelve hours a day has no connection to risk. I've heard the claims, and initially they seem so plausible that one might believe they have a basis in fact. I repeatedly hear two schools of thought. One involves stating that tight bras compress the lymphatic system of the breast, which leads to toxins building up within the breast tissue itself, deleteriously altering the cells. This has no grounding in breast anatomy or physiology. We treat breast lymphedema (a blockage of lymphatic fluids within the breast that infrequently occurs after cancer surgery and radiation) with, among other strategies, *breast compression*.[13] The other smart-sounding hypothesis proposes that the underwire itself conducts environmental electromagnetic fields (EMFs). As you will read in a minute, even if this antenna theory were true, EMFs don't cause breast cancer.

A 2014 study compared bra-wearing habits between postmenopausal women with and without invasive breast cancer. Researchers found that details such as cup size, underwire presence, age first beginning to wear bras, and average hours worn were not associated with an increased risk of breast cancer.[14] So, ladies, whatever you feel is appropriate in terms of chest support, I support you.

Next up: antiperspirants and deodorant. You can officially slow your search for the ultimate natural substitute because no scientific evidence backs the claim that antiperspirants or deodorants cause breast cancer due to toxin buildup or aluminum exposure or parabens.[15] As a reminder, antiperspirants block the pores with astringents such as aluminum chlorohydrate so that they can't release sweat, thereby preventing bacterial buildup and odor. On the other hand, deodorants don't prevent sweating but rather neutralize the smell of excess bacteria by combining fragrances that mask odor with propylene glycol that creates an environment where bacteria can't grow.

One cancer-linking theory purports that pore-plugging aluminum compounds absorbed near the breast contain estrogen-like activity.[16] As we will review later, estrogens feed and fuel the majority of breast cancer cells. Therefore, the presence of estrogen-behaving compounds might increase the division of cancer cells. A second study suggests that aluminum itself directly negatively affects breast tissue cells.[17] But a 2014 systematic review of peer-reviewed literature regarding these two potential health risks posed by aluminum concluded that no such relationships exist.[18]

Maybe it's not the aluminum? One publication found traces of a preservative called parabens inside a tiny sample of twenty breast cancer tumors.[19] As "endocrine disrupters," parabens demonstrate weak estrogen-like properties, but the study in question made no cause-and-effect connection between parabens and breast cancer, nor did it conclusively identify how they got there in the first place. Parabens have even been found inside tumors when women don't use underarm products at all.[20] Besides, the dose of parabens required to initiate a mutation in a human breast would be much higher than that absorbed through the application of a stick or spray. Additionally, most brands no longer use parabens, but if you're still worried about this, choose a product that specifically says *paraben-free* on the packaging.

Another widely circulating rumor claims that antiperspirant prevents you from sweating out toxins, which can then accumulate in the lymph nodes and cause breast cancer. To draw conclusions that wipe the sweat off our concerned brows (and pits), we need epidemiologic studies that compare two groups of people who are alike except for one deodorant factor. Luckily we have a few. In 2002, researchers at the Fred Hutchinson Cancer Research Center in Seattle conducted an epidemiologic study to address the sweat issue and other antiperspirant-related toxicity theories. They compared 1,600 women with and without breast cancer and found no link between breast cancer and antiperspirants, with or without shaving.[21] A similar but smaller Iraqi study of 104 women with and without breast cancer also showed no link.[22]

The only published epidemiologic study with a competing point of view observed 437 Chicago-area breast cancer survivors and divided them according to underarm habits.[23] The author found that women who used antiperspirant/deodorant earlier in life and more frequently and with underarm shaving were statistically more likely to develop breast cancer at an earlier age. He theorized that aluminum salt substances found in these products entered the lymphatic system through nicks in the skin caused by shaving. However, this study did not demonstrate a conclusive link between underarm hygiene habits and breast cancer. Furthermore, a major study no-no existed: the omission of a control group of women *without* breast cancer. The studies with the most research cred always have a control group. And one more thing: girls who use deodorant and shave earlier than others probably went through puberty sooner. Strong evidence shows that the earlier periods start (menarche), the higher the breast cancer risk.

The National Institutes of Health (NIH), American Cancer Society (ACS), National Cancer Institute (NCI), and the US Food and Drug Administration (FDA) report that no conclusive evidence links the use of underarm antiperspirants or deodorants to the development of breast cancer. On the flipside, some argue that we see a lower prevalence of breast cancer in developing countries where women don't use these products. But in Europe, where antiperspirants are not widely used, the rate of breast cancer is *higher* than in the United States,[24] so it seems that factors much more influential than sweat-stopping antiperspirants and odor-eating deodorants are at play.

While we're talking chemicals, let's move on to hair relaxers, particularly those feared to cause cancer in African American women. No doubt about it: cancer-causing compounds abound in hair products, but luckily for African American women who sport straight and silky hair, hair relaxers don't make a cancer connection. Hair relaxers or straighteners, in the form of lotions or creams, chemically straighten curly hair by altering the hair's internal structure. Product ingredients can enter the body through scalp burns or open cuts and sores. Since millions of African Americans use relaxers to reduce curl—one study found that 94 percent of African American women surveyed under age forty-five had used them at some point in their lives—these products have become the subject of much scrutiny, particularly as they may or may not relate to causing breast cancer.[25] Funded by the National Cancer Institute (NCI), researchers followed over 48,000 African American women for six years in the Black Women's Health study.[26] A number of parameters were evaluated with respect to health and habits. Participants included women who had used hair straighteners seven or more times a year for twenty years or longer. When analyzing the 574 new cases of breast cancer that occurred during the study, researchers could not find any association between breast cancer risk and the duration of hair relaxer use, frequency of use, age at first use, number of burns experienced during use, or type of hair relaxer used.

Perhaps what we should be focusing on isn't straighteners specifically, but the fact that there are numerous and potentially cumulative health hazards hiding in our self-care products—particularly in African American communities. Specifically, hair products, including shampoos, conditioners, oils, dyes, relaxers, and root stimulators, containing estrogens and placental extracts can mimic estrogen in our bodies so much that use of these hair products in early life has been considered a major contributor as to why the proportion of girls at age eight who experience early puberty (precocious puberty) is nearly four times greater for African Americans than for whites (48.3 percent and 14.7 percent, respectively).[27] Check hair product labels and avoid using ones that contain estrogens, other hormones, and placenta, particularly for young children or while pregnant.[28]

PIERCINGS AND TATS

If you're worried about the nipple piercings and body tattoos you got during your punk phase in college, let me put your mind at ease. Nipple piercings don't cause breast cancer. Studies show that nipple piercings can cause breast infections, or theoretically create difficulties with breastfeeding, but they don't cause breast cancer.[29]

Tattoos also can cause infection and allergic reactions; sterile needles and uncontaminated ink minimize that risk. Unlike piercings, tattoos fall under the "not sure, probably fine" cancer category. Studies show that skin cancers do *not* occur any more frequently than would be expected at the location of a tattoo,[30] which should reassure breast cancer patients recreating a 3-D–appearing nipple and areola on mastectomy skin, or tattooing makeup in anticipation of chemotherapy-induced eyebrow and eyelash loss. On the other hand, when I remove lymph nodes during a cancer operation on someone with upper body art, the pathologist usually identifies tattoo pigment trapped within a node or two because the skin lymphatics drain ink to that location. No reports find that tattoos increase breast cancer risk, or that nodes with ink are more likely to contain metastatic breast cancer; however, ink does contain phthalates, hydrocarbons, and a number of other potential carcinogens and endocrine disruptors,[31] which, as part of a larger whole, possibly impact breast cancer risk (see chapter 5). For mastectomy patients who worry about FDA warnings to "think before you ink," pretty real-looking silicone reusable nipple prostheses come in a shade that matches skin tone; they just stick in place. An option: pinklotus.com/adhesivenipple.

RADIATION REBUKES

In our increasingly tech-reliant world, a lot of patients worry about radiation affecting breast cancer risk—specifically from mobile (cell) phones and power lines. Based on the studies available, this doesn't appear to be a concern. *Phew.*

In 2018, the number of mobile phone subscriptions (6.8 billion) approached the number of people on Earth (7.5 billion). Since these devices emit radio-frequency (RF) signals and electromagnetic fields (EMF), their ubiquity has generated public concern over possible adverse health effects. The real controversy centers on cell phone use and the risk for brain cancer, but breasts have a way of getting attention too.

From what we can tell, mobile phones can't cause breast cancer, even if you tuck them in your bra, because they do not emit the right type of energy (or a high enough amount of energy) to damage the DNA inside breast cells. In order to communicate with service towers, cell phones emit EMF. Body tissues absorb some of this radiation during regular phone use; usually those nearby tissues would be your face and brain, not your breast, but in the quest to be hands-free, many women tuck that smart box into a bra or shirt pocket. Here's the key concept: mobile phone EMF is nonionizing, and as such, the energy waves are too wimpy to break DNA and other biochemical bonds. Besides your phone, other nonionizing sources of radio-frequency signals include microwaves, television, radio, and infrared.[32]

In contrast to nonionizing EMF, X-rays, gamma rays, and ultraviolet (UV) radiation emit ionizing EMF. These do create enough energy to mutate DNA, which can potentially lead to cancer. Common ionizing sources include sun exposure (UV rays) and medical X-rays like CT scans and mammograms. For a cell phone's energy to go from nonionizing to ionizing, it would have to get 480,000 times stronger than it currently is.[33]

Several notable studies have examined the cell phone/cancer connection as it relates to brain tumors.[34] Only one of these authors observed an increase in brain tumors with the use of mobile phones, and all the other studies could not reproduce the correlation.[35] No study has postulated that cell phones cause breast cancer. If you carry your phone in your bra, I'd be more concerned about accidentally texting a photo of your breast to your boss than causing cellular damage to your breast DNA.

Living near power lines can't cause cancer either. Power lines emit both electric and magnetic energy that's too muted to damage breast DNA. Additionally, walls, cars, and other objects shield and weaken the energy from power lines. When rates of female breast cancer on Long Island ranked among the highest in New York State, a 2003 study set out to explain possible environmental reasons why.[36] One theory was that EMF caused the hike in cancer. Rather than using indirect measurements of EMF exposure (such as occupation or distance from power lines), investigators performed comprehensive in-home assessments of magnetic field exposure and only looked at women living in the same home for at least fifteen years. They compared these data between almost six hundred local women with and without breast cancer; in the end, they found no link between the disease and EMF emitted by power lines. A nationwide Finnish study and a Seattle-based study also concluded that typical residential EMF generated by high voltage power lines do not elevate overall cancer risk in adults.[37]

Similar to the EMF from cell phones, magnetic energy from power lines produces a low-frequency, nonionizing form of radiation that doesn't mess with the breast. Maintaining that the weak EMF derived from power lines could have a catastrophic biologic effect sounds plausible to most of us because we don't readily understand physics; but to a physicist, it's a laughable proposition.[38] Consider this factoid: the magnetic field from the earth itself is 150 to 250 times stronger than ones from power lines. If a power line's small magnetic field could cause breast cancer, then just inhabiting Earth for a few years should lead to a total body cancer transformation.

HORMONE-RELATED HEALTH WORRIES

A lot of women express concern that certain health habits increase their risk—most of which circle the topic of affecting their estrogen levels, since estrogen feeds the majority of breast cancers. However, a bunch of these worries are, in fact, myths.

I've repeatedly heard the popular rumor that oral contraceptive pills (OCP)—birth control pills—cause breast cancer. But if you are at normal risk for breast cancer, an unexpected pregnancy will add a lot more worry to your life than OCPs. Strong evidence from fifty-four studies concludes that current OCP users have a tiny 24 percent increase in the risk of having breast cancer diagnosed *while* they are taking OCPs and then the risk becomes 16 percent one to four years after stopping, 7 percent five to nine years after stopping, and no risk ten years out.[39] Why do I call that "tiny"? Let me make this brilliant point: if you are twenty, the probability of developing breast cancer by age thirty is 1 in 1,567, so it only takes *one more* breast cancer case (2 in 1,567) to suddenly proclaim that rates went up 100 percent. And since studies say it's 24 percent, your new risk will actually be 1.24 in 1,567 on OCPs. Pretty tiny, right?

Depending on your personal risks, the bump in breast cancer might be offset by the fact that OCPs reduce colorectal cancer by 14 percent and endometrial (uterine) cancer by 43 percent.[40] And if you're a BRCA gene mutation carrier, there's OCP good news for you too. After six years of use, OCPs reduce the risks of ovarian cancer by 50 percent for BRCA-1 and 60 percent for BRCA-2—with no increase in breast cancer.[41] All premenopausal BRCA carriers with ovaries who are not trying to get pregnant should take OCPs to slash ovarian cancer risk.

Women who have had or are considering in vitro fertilization (IVF) also shouldn't fret that it causes breast cancer. Given the causative connection between hormones and breast cancer, fertility treatments have come under suspicion since they involve ten times the normal exposures of estrogen and progesterone each time the ovaries are stimulated.[42] No evidence strongly connects fertility drugs with increased risk. A multitude of studies conclude that prospective moms using any of the ovarian stimulation medications associated with IVF, including clomiphene citrate (Clomid), gonadotropin-releasing hormone (GnRH antagonist, Lupron), human chorionic gonadotropin (hCG), follicle stimulating hormone

(FSH), luteinizing hormone (LH), and progesterone, do not have a higher risk of breast cancer.[43] In fact, works published since 2012 on the matter not only suggest a lack of interaction, but even a protective role of ovarian stimulation, as emphasized in two meta-analysis studies that pool the results of over 1.5 million infertile women who underwent IVF.[44] And for those of you who have endured over seven cycles of IVF, I have reassuring news: the largest, most comprehensive study to date followed over 25,000 infertile Dutch women for twenty-one years, and guess what? Your tenacity paid off (I hope with a baby too): breast cancer risk was significantly *lower* in women undergoing seven or more cycles compared to those receiving one to two cycles.[45] For all the twenty-one years they were followed, breast cancer risk among IVF-treated women was no different from that in the general Dutch population. There are exceptions, naturally, but they're few. For example, one notable study from Australia did find an increased rate in women starting IVF under the age of twenty-four, but that's an unusually young group to undergo IVF, and the study otherwise showed no overall increase in risk.[46]

Abortions and stillbirths don't cause breast cancer either, though a link has often been suspected due to the estrogen surges that occur with pregnancy. I want all of you affected personally by any type of terminated pregnancy to read on and know this good news applies to *you*! When most women hear the word *abortion*, they commonly consider that word to mean an *induced* abortion, a medical procedure performed to voluntarily end a pregnancy. But there's also the natural event of a *spontaneous* abortion, usually referred to as a miscarriage, which means the loss of a fetus before five months (twenty weeks) into the pregnancy. These generally result from genetic issues with the fetus that are incompatible with life, or from problems with the environment in which the unborn child is growing. And then there's a *stillborn* birth, which refers to the death of a fetus after five months' gestation while still in the uterus. While the cause is usually unknown, common identifiable reasons include nicotine, alcohol, or drugs taken by the mother, physical trauma, umbilical cord problems, Rh disease, and radiation poisoning.

Research examining whether abortions cause breast cancer should relieve any concerns you have. Data from fifty-five studies spanning sixteen countries and including 83,000 women with breast cancer show no connection between breast cancer and spontaneous or induced abortions.[47] A panel of over one hundred leading world experts convened by the National Cancer Institute (NCI) in 2003 performed a rigorous review of the scientific evidence regarding abortions and breast cancer risk.[48] They concluded that no correlation exists between breast cancer and abortion, either spontaneous or induced. They deemed the level of scientific evidence for these findings as "well established," which is the highest level achievable.

With such an important and charged issue as abortion, we must be right when declaring a connection or not. We must rely upon data that is free from responder bias. We deserve and have the highest level of evidence from which to draw conclusions. Hence the consensus statements of both the 2003 NCI report and the concurrent American College of Obstetricians and Gynecologists (ACOG) Committee on Gynecologic Practice report rely upon only the most rigorously conducted research. Ethical and political disputes aside, let's hear this good news clearly: "the totality of worldwide epidemiological evidence indicates that pregnancies ending as either spontaneous or induced abortions do not have adverse effects on women's subsequent risk of developing breast cancer."[49]

DOES CHANGING YOUR ANATOMY CAUSE CANCER?

Making changes to your natural anatomy doesn't cause breast cancer, though you might worry it would based on misinformation that trauma (accidental or surgical) upsets the natural state of things.

Let's first talk breast implants: if you have them, should you have regrets too? Whether saline or silicone, above or below your chest muscle, decades old or brand new, textured or smooth, round or shaped, implants do not cause breast cancer.[50] In fact, a study of 3,139 women who got an augmentation between 1953 and 1980 shows that, after an average of 15.5 years, these women have 31 percent *less* breast cancer than would be expected.[51] And this isn't the only such study. A meta-analysis of seventeen studies also showed a significant decrease in cancer incidence among those with cosmetic implants by one-third.[52] Before you rush out to protect your breasts with implants, the decrease in risk likely corresponds to the facts that women with implants generally have a lower body mass index (BMI) than those without implants, and have their children prior to age thirty, two known factors that decrease breast cancer.[53] That being said, implants can complicate the detection of an *existing* breast cancer, so I do recommend more rigorous screening for those who have them. Generally speaking, women with breast implants in whom breast cancer develops are diagnosed at similar stages and have equivalent survival rates as compared with breast cancer patients without implants.[54]

It's important to note, however, that the World Health Organization has confirmed a probable association between breast implants and the rare development of anaplastic large cell lymphoma (ALCL), a cancer of the immune system, but that is not the breast, and ALCL is not breast cancer.[55] Implant-associated ALCL occurs in approximately 1 per 5,000 women with textured implants (rarely with smooth implants) and presents with fluid forming around the implant an average of eight years after placement. Thankfully, just removing the implant and the capsule that forms around it completely cures 97.5 percent of women. If needed, those affected can receive a targeted antibody-drug called brentuximab; chemotherapy and radiation are rarely indicated.

We also know that while implants don't cause cancer, augmentation and implants after mastectomy can present long-term complications, including changes in nipple or breast sensation, undesirable implant positioning, implant rupture, tight scar tissue around the implant (capsular contracture), or persistent pain.

On the other end of the spectrum, you should also know that no link exists between breast *reduction* surgery (reduction mammoplasty) and breast cancer. In fact, you may actually see a *decrease* in breast cancer risk. Medical literature supports the notion that breast reduction surgery decreases risk consistently around 30 to 40 percent, with even higher numbers reported when removing two cup sizes (over six hundred grams) of tissue per breast.[56] By removing additional ducts and lobules that carry the potential to become cancerous, there aren't as many around to cause trouble.[57] Another prevailing theory as to why reductions help suggests that removing fat (i.e., adipose tissue) favorably changes the world where breast cells live, called the *microenvironment*.[58]

While we're on the topic, you should know that breast size doesn't directly affect risk either; small-breasted women don't have less risk of breast cancer than large-breasted ones. However, there's one connection between breast size and cancer when analyzing the *composition* of your breast tissue.[59] Remember, the more ducts and lobules you have (as opposed to adipose tissue), the more cells you possess that can become cancerous. To demonstrate, a prospective study compared self-reported bra size and cancer risk among of 88,826 premenopausal women followed for eight years.[60] They held a number of factors constant so as to isolate the effect of breast size. After stratification by body mass index (BMI), they found a significant trend for increasing bra cup size and greater breast cancer risk in one and only one group—the leaner women. Among overweight or obese women, no association between bra cup size and breast cancer was found.

In other words, leaner women with generous breasts have more breast cancer precisely because they have very little fat, and therefore, a lot more glandular tissue. More glandular tissue simply equals more breast cancer risk. In this group of 420 leaner women with breast cancer, 96 percent wore smaller than a D-cup, so the subgroup of large-breasted lean women at risk due to size alone is small. The vast majority of large breasts are large because of all the fat surrounding the glandular tissue (and as stated, this fat is very unlikely to become cancerous). Conversely, small breasts generally have less fat, and potentially have the same net volume of glandular tissue as many larger breasts. Therefore, in the final analysis, women should have a similar incidence of breast cancer risk irrespective of their breast volume. The majority of studies attempting to correlate size to risk conclude that no such association exists.[61]

ACHOO! CAN YOU "CATCH" BREAST CANCER?

Wondering if you can catch breast cancer or give it to someone else—whether it's by breathing it through the air, or from exposure to bodily fluids such as breast milk, blood, and saliva, or from sharing utensils, kissing, or having sex—might at first seem ridiculous. But this is actually a real question I'm asked. So here's your real answer.

When the DNA within a breast cell mutates, that cell starts to grow and divide and spread without control or order; that's how cancer happens. And that's the only way it starts. Exposure to someone else's mutated breast cell doesn't do anything to your own cells' DNA. Yet several studies have shown that many people believe breast cancer to be contagious; these findings suggest a pressing need to develop breast cancer educational programs.[62]

What's encouraging is that in 1964, 20 percent of residents interviewed in Perth, Australia, believed that cancer is contagious; however, when that same interview was repeated forty years later, only 3 percent expressed that same belief.[63] In other words, improved education about health issues can impact beliefs. We need effective community-based interventions that target the demographics most vulnerable to these faulty myths, which tend to be recent immigrants and those of lower socioeconomic status. Busting myths can change behavior and, in turn, improve cancer outcomes.

SEND ME YOUR BREAST MYTHS!

Heard of another myth and you just can't figure out the truth? I want to hear about it! Head on over to pinklotus.com/breastmyths and tell me more. I choose the best myth submissions and debunk them for you on our *Pink Lotus Power Up* blog.

PART 2

REDUCING CANCER RISK

CHAPTER 3

Eat This

"Hey honey, can you run over to aisle five and grab a jar of flavonoids? You'll see it next to all the polyphenols . . ." Though your ability to track down such cancer-kicking, life-giving antioxidants isn't *this* obvious, I am about to make your life easier by showing you where to find the best food-based nutrients to support your breasts and body. I think you'll love that they're not found in obscure, disgusting, or pricey foods. They're yummy, affordable, and located in every grocery store around the world.

When eating food, as opposed to supplements, we don't consume individual nutrients, like swallowing a spoonful of one essential amino acid. We eat meals and snacks with combinations of ingredients inside a variety of foods. Therefore, an obvious difficulty arises when trying to arrive at a definitive, "Yes, consuming 5 milligrams of *this* decreases breast cancer risk by 50 percent." Nonetheless, trends do emerge when one examines the body of literature related to this topic, so let's be trendy, shall we?

THE MIGHTY PHYTOCHEMICAL (A.K.A. PHYTONUTRIENT)

The key to using food to protect yourself from breast cancer is to understand that food holds the power to alter the following factors inside of you: estrogen levels, growth factors, new blood vessel formation (angiogenesis), inflammation, and immune system function.

Each of these factors affects what we call a tumor's microenvironment—the fluids and cells that bathe, support, and fuel cancers . . . *or seek and destroy them*. You choose. When your microenvironment cries out, "Pro-cancer!" cancer cells can form and multiply. I want you to regularly ingest foods that make your breast microenvironment unpleasant to tumors by shouting out, "Anticancer!" The ones that do so the loudest come naturally packed with phytochemicals. Phytochemicals are plant-derived molecules (*phyto* means "plant" in Greek) known to possess profound anticancer and anti-inflammatory properties that directly target the very processes that cancer cells use to develop a tumor.

Imagine a normal cell happily humming along when, unexpectedly, in a matter of days, what was normal becomes mutated by factors like the sun's UV rays, cigarette smoke, or carcinogenic foods. This mutated cell transforms into a cancer *seed*. Whether or not that seed takes root and blooms into a full-blown cancer capable of destroying your life depends on the microenvironment—the *soil* in which cancer seeds either flourish or fail. In 1974, the National Institutes of Health (NIH) funded a study that showed that breast cancers implanted into female rats shed tumor cells into the bloodstream at dizzying rates. From one cubic centimeter of breast cancer—the size of a peanut M&M or sugar cube—cancers will shed 3.2 million malignant cells into the bloodstream every twenty-four hours.[1] Kind of makes you catch your breath, doesn't it? How, then, doesn't every cancer story have a fatal ending? The majority of these cells are rapidly cleared from the blood by a functional immune system, and if breast cells do arrive in a foreign land like the liver, they usually stop dividing and perish—unless they find that soil conducive to growth.

How do we engineer soil that stops cancer seeds from sprouting? In the most comprehensive study of human nutrition ever conducted in the history of science, the China Study, the authors observed that *nutrition* is infinitely more important in controlling cancer growth (the soil) than the dose of the initiating carcinogen (the seed maker).[2] In other words, healthy cells can wear nutritional armor that protects against mutations when they get exposed to bad things, so they don't become seeds. Furthermore, even if some cells mutate into malignant seeds, by maintaining an anticancer microenvironment, seeds wither away. But in a pro-cancer body, that mutated cell multiplies and divides over and over again, as weeks turn to years, becoming *decades of growth* without the body's ability to control these cells the way it controls normal aging cells. Eventually, that little zombie creates its own blood supply to bring itself even more of the nutrients it needs to now rapidly progress into a cancerous mass that you suddenly feel in your breast, making you gasp and say, "What? That was not there yesterday."

Let me introduce you to some of the powerful plant compounds that block carcinogenic action—like sulforaphane and indole-3-carbinol (broccoli, kale), genistein (soy), diallyl sulphide (garlic), and ellagic acid (berries, walnuts)—and can save your life. Plants preceded humans on this earth, and they developed some awesome weaponry to protect themselves against adversaries like the sun's UV rays, microorganisms, and insects.[3] So we are going to pay serious attention to them, just as scientists have for many years. Plants behave like little pharmacies, auto-dispensing molecules that kill off bacteria, viruses, and fungi before these attackers kill them. Let me ask you this: If you were to *eat* plants, would their protective powers extend to you as a human? Of course they would! Folk medicine isn't folklore. The medicinal gifts of the Amazonian jungle provide the basis for countless medications sold by pharmaceutical companies.[4]

A number of natural chemicals known to actively block the birth and growth of cancer cells (carcinogenesis) have been isolated from fruits and vegetables. When cancer seeds do form, these same phytochemicals enable or disable the soil's microenvironment *everywhere* in your body—in the breast, yes, but also in the liver and lung and bone and brain—in all the places where breast cancer likes to travel. Phytonutrients include curcumin (turmeric), epigallocatechin gallate (EGCG, in green tea), resveratrol (grapes, wine), omega-3 fatty acids (flaxseeds, avocado), procyanidins (berries), genistein (soy), lycopene (tomatoes), anthocyanidins (apples), and limonene (oranges). Research reveals that phytochemicals exude serious anticarcinogenesis powers by[5]

- providing antioxidant activity and scavenging free radicals, which stop harmful things we consume and encounter (i.e., carcinogens) from becoming cancer cells in our bodies
- preventing DNA damage
- repairing broken DNA
- destroying harmful cells in our body
- tempering the growth rate of cancer cells
- inhibiting new blood supply to tumor cells (anti-angiogenesis)
- stimulating the immune system
- regulating hormone metabolism
- reducing inflammation
- supplying antibacterial and antiviral effects

THE ACCLAIMED ANTIOXIDANT

The most famous phytochemicals behave as antioxidants, such as vitamins C and E, beta-carotene, and lycopene. But what are antioxidants, and what do they do? Don't worry, this won't become a biochemistry lesson, but you need to understand the battlefield we call *oxidative stress*. Free radicals are bad oxygen molecules, acting like a dog without a bone. Because they need an electron to make themselves stable and happy, they steal it from any cell next to them, and this now makes the adjacent cell unhappy, so it steals from its neighbor, and so on and so on. What-oh-what can stop all the oxidative madness? Antioxidants can halt this cascade of free radical formation and ravaging cell damage. A kind-hearted, life-giving molecule, the antioxidant says to the oxidant, "Hey dog, take my electron. I'm super stable even without that bone. You need it, and I don't."

Free radicals are actually necessary to some degree in that they help us breathe (useful, I would say); they combat infection and can actually kill the cancer cells they help cause (ironic, but also useful); and they start the inflammatory response to injury so that your body can repair itself (that's nice).[6] But if more "bad" hangs around than there is "good" to stop it, then oxidative stress results, and when this imbalance persists day after day, year after year, your body's cells and DNA get too beat up. Sickness results. Basically, whichever organs these free radicals injure the most frequently determines what diseases you'll get. If it's your blood vessels, hello heart disease. If it's your muscles, you're chronically fatigued or have fibromyalgia. If it's your brain, I forgot what happens—oh wait, dementia and Alzheimer's. If it's your gut, bowels get irritable. If there's excessive free radical damage in your breast tissue, well . . . Eliminate oxidative stress, and you just might live forever.

The role of antioxidants in tempering oxidative stress only scratches the surface of the anticancer abilities of phytonutrients, as evidenced by antioxidant activity being just the first of our ten bullet points above. If you really want to defeat cancer, then eat like you mean it.

I have something to share that will transform your eating forever. Every meal creates damaging free radicals in an effort to digest food; that is, oxidative stress rules what's called the *postprandial*—after a meal—*state*. In fact, harmful oxidation is so high with the standard American diet (a.k.a. SAD) that most people go to bed every night with fewer antioxidants than when they woke up. How can you reverse this? Well, a study gave people a standard breakfast and measured their oxidized LDL cholesterol levels hourly.[7] Cholesterol tracked up and up, and by noon, the participants were in a hyperoxidized state, ready to chow down their next SAD meal. What happened when people ate the same meals with one change: they added a cup of strawberries? All it took was *one cup of antioxidant-packed strawberries* with that same breakfast, and oxidative stress levels returned to baseline by noon! I hope your eyes just widened and nearly popped out of your head. Imagine if the meal weren't pancakes and bacon, or steak and eggs plus that strawberry cup, but rather, steel cut oatmeal plus berries? Wow—then you would be building up health instead of staying neutral. The take home point: eat antioxidants with every meal (not just a cup of blueberries in the morning, and you're done for the day). Every meal creates an oxidation battle—fight back with antioxidant-rich plant-based foods every time you lift fork to mouth.

The Mediterranean diet (MedDiet) comes up often as a healthy way to eat, and not surprisingly, it makes phytonutrients a priority, emphasizing fruits, vegetables, whole grains, olive oil, fish, and red wine in moderation. The MedDiet theoretically creates a microenvironment that cancers should consider hostile . . . so what happens when you put it to the test? Recently, nineteen studies unanimously showed strong benefits of the MedDiet to reduce the risk of total mortality from all the illnesses we fear: heart attacks, strokes, cognitive decline, and cancer.[8] Could the MedDiet be the reason why breast cancer rates have been lower in Mediterranean countries (such as Spain, Italy, Greece) than in the United States, and northern and central European countries (such as Scotland, England, Denmark)?[9] In a multicenter study from Spain, adherence to a MedDiet decreased the occurrence of *all* breast tumor subtypes, but most notably, the aggressive triple-negative breast cancers (TNBC) dropped by 68 percent.[10] A Dutch study of over 62,000 women tracked for twenty years showed a 40 percent drop in TNBC on the MedDiet.[11] Finally, a ten-country European study followed a whopping 330,000 women for eleven years and found 20 percent less TNBC with a MedDiet.[12] Well, I'd say the MedDiet passed the longevity test with flying (antioxidant-rich) colors.

THE PERFECT PLATE

So what does a plate loaded with antioxidants and other cancer-fighting nutrients look like? The ideal meal is largely plant-based with an abundance of fresh fruits and vegetables, healthy fats, whole grains, legumes, occasional fish or lean meats (or not, as we later discuss), with a cup of green tea—and sometimes wine—on the side.

VEGETABLES

Limitless consumption of leafy greens (kale, spinach, collard). Vary colors to capture more phytonutrients: green broccoli, red tomatoes, white mushrooms, orange butternut squash, purple potatoes.

FRUITS

Eat whole fruits, including edible skins. No juice. Berries, apples, bananas, citrus.

FLUIDS

Water—plain, fizzy, natural flavors (citrus, mint, cucumber). Tea. Coffee. Substitute almond and soy milk for animal milk. Do not exceed one alcoholic drink a day. No juice. No added sugars. Sorry, soda.

WHOLE GRAINS

100 percent whole grains say so on the ingredients and must list the whole grain first: whole wheat bread, pasta, rice, oats, quinoa, barley, couscous. Wave bye, white bread.

HEALTHY PROTEIN

Soy (tofu, tempeh, edamame), seitan, lentils, beans, peas, nuts, quinoa, wild rice. Cut way down on all meat, poultry, fish, dairy, and eggs. Eliminate processed meat (sausage, deli slices). Later, bacon.

HEALTHY FATS

Healthy fats come from whole foods: avocados, nuts, seeds, nut and seed butters, olives. When using oil, prioritize extra virgin olive oil and expeller pressed canola oil.

Your plate at any given meal should be 70 percent full of fresh fruits, vegetables, and leafy greens (kale, spinach, collards), and 30 percent packed with whole grains and protein (legumes and soy). Don't fear starchy veggies like sweet potatoes and butternut squash; go for a deep-colored rainbow of foods, since the *color* contains the phytonutrients (chlorophyll makes a mean green; carotenoids create yellow and orange; flavonoids equal blue, red, and cream). For example, red jasmine rice extract reduced the migration and invasion of human breast cancer cells in a petri dish; the same thing happened with bran extract from brown rice dripped onto breast cancer cells. But white rice extract did nothing; what's more, black rice extract fed to mice with human breast cancer grafts (I know, science can be cruel) clearly suppressed tumor growth and angiogenesis.[13] So be colorful. And FYI, sprouting, soaking, and fermenting whole grains forms a more digestible carbohydrate.

A typical meal for me follows the 70/30 rule. I'll eat a huge salad with a thick, delicious whole grain base across half the bottom and legumes on the other. I pile kale, arugula, and broccoli sprouts atop this layer, and then I vary what gets thrown on next among about five to ten different foods that suit my mood: raw broccoli (always), cherry tomatoes, artichoke hearts, sweet yellow peppers, fresh blueberries, avocado, a heap of hummus, and pumpkin seeds. My dressing involves a blend of apple cider vinegar, crushed garlic, ground pepper, and herbs. But honestly, if this concept is new to you, and you need a little Thousand Island or creamy ranch to enjoy it, go ahead. I'm so psyched that your plate has all those antioxidants, you won this meal's oxidative stress battle already.

MY IDEAL MEAL, DECODED . . .

We all know our fruits and vegetables, and we even have a number of go-to faves, but when I got started eating a whole food, plant-based diet and wanted to find hearty replacements for my butter, eggs, and salmon fillet, I ran into quite a few delicious discoveries. So may I introduce to you . . .

- Healthy fats: Avocados, nuts (walnuts, pecans, pistachios, cashews, macadamia, almonds), seeds (ground flax, chia, sunflower, sesame), nut and seed butters (almond, cashew, sunflower), olives, tofu, edamame, at least 70 percent cacao dark chocolate, extra virgin olive oil, organic expeller-pressed canola oil.
- 100 percent whole grains: Whole wheat and whole grain bread and pasta, brown/wild/black/red rice, whole oats, quinoa, freekeh, farro, popcorn, whole rye, whole barley, buckwheat, whole wheat couscous, bulgur, amaranth, sorghum, teff.
- Legumes: Beans (kidney, garbanzo, lima, fava, mung, black, soy), peas (green, snow, snap, split, black-eyed), special nuts (peanuts, soy nuts), and lentils (brown, green, red, black, yellow).

RELATIVE WHAAA?

Before we chase a rainbow of healthy foods, we need a stat course in statistics. I want you to understand two important terms, *relative risk* and *absolute risk*, so you have a way of digesting the numbers I use to explain how your diet and lifestyle choices impact cancer risk.

Relative risk compares the chance of getting a particular disease when people are exposed to a certain factor with the chance of people getting the disease who are *not* exposed to the same factor. The easiest analogy is smoking and lung cancer; no one will be surprised to hear that the relative risk for those who smoke is way higher than for those who don't. So now, let's talk breast cancer and compare not eating enough fiber to chowing down plenty of fiber. Fact: if you don't eat at least 30 grams of fiber per day, your breast cancer risk goes up 50 percent. This means you have a 50 percent increase in breast cancer *relative* to the high-fiber consumer. But what you really want to know is how this affects absolute risk. Absolute risk takes you out of the one context of fiber and puts you back into the context of all women, including your fiber factor. The numbers show that women have a 1 in 8 risk of developing breast cancer by the time they reach age eighty, so how does "50 percent" alter this risk in a low-fiber consumer? Well, 50 percent of 1 is 0.5. So a 50 percent increase in relative risk takes your absolute risk from 1 in 8 to 1.5 in 8.

Indulge me as I share two more interesting ways to assimilate this statistical information. First, the other person in our example—the fiber lover—had 50 percent *less* breast cancer, yes? Again, 50 percent of 1 is 0.5, but this time a *decrease* in relative risk takes absolute risk from 1 in 8 to 0.5 in 8. As we dive into all that I have learned and plan to show you, we will use these powerful additions and subtractions to our lifetime risk of breast cancer to try to optimize health. Second, risks may come and go, especially if we step up our anticancer game and change our behavior. Sometimes it's reassuring if you look at your absolute risk over a shorter period of time than an entire lifespan. For example, if you are currently forty-two years old, it turns out that your absolute risk of developing breast cancer *this year* is 1 in 680.[14] If you don't consume lots of bran cereals and fiber-rich fruit, your risk becomes 1.5 in 680—see, a "50 percent increase" barely moved your absolute risk at the age of 42.

When you read about a risk factor, and it says you are 300 percent more likely to have breast cancer because you *drank something*, remember to relate it to absolute risk. A 300 percent increase means a forty-two-year-old with a 1 in 680 chance without the *drink of something* now has a 4 in 680 chance. I doubt you'd take those odds to Vegas. So nobody panic, but remember that *eventually* all the little trees of relative risk (all the daily choices about each food or habit) add up to a forest, which determines the health of your breasts.

KNOW YOUR PHYTOS

As difficult as it may be to pinpoint a single nutrient and confirm its cancer-fighting capacity, scientists have identified tens of thousands of phytochemicals and continue to study their complex functions. So far, these nutrients appear to be little masterminds at playing the anticancer game. The exquisite and truly unknowable power packed into foods like broccoli and berries, and then the complex cascade of events that follow from your stomach to the insides of your every cell . . . it's dazzling. If the starring role of that movie goes to a Big Mac, it's more horrifying than dazzling, but that's the next chapter.

The following cast of characters represents the A-listers, the most fabulous phytonutrients in town, and they should make daily appearances in the story of your life. Start including these foods in your grocery cart *today*.[15]

THESE PHYTONUTRIENTS	ARE FOUND IN THESE FOODS	AND THIS IS WHY YOU CARE
Isothiocyanates, indoles, carotenoids, flavonoids	All cruciferous vegetables: broccoli, cauliflower, leafy greens (kale, spinach, bok choy, collard greens, watercress, arugula), brussels sprouts, cabbage, radishes, rutabaga, turnips	• Reduce breast cancer • Decrease inflammation • Neutralize carcinogens • Slow cancer cell growth • Stimulate cancer cell suicide • Limit free radical damage • Preserve memory • Lower heart disease

THESE PHYTONUTRIENTS	ARE FOUND IN THESE FOODS	AND THIS IS WHY YOU CARE
Flavonoids, lignans, phenolic acids, phytic acid, protease inhibitors, saponins	100 percent whole grains: brown rice, wild rice, whole oats, quinoa, whole rye, whole barley, whole wheat pasta, popcorn, buckwheat, whole wheat couscous, millet, bulgur, freekeh, amaranth, sorghum, teff	• Reduce breast cancer • Slow cancer cell growth • Lower heart disease
Ellagitannins, flavonoids (anthocyanins, catechins, kaempferol, quercetin), pterostilbene, resveratrol	Blackberries, blueberries, raspberries, strawberries, grapes, wine	• Reduce breast cancer • Decrease inflammation • Slow cancer cell growth • Stimulate cancer cell suicide • Limit free radical damage
Carotenoids: beta-carotene, lycopene	Tomatoes	• Reduce breast cancer • Slow cancer cell growth • Stimulate cancer cell suicide • Limit free radical damage
Carotenoids: alpha-carotene, lutein, beta-carotene, zeaxanthin, beta-cryptoxanthin	Everything orange: winter squash (butternut, acorn, pumpkin, spaghetti), carrots, sweet potatoes, apricots, cantaloupe, mango	• Reduce breast cancer • Neutralize carcinogens • Slow cancer cell growth • Stimulate cancer cell suicide • Limit free radical damage
Allium compounds (allicin, allyl sulfides), flavonoids	Garlic, onions, leeks, shallots, chives, scallions	• Reduce breast cancer • Neutralize carcinogens • Slow cancer cell growth • Lower heart disease
Isoflavones (daidzein, genistein, glycitein), phenolic acids, protein kinase inhibitors, sphingolipids	Soy: tempeh, miso, nattō, soybeans, edamame, soy milk, tofu	• Reduce breast cancer • Slow cancer cell growth • Reduce hot flashes • Lessen breast pain
Lignans	Ground flaxseed	• Reduce breast cancer • Decrease inflammation • Slow cancer cell growth

THESE PHYTONUTRIENTS	ARE FOUND IN THESE FOODS	AND THIS IS WHY YOU CARE
Inositol, flavonoids, lignans, polyphenols, protease inhibitors, saponins, sterols, triterpenoids	Beans (kidney, pinto, black, white, green, garbanzo), peas (green, snow, snap, split, black-eyed)	• Reduce breast cancer • Decrease inflammation • Slow cancer cell growth • Stimulate cancer cell suicide • Lower cholesterol
Flavonoids (beta-carotene, naringenin, lycopene), carotenoids, limonoids	Citrus fruits: grapefruit, orange, tangerine, clementine, tangelo, lemon, lime	• Reduce breast cancer • Slow cancer cell growth • Stimulate cancer cell suicide • Limit free radical damage • Protect vision • Lower heart disease
Flavones, isoflavones, polyphenols, L-ergothioneine	Mushrooms: shiitake, oyster, portabella, maitake, crimini, white button	• Reduce breast cancer • Decrease inflammation • Boost immune function • Slow cancer cell growth
Ellagitannins, flavonoids, phenolic acids, phytosterols	Walnuts	• Reduce breast cancer • Neutralize carcinogens • Slow cancer cell growth • Stimulate cancer cell suicide • Limit free radical damage
Flavonoids (anthocyanins—red apples, epicatechin, quercetin), triterpenoids	Apples	• Reduce breast cancer • Slow cancer cell growth
Caffeine, flavonoids (epigallocatechin gallate—non-herbal tea)	Tea: green, matcha, hibiscus, black, white, rooibos, chai, chamomile	• Reduce breast cancer • Neutralize carcinogens • Slow cancer cell growth • Stimulate cancer cell suicide • Limit free radical damage
Caffeine, diterpenes, phenolic acids (chlorogenic acid, quinic acid)	Coffee	• Reduce breast cancer • Decrease inflammation • Neutralize carcinogens • Slow cancer cell growth • Stimulate cancer cell suicide • Lower heart disease

In 2009, researchers used data from surveys that capture what Americans eat on a daily basis (the National Health and Nutrition Examination Surveys, NHANES), as well as data about nutrient content from the United States Department of Agriculture (USDA) and other published literature to estimate "the phytonutrient gap"—that is, how far we fall short of the recommended five to thirteen fruit and vegetable servings a day.[16] They grouped our phytonutrient A-listers above into one of five *color* categories depending on the primary pigment of the foods in which they are found. Based on this report, here's your fun and informative breakdown of the rainbow we eat (or don't eat, as the case turns out):

- **Green:** 69 percent fall short (kiwi, honeydew melon, broccoli, kale, spinach, avocado, peas)
- **Red:** 78 percent fall short (apples, grapefruit, raspberries, tomatoes, beets, kidney beans)
- **White:** 86 percent fall short (pears, cauliflower, chickpeas, garlic, onions, mushrooms)
- **Purple/blue:** 88 percent fall short (plums, grapes, blueberries, eggplant, turnips)
- **Yellow/orange:** 79 percent fall short (banana, pineapple, peach, lemon, carrots, yams)

Yowza—a phytonutrient gap exists in 8 out of 10 Americans. Ideally, you should consume ten servings of fruits and vegetables daily (this quantity averages about five cups). While we could debate the exact balance of servings per color, a simple goal should be to eat two servings from each color each day. Choose the richest, most vibrantly colored foods whenever possible, since color generally reflects phytonutrient content.

THE TEN BREAST SUPERFOODS

Ready for the ten most powerful superfoods that just might stop breast cancer cold in its tracks?

#1: Cruciferous Vegetables and Leafy Greens

These include broccoli, cauliflower, cabbage, brussels sprouts, turnips, radish, watercress, kale, arugula, collards, bok choy, and Swiss chard. The high isothiocyanate exposure from cruciferous vegetables may be the primary reason for breast cancer reduction.[17] In order to get the most bang for your broc, eat it lightly steamed or raw, and chew it thoroughly to break down the cell walls, which then allows the molecules to mix together, creating (yes, it was not there before) sulforaphane, the superstar of all isothiocyanates. Sulforaphanes display ridiculous talent when it comes to seeking out and destroying breast cancer cells.[18] And broccoli sprouts contain one hundred times the sulforaphane of broccoli. If that weren't enough, greens also provide indole-3-carbinols, which exit excess estrogen out the urinary door.[19] A study following nearly 52,000 African American women for twelve years analyzed food consumption and found that cruciferous veggies cut breast cancer by 41 percent among premenopausal ladies consuming more than six servings a week.[20]

#2: Dietary Fiber

Think whole grains, beans, and veggies. Estrogen feeds and fuels 80 percent of all breast cancers. Unfortunately, most women don't know this fact, or that estrogen can be suppressed with a targeted diet. Fiber crushes cancer's dreams when it binds estrogen and toxins in your gastrointestinal tract (you poop them out!), improves insulin sensitivity, and releases a litany of antioxidant vitamins and anticancer compounds.[21] High vegetable intake even quells the more aggressive estrogen-negative tumors.[22] Strive to consume more than 30 grams of fiber per day to decrease breast cancer risk by as much as 50 percent.[23] Even just 20 grams gives you a 15 percent cancer reduction.[24]

What does 30 grams look like? It's three to five servings a day of high fiber foods, such as the following:

- one cup of boiled split peas, lentils, black beans (15 grams), lima beans (13 grams), baked beans (10 grams), green peas (9 grams)

- one avocado (13.5 grams)
- one half cup of passion fruit (12 grams)
- one medium artichoke (10.3 grams)
- one cup of raspberries (8 grams)
- one cup whole wheat spaghetti (6.3 grams) or pearled barley (6 grams)
- one medium pear (5.5 grams)
- three-quarters cup bran flakes (5.5 grams)
- one cup of broccoli (5 grams)

How many American adults fail to consume enough daily fiber? Ninety-seven percent.[25] You and I will be in the 3 percent. Long live legumes (and us)!

#3: Berries

In decreasing order of antioxidant/free radical scavenging power, please meet and greet the wild blueberry, cranberry, blackberry, raspberry, strawberry, and cherry. Compounds like ellagic acid, anthocyanidins, and proanthocyanidins interfere with cancer cell signals, encourage cancer cell suicide (apoptosis), and inhibit angiogenesis.[26] Frozen berries more rapidly release these polyphenol heavyweights than fresh berries, but either fresh or frozen, throw them into oatmeal, smoothies, and salads—nobody's looking, go ahead and just pop them straight into your mouth. I also love the Indian gooseberry, which has 124 times the antioxidant power of a blueberry, and works synergistically within the body to extinguish oxidative damage from free radicals.[27] You can use it in the powdered form, *amla*, as I do in my Antioxidant Smoothie recipe at the end of this chapter.

#4: Apples

Can an apple a day keep breast cancer away? Seems so! The flavonols and catechins in all apple peels and the anthocyanins in *red* apples work against every metabolic pathway cancers try to take, at least in animal models.[28] Daily apple eaters (not pie, people) have 24 percent less breast cancer than those eating fewer apples.[29] Extracts from the peel stop cancer cells in the lab ten times more effectively than from the flesh of the same apples, so eat them whole or blended, but not juiced.[30]

#5: Tomatoes

One of the carotenoids, lycopene, colors tomatoes bright red and is most concentrated in the skin. As a powerful antioxidant, lycopene exhibits anti-inflammatory and anti-angiogenesis abilities, both plausible reasons for the reported decrease in breast cancer among women with high tomato intake.[31] Unlike most phytochemicals, which are best consumed in their raw state, heating tomatoes for fifteen minutes increases the lycopene bioavailability by 300 percent.[32] They are fat-soluble, so bump up absorption even more by sautéing or roasting them in a touch of olive oil.

#6: Mushrooms

Mushrooms aren't technically fruits, vegetables, or even plants—they're fungi, but they're also delicious and nutritious. Who would've guessed that fancy mushrooms like portobello, chanterelle, and oyster have fewer flavones and isoflavones than the little ol' white button?[33] True, the buttons carry the highest estrogen-blocking abilities of all these mushrooms and inhibit an enzyme, aromatase, which normally converts precursors of estrogen to its cancer-causing active form. A daily intake of 10 grams or more—the equivalent of *half* a button mushroom—dropped breast cancer rates in Chinese women by 64 percent compared with age-matched "no mushroom" eaters, and by 89 percent when they sipped a halfcup of green tea to boot.[34] Medicinal mushrooms such as reishi, turkey tail, shiitake, and maitake are used extensively and successfully in Asia to treat various cancers. Studies credit polysaccharides in medicinal mushrooms with stimulating immune response pathways and exhibiting direct antitumor ninja skills.[35]

#7: Garlic, Onions, Leeks, Shallots, Chives, Scallions

Crush, chop, or chew them, but these immunity-boosting bulbs need to be fresh to unleash the antiproliferative and antioxidant protection of the phytochemical allicin.[36] A French study showed an astounding 75 percent drop in breast cancer with eleven to twelve weekly servings of the allium vegetables such as garlic and onions.[37] Vampires were also reported missing.

#8: Turmeric and Spices

Could curcumin, the most active ingredient in the pungent yellow herb turmeric be the reason breast cancer rates in India are five times less than in Westernized countries? Curcumin decreases estrogen, induces cancer cell apoptosis, suppresses inflammation (COX-2 inhibition), and inhibits free radicals.[38] In fact, human blood samples were exposed to free radicals in a lab one week, and when this exposure was repeated on fresh samples from the same people the following week, they sustained *half* the oxidative DNA damage. What changed in one week? The study subjects merely consumed one daily pinch of turmeric.[39] Piperine, found in black pepper, increases the bioavailability of curcumin from barely detectable to 2,000 percent higher.[40] In its own right, piperine has been found to suppress breast tumor growth and metastatic spread in animal models.[41] Mixing 1/4 teaspoon of turmeric powder or a quarter inch fresh turmeric root with 1/4 teaspoon of black pepper and one tablespoon of fat like ground flaxseeds helps with absorption and avoids elimination by the liver—and makes a great topping for salad, rice, or vegetable dishes. While straight curcumin is powerful, it shows less cancer inhibition than turmeric when the two go head-to-head against breast cancer cells in a petri dish, so you may as well reap all the benefit you can from turning things ochre yellow (like I did the inside of my blender) and choose turmeric.[42] Avoid turmeric if you have gallstones; it stimulates gallbladder contraction, which can lead to a painful gallbladder attack.[43]

Spices contribute far more than color and flavor to food; they beneficially affect inflammation, free radical formation and cancer cell proliferation, apoptosis, angiogenesis, and immune function.[44] So while we're feeling spicy, let me also suggest anticancer cooking with clove (second only to that gooseberry in antioxidant potency), ginger, paprika, cumin, cinnamon, sage, rosemary, oregano, thyme, and anything else inside the box below that you think adds zest and zing.[45] Incidentally, cassia cinnamon contains much more of the blood thinner, coumarin, than does Ceylon cinnamon; coumarin can also be toxic to the liver at doses of 1 teaspoon a day, so favor Ceylon if you consume cinnamon regularly.[46]

HEY, HERB, LET'S SPICE IT UP

A pinch of this and a dash of that can transform bland and boring into "Yummy yummy, seconds, please!" Over 180 spice-derived phytonutrients have been explored for their health benefits, so the most impressive of these deserve some shelf space, please.[47] If salt and pepper is your idea of a spice rack, try incorporating these breast-friendly herbs and spices into your cooking and experience the flavorful taste of cancer fighting:

- allspice
- barberries
- basil
- bay leaves
- black pepper
- caraway
- cardamom
- chili pepper
- chili powder
- chives
- cilantro
- cinnamon (Ceylon)
- clove
- coriander
- cumin
- curry powder
- dill
- fennel
- fenugreek
- garlic
- ginger
- horseradish
- kokum
- leeks
- lemongrass
- marjoram
- mint
- mustard powder
- onions
- oregano
- nutmeg
- paprika
- parsley
- rosemary
- sage
- saffron
- scallions
- shallots
- thyme
- turmeric / turmeric root

#9: Seaweed

Seaweed reduces the estrogen burden in the body by promoting urinary excretion and altering the gut bacteria.[48] A Korean study showed that daily consumption of *gim* (like a sheet of nori, the sushi wrap) drops breast cancer by over 50 percent.[49] Common seaweeds include nori, wakame, arame, mekabu, kombu, dulse, Irish moss, and spirulina. Try snacking on sheets of nori instead of chips, or roll up veggies and colored rice in a nori wrap. Throw a teaspoon of powdered spirulina into a smoothie or salad dressing, or shake seaweed flakes (found online or in Asian markets) instead of salt onto any meal.

#10: Cacao

Packed with flavonoids and procyanidins, cacao powder (not Dutch-processed) can be added to berry smoothies to satisfy a sweet tooth.[50] Consuming 1.5 ounces (40 grams) of more than 70 percent cacao solid dark chocolate gets an anticancer thumbs up, as it delivers antioxidants more than it does cocoa fat and sugar.[51]

THERE'S SOMETHING SPECIAL ABOUT SOY—NO, REALLY

It's time to set the record straight on this healing ingredient because it gets an unfair bad rap. Soy contains isoflavones, some of which act as phytoestrogens (plant-based estrogen-like compounds), and estrogen fuels most breast cancers, so I'll bet somebody somewhere told you, "Say no to soy!" and you spit that miso soup right out of your mouth. Most physicians believe this to be unchartered territory, so they err on the side of caution and advise you to avoid all phytoestrogens. I guess they haven't seen the evidence, so let me show you.

First of all, we have two totally different estrogen receptors (ER) in our bodies: ER-alpha and ER-beta. When estrogen from any source stimulates these receptors, the cells respond according to their programmed function. In the breast, ER-alpha sends signals to cancer cells to multiply and divide, whereas ER-beta actually exerts an *antiestrogen effect*. It turns out our natural estrogens love ER-alpha (yes, the ones implicated in cancer); but soy phytoestrogens, like genistein, bind 1,600 percent more to *ER-beta* than alpha.[52] When bound to its ER-beta throne, soy actually blocks estrogen from sitting in the alpha chair. And if soy should land in ER-alpha, it has about one-tenth to one-hundredth of the signaling capacity of real estrogen, so soy essentially behaves like tamoxifen, a drug given to cancer patients that occupies but inactivates ER-alpha receptors.[53] On top of that, soy stops the conversion of other steroids *into* estrogen.[54] Okay, if that's true, then people who consume soy should drop their circulating estrogen, right? Right. A group of premenopausal women in Texas drank three twelve-ounce cups of soy milk a day for one month. Depending on where they were in their menstrual cycles, blood levels of estrogen dropped between 30 to 80 percent in *all of them*, and estrogen levels stayed lower than baseline for another two to three months.[55] Wow, so soy really does slow down estrogen production.

With less estrogen from a few daily servings of soy, should we then expect to see less breast cancer forming? Yes. One study examined the dietary intake of over 73,000 Chinese women and concluded that consuming soy during childhood, adolescence, and adult life protects against breast cancer, especially when consumed in youth.[56] Early soy intake (more than 1.5 times per week, not much) during childhood reduced adult-onset breast cancer by 58 percent in a study of Asian women in California and Hawaii, so tell your daughters to soy it up.[57] Even among Korean BRCA gene mutation carriers, largely considered to be at the mercy of their DNA breaks, a reduction in breast cancer up to 43 percent was noted in high soy consumers.[58]

Okay, so far soy blocks estrogen effects on ER-alpha; it lowers estrogen levels in the blood; it protects against making breast cancer; but . . . what if you already had an estrogen-driven cancer, and now you're on a drug that blocks estrogen's actions in your body, like tamoxifen? Will the isoflavones in soy interfere with these drugs? Until 2009, we weren't sure.

In the Life After Cancer Epidemiology Study, 1,954 multiethnic survivors on tamoxifen (estrogen-driven cancers) were followed over six years; those eating the most tofu and soy milk products had a 60 percent *reduction* in breast cancer recurrence compared to women ingesting low soy amounts.[59] Isoflavones not only deal favorably with estrogen, they exhibit antiproliferative, antioxidant, anti-angiogenesis, and anti-inflammatory properties such that soy even keeps estrogen-*negative* tumors at bay.[60] The largest soy study to date in breast cancer patients followed over 6,200 multiethnic women from the United States and Canada for 9.4 years.[61] For those consuming merely 0.5 to 1.0 servings of soy *a week*, researchers observed a 21 percent decrease in all-cause mortality compared to lower soy consumption; this increased to 51 percent for estrogen-negative cancers, and 32 percent for those estrogen-positive cancer patients not taking antiestrogen therapy. Another study with over 5,000 breast cancer patients found a 29 percent decrease in death and a 32 percent drop in recurrence for high soy consumers, independent of receptor status.[62] Even just one cup of soy milk a day provides enough phytoestrogens to reduce recurrence by 25 percent.[63] So soy consumption after breast cancer is safe and protective.

Soy does not increase breast cancer but in fact decreases the occurrence, recurrence, and death rates in every single study exploring this matter since 2009.[64] What's a safe soy to consume? Choose soy products specifically labeled USDA organic, 100 percent organic, or non-GMO. Although 94 percent of soy comes from genetically modified organisms (GMOs), non-GMO products shouldn't be hard to find; most GMO-soy is fed to livestock and not you (unless you eat the livestock).[65] Soy is a "complete protein," meaning it contains all of the essential amino acids necessary for biological function. Strive to consume two to three servings of soy food every day; whole food soy far outranks processed, and fermented whole soy products like tempeh, miso, tamari (a fermented soy sauce), and nattō are the best. The natural fermentation process accomplishes two things: it lessens gas and bloating with good-for-your-gut probiotics, and it converts soy's powerful isoflavones into their most active form, making this superfood even more super. Tofu, soybeans (edamame), roasted soybeans, and soy milk are great ready-to-consume options. Avoid soy milk made from soy protein or soy isolate; you want to see *whole organic soybeans* written as the first ingredient on your milk label. Processed soy products lose some of the nutritional value found in whole foods but provide great substitutes for meat, sauces, cheese, eggs, yogurt, and milk.

ESSENTIALS: VITAMINS, MINERALS, AND A LITTLE SUPPLEMENTAL INFO

If your cells could write an editorial, "A Day in the Life of a Body," they'd gush about how they hold in high esteem around thirty different essential vitamins and minerals that they cannot produce on their own. Cells use these raw materials to perform hundreds of life-sustaining functions. Your cells would say that consuming whole foods, and not supplements or pills like a single vitamin, exposes them to at least 25,000 phytochemicals, the complexities of which we only poorly understand. These bioactive food constituents can work individually, like what you get from a supplement, but I don't want you to miss out on all the additive and synergistic ways this vast community of chemicals comes together to thwart disease development. For instance, sure, vitamin C is an antioxidant, but eating a whole orange unlocks other weapons, like limonene, which accumulates inside breast cells where it exerts *chemotherapy-like* activity.[66] Your chewable vitamin C didn't know about limonene-flavored chemo! With rare exceptions—noted in the B_{12}, folate, and vitamin D sections below—balanced eating remains the safest and most efficient way to get adequate amounts of the vitamins and minerals you need. Here are the biggies:

Vitamin A: Fenretinide (200 milligrams per day), an analogue of vitamin A, promises a 35 percent reduction in recurrent or new breast cancers in premenopausal women.[67] It's found in carrots, sweet potatoes, kale, spinach, broccoli, and yellow squash.

Beta-carotene: An eleven-study meta-analysis showed an 18 percent breast benefit from beta-carotene.[68] It becomes vitamin A in your body, so add apricots, cantaloupe, and sweet red peppers to our vitamin A-rich foods listed above.

Vitamin B$_6$: Vitamin B$_6$ confers a 30 percent reduction.[69] Eat avocado, pinto beans, molasses, sunflower seeds, sesame seeds, and pistachios; if you consume meat, you can find B$_6$ in tuna, chicken, and turkey breast.

Vitamin B$_{12}$: B$_{12}$ exerts a 64 percent breast advantage in premenopausal women.[70] Find it in shellfish, fish, meat, poultry, liver, dairy, eggs, fortified cereals. For vegans and adults under age sixty-five who do not consume adequate amounts of the stated B$_{12}$ sources, take *cyano*cobalamin (not *methyl*cobalamin) 2,500 mcg weekly supplements,[71] and for those at or over sixty-five, ingest *cyano*cobalamin 1,000 micrograms a day.[72]

Folic Acid (Folate): Folate works alongside B$_6$ and B$_{12}$ to engineer glutathione, the most powerful of all intracellular antioxidants, which detoxifies and eliminates carcinogens.[73] You'll find folate in foods like peas, beans, nuts, spinach, collard greens, asparagus, and fortified whole wheat sources. In the Nurses' Health Study, high levels of serum folate led to 27 percent less breast cancer.[74] Among those in this study averaging one glass or more of alcohol a day, the drinkers who consumed the most folate from food or supplements plummeted their cancer risk by 89 percent compared to drinkers who had low folate. You see, alcohol inhibits the conversion of folate into its helpful DNA-repairing form called methylfolate. Therefore, moderate drinkers (one or more drinks a day) should consider taking methylfolate (not folic acid), 800 micrograms once a day—or stop drinking so much.

Vitamin C: When you think vitamin C, you may think orange juice, yet citrus fruits—oranges, tangerines, grapefruits, lemons, and limes—bestow a modest 10 percent reduction in breast cancer.[75] When you add other vitamin C sources (and therefore multiple phytonutrients), like carrots, sweet potatoes, greens, and broccoli, you amp up the protection to 31 percent.[76]

Vitamin D: The sunshine vitamin deserves the spotlight it's stolen.

At proper doses, vitamin D exerts protective effects: more than 800 IU (International Units) per day confers a 34 percent decrease in breast cancer among postmenopausal women.[77] Bump it to 50 percent protection with dietary doses of 2,000 IU a day combined with approximately 3,000 IU synthesized in your skin after twelve minutes of daily sunlight exposure without sunblock.[78] Once diagnosed with cancer, adequate vitamin D cuts the death rate from breast cancer in half.[79] Excellent vitamin D sources include fortified milk and soy milk, fortified tofu and cereals, UV-exposed mushrooms (stick them in the sun for two days), sardines, salmon, and the very best source: you + sunshine.

If you live anywhere in the world north of 40 degrees latitude (New York, Barcelona, Rome, Toronto, Budapest, Zurich, Vienna, Munich, Paris) or south of 40 degrees latitude (Queenstown, Sydney, Cape Town, Buenos Aires), if you are over sixty years old, or if you have darker skin and spend less than thirty minutes a day in the sun, you need a vitamin D boost. Take 4,000 IU daily during winter months when the sun doesn't shine.[80] The latest research suggests that you reduce cancer the most with a serum level of 40 to 80 nanograms per milliliter, which often requires 5,000 IU or more, so at your next doctor visit, get your vitamin D blood level checked and ask your physician to optimize your supplement strategy if you need one.[81]

Calcium: Dietary calcium, 1,250 milligrams per day, reduces breast cancer by 20 to 50 percent, and up to 74 percent for premenopausal women,[82] probably by decreasing fat-induced cell proliferation, neutralizing fatty acids, and binding mutagenic bile acids.[83] You'll find it in kale, broccoli, all dark leafy greens, yogurt, cheese, milk, soybeans, fortified cereals, and grains.

Long-Chain Omega-3 *Alpha*-Linolenic Acid (ALA): For those who do not consume fish, you might not generate enough long-chain ALA from your intake of short-chain ALA (see the next section on fats). Be sure you get enough of this essential fatty acid for optimal brain health, and supplement with either omega-3 fish oils or with fish-free yeast- or algae-derived long-chain ALA, 250 milligrams daily.[84]

SPEAKING OF FATS . . .

Fat used to be a dirty word, remember? We thought that if you don't eat fat, you won't *be* fat. Turns out that if you don't eat fat, you will be dead. Fat efficiently stores energy, supplies energy, and regulates body temperature; fat surrounds your nerves, brain tissue, and eyeballs like teacups in bubble wrap; fat transports vitamins, makes steroids, supports cell growth and function, and keeps your skin from looking like a shar-pei.[85] But do you know the difference between friendly fat and foe fat? Let's talk friendly fats here.

What's the healthiest fat? An unsaturated fat. These contain poly-unsaturated fatty acids known as PUFAs, or as I like to say, "PUFA! There goes a cancer cell." PUFAs are liquid at room temperature. They are *essential*, which means your body can't make them, and you can only find them in food. You need them if you plan to do things like move your muscles or stop bleeding when you're cut. You find omega-3 PUFAs, also called *alpha*-Linolenic acid (ALA), in flaxseed, walnuts, canola oil, unhydrogenated soybean oil, and oily fish like salmon, herring, sardines, and mackerel.

Beneficial fats also include monounsaturated fatty acid or MUFA, as in "MUFA! More Fa me!" (I'm hoping my goofy mnemonics help you with label reading, which we discuss soon.) Find MUFAs in oils like olive, canola, sesame, walnut, peanut, almond, flaxseed, borage, and high-oleic safflower or sunflower oils; whole food sources include avocados, olives, almonds, cashews, pecans, macadamias, and nut butters. By the way, oils can contain blends of different PUFAs and MUFAs *and* saturated fat, so they can be in three places at once.

Pick the purest unsaturated fats, and minimally consume or elimi-nate saturated fats from sources like meat, chicken, oil (avoid safflower, sunflower, hydrogenated soybean, corn, coconut, and palm oils, further discussed in chapter 4), butter, and cheese. A number of studies confirm the benefits of MUFAs and omega-3 PUFAs.[86] In the largest study to look into the fat-cancer connection, European researchers followed

337,327 women in ten countries over eleven years.[87] They found that women who ate the most saturated fat were about 30 percent more likely to develop breast cancer.

Remember when Mama told you to eat your vegetables? Mama's always right. Emerging evidence confirms that eating more vegetable fat (PUFA, MUFA) and nuts at ten to fifteen years old significantly decreases postmenopausal breast cancer many years later.[88] The Nurses' Health Study II showed a 42 percent reduction for increased vegetable fat consumption during high school years.[89]

For more insight into a friendly fat's power, consider flaxseeds (a MUFA). They offer the most concentrated source of omega-3 fat *on the planet*, and over one hundred times the lignan phytonutrient content of most other foods.[90] Lignans exhibit all kinds of anti–breast cancer virtues related to lowering estrogen and stopping cancer cell growth.[91] In one study, forty-five women got a breast biopsy that showed precancerous cells. This put them at high risk. They simply ate one teaspoon of ground flaxseed a day for a year, and then repeated the biopsy. Precancerous cell changes reverted to normal in 32 percent, and a biomarker for cell division called Ki-67 went down in 80 percent of the women.[92] Toss a spoonful of ground flaxseed onto your salad at lunch today (whole flaxseeds go straight out the other end), or blend into a smoothie as I do. If there's only one thing you change after reading this chapter, may it be in the form of one to two tablespoons of ground flaxseeds daily. True that.

Not All Oil Is Evil: Extra Virgin Olive Oil

Just like wine, the quality of olives varies from region to region, and the processing of olives leads to different qualities of oil. Extra virgin olive oil (EVOO) ranks supreme, for the sole reason that it contains the highest oil levels of cancer-kicking antioxidants: phenols, polyphenols, and lignans. It also gets bragging rights about its high squalene content, a molecule that inhibits the ras oncogene.[93] The phytonutrient oleocanthal swims abundantly in this golden oil and bears a striking chemical similarity to ibuprofen, which decreases inflammation in your body.[94] Besides taking away inflammation,

EVOO also regulates insulin secretion and lowers blood-sugar levels, which really annoys cancer cells (remember the microenvironment?).[95]

Most studies investigating whether EVOO exerts protective effects against breast cancer conclude YES in all caps.[96] In the only prospective randomized trial (the best type) looking at the MedDiet, 4,152 women (no personal cancer history) aged sixty to eighty were randomly allocated to a MedDiet supplemented with EVOO, a MedDiet with mixed nuts, or a control diet (advised to reduce dietary fat).[97] At 4.8 years follow-up, thirty-five breast cancers developed (eight in the oil group, ten in the nuts group, seventeen in the control group). The MedDiet plus EVOO group was 68 percent less likely to have breast cancer than the control. There's one oil-slick caveat to all this I must mention: as an isolated, concentrated nutrient entirely stripped of its vitamins, minerals, fibers, and other phytochemicals, EVOO becomes simply fat without the power and function it once had back in its oval olive days. Always prioritize whole foods, as they are best for the breast.

Don't cook with EVOO, because you will destroy all its awesomeness; use organic canola, or try broth, vinegar, or water to keep food from sticking while you cook. Store your oil away from light to keep from degrading nutrients, and replace open olive oil every three months. Use in salad dressings, sauces, pesto, smoothies, drizzle onto already cooked foods, and substitute it for butter or margarine. And trust me, not all fat makes you fat; in fact, extra virgin olive oil consumption aids in weight loss.[98]

READY TO WASH IT ALL DOWN?

Let's start this off with a pop quiz. What's the most common beverage enjoyed by centenarians, a.k.a. people over one hundred years old? Water, grapefruit juice, tea, or red wine?

If you guessed tea, you're a smart crumpet.[99] And when it comes to breast health, your beverages of choice should include tea, coffee, and the ever-clear winner, water.

Tea's Not Teasing

To me, tea is liquid gold. It inhibits cell-damaging free radicals and sends polyphenols coursing through the bloodstream to stop tumor production, invasion, and metastases.[100] The high epigallocatechin gallate (EGCG) antioxidant content fights cancer and often wins. You derive a number of health benefits from all types of tea—green, black, white, oolong, and pu'er—so enjoy your favorite, but know that *herbal* tea does not come from the powerful tea plant, *Camellia sinensis*. As such, herbal tea lacks tea catechin flavonoids like EGCG, but it still gets a high-five for cancer-fighting phenolic compounds and antioxidant activity.[101] When it comes to the breast, green surpasses all other tea. Three cups of green tea a day can reduce breast cancer by as much as 50 percent![102]

Researchers go gaga over green tea. Over 500 Asian American women in Los Angeles County with breast cancer were compared to 594 without cancer. Women who drank less than 85.7 milliliters (one-third cup) of green tea daily were 29 percent less likely to have breast cancer, and those who drank more than 85.7 milliliters (one-third cup) were 47 percent less likely to have breast cancer, as compared to women who did not drink green tea at all.[103] A meta-analysis combining seven studies of cancer incidence between green tea drinkers and nondrinkers echoes these findings.[104] Then there's the question of cancer recurrence: can green tea decrease the chances of cancer coming back again? A striking study showed that Japanese women with stage I breast cancer who drank more than three cups of green tea a day were 57 percent less likely to recur, and stage II cancer patients were 31 percent less likely to recur than women in both groups who drank less green tea.[105] Among premenopausal women with breast cancer, more tea correlates to fewer positive nodes and improved survival.[106] This effect might be especially true in aggressive subtypes of cancers expressing HER2 receptors.[107]

The brewing of black and oolong teas destroys catechins like EGCG, so gulp down the green variety when combating breast cancer.[108] If you're not a huge fan of green tea, I still want you to reap the rewards from it, so just plug your nose and chug down three cups or add it to a smoothie

(I put matcha—green tea powder—in mine and consume the entire leaf). Three cups of green tea equals the caffeine content of one cup of coffee; although decaffeinated green tea has one-third the antioxidants of caffeinated, drinking *some* tea is better than none, even if you prefer decaf. In high to low polyphenol concentration, brewed hot green tea far outweighs instant preparations, iced, and ready-to-drink green teas.[109] Tea aficionados will tell you that tea bags literally contain the bottom of the tea barrel, the lowest quality tea known as *fannings* or *dust*. It all boils down to freshness, flavor, and cost, but nowadays you can also find whole leaves in a tea bag. To see what all the fuss is about with loose-leaf tea, place one teaspoon of green tea leaves in a cup, pour in four ounces of hot water, cover and steep for three minutes, then pour through a kitchen strainer into your mug. Whether you dunk and dash, or steep then strain, you will receive that precious EGCG either way you brew it. Always add a squeeze of lemon, since citrus quintuples the antioxidant absorption of your green tea.[110] PS: green tea also treats atherosclerosis (clogged arteries) and burns fat.

The Scoop on Coffee

Coffee is another powerful beverage, though it comes in second to tea because the data isn't as impressive as my matcha. Coffee was falsely implicated in playing a role in breast cancer in the 1970s and 1980s because caffeine could cause benign breast diseases such as cysts, pain, and fibrocystic changes. Since that time, however, animal studies have shown that caffeine both stimulates and suppresses breast tumors, depending on the rodent species and cancer phase of caffeine administration.[111] So is it safe for humans? Study results vary as to whether women experience cancer reduction, with most showing no effect,[112] but studies convincingly showing protective effects average a 40 percent reduction at high levels of coffee consumption.[113]

Decaffeinated coffee does not carry any cancer-reducing powers, although it's unclear if the caffeine itself protects us, or if the decaffeination process removes another essential factor.[114] We do know that coffee is rich in anticancer phenolic compounds, including substantial amounts of several lignans, which convert into substances with antiestrogen properties.[115] Consequently, less estrogen floats around trying to stimulate breast cell receptors. However, the protective effect extends to all tumor subtypes, both estrogen-driven and not, so the main mechanism of defense remains unclear.[116]

To enjoy these coffee-induced benefits, it takes five cups a day to achieve a 59 percent reduction in estrogen-negative tumors, and a 37 percent drop in all postmenopausal cancers.[117] For BRCA gene mutation carriers, one study identified a 69 percent cancer reduction in those drinking six cups a day.[118] The results from 14,593 Norwegian women suggested that five cups a day reduces the risk of breast cancer in lean women by 50 percent, whereas coffee *doubled* the cancer risk in relatively obese women.[119] These authors suggested that methylxanthines in coffee might interfere with the protective interactions postulated between premenopausal obesity and the ovary, thus increasing breast cancer. Another study of over 35,000 Singaporean Chinese women found that coffee intake more than doubled the development of advanced breast cancer, but *only* among heavier women with a body mass index (BMI) greater than 23 (see chapter 5 to understand BMI).[120] And if you're worried about dehydration, drinking three to six cups of java daily actually contributes to your daily water consumption.[121] Speaking of *agua* . . .

It's Crystal Clear

Water makes up 60 percent of the human body, so consuming the right amount keeps blood flowing freely through your vessels and into all of your organs and cells. Water also moves all the toxins and cellular by-products into the lymph system and out the doors of excretion via stool and urine. In and of itself, water doesn't contain cancer-fighting constituents, but we all know it's vital to life; a few too many days without it, and that's the end of you.

How much water is enough? Based on institutions in Europe and the United States, and the World Health Organization, women need about five twelve-ounce cups a day, once you factor in that we ingest four cups a day from food sources.[122] Consume seven cups if you live in a warm climate, are pregnant or nursing, or vigorously exercise. Restrict water if your physician advises you to do so, perhaps due to having heart or kidney disease. The US Beverage Guidance Panel convened in 2006 to advise us about the best and worst beverages to consume. All liquids are hydrating, except for wine and liquor, which leave you high and dry. Water ranks supreme, followed by tea and coffee, with Coke as a distant last.[123] (Sugary sodas win all the "worst" awards.)

What kind of water is best then? Plain ol' tap water, because it avoids the carcinogenic estrogen-mimicking effect of BPA in plastic and the negative environmental impact of bottled (Americans throw sixty million plastic bottles away *a day*). Tap also contains fewer chemicals, molds, and microbial contamination when tested against bottled.[124] Want to know what's coming from the kitchen sink? Tap water suppliers publish their water-quality results (bottled water companies don't). Enter your zip code and learn what's in the water using the Environmental Working Group's National Tap Water Atlas at ewg.org/tap-water. If you don't like what you see, invest in a high-quality home water filter, which offers the most practical and affordable long-term solution for those concerned about contaminated drinking water or those living where water is unfit for drinking. Reverse-osmosis filters will give you the taste you most likely enjoy from bottled water. Which reminds me, according to the Natural Resources Defense Council (NRDC), 25 percent of bottled water is nothing more than tap water (e.g., Aquafina, Dasani, Nestlé Pure Life). We often pay good money—$61.4 billion globally each year—for what could be free. It's amazing what tidy profits come from our municipal water supply, a few purification tricks, and sexy packaging that connotes the most refreshing drink in town.

Rethink your drink. Add bubbles or buy it fizzy and flavored for fun. Zest it up with cucumber, lemon slices, and mint. Pop in a few berries. You don't need a green thumb or much effort to grow some tasty water additions for the price of seeds. My eight-year-old son, Justin, decided to grow mint in a little patch of dirt—and he transformed the entire backyard into a mint mine! If he can do it, you can too. (I suggest using a small pot to control the mint madness.)

YOU'RE SO SMOOTHIE

Juiceries are popping up on every corner lately, and while I hear patients swear by the anticancer, detoxifying powers of juicing, I am not a fan. The main problem with juicing is that you miss out on all the fiber from the pulp and skins that otherwise remain when blending or consuming whole foods. Many mistakenly think of fiber as just an insoluble stool-bulking agent. Not so, friends! This isn't about regular bowel movements. Remember, fiber yields protective benefits against breast cancer; phytochemicals bind inextricably to the skins and pulp that juicing discards. The good bacteria in your gut liberate these bound polyphenols and send them streaming through your body to relieve oxidative stress.[125] That's also why fruit *juice* spikes blood-sugar levels and exacerbates existing insulin resistance and diabetes, but eating the same thing in whole fruit form lowers these conditions.[126] Every time you drink juice, you miss an opportunity to drink or eat the whole food. We only have 1,600 to 2,000 calories to consume a day, so make them work as completely as possible. Blended smoothies, as opposed to juice, combine delicious *whole* fruits and vegetables, maximizing your intake of plant-based health secrets. You can almost hear the cancer cells crying out, "Oh no, not more turmeric and blueberries!"

In my home, the jarring sounds of pulse/puree/liquefy/chop waken three little boys who, every morning, shuffle sleepy-eyed into the kitchen and plop down at the table. I pour each one a portion of my Antioxidant Smoothie (recipe below), the ingredients of which I've been tweaking since 2012. I am pretty sure it contains the most cancer-kicking compounds found in one single glass of goodness on Earth. The boys devour it, and I head to work knowing they downed a morning dose of phytonutrient fabulousness.

To make this nutrient bomb, you will need a high-quality blender to mash through frozen antioxidants and mix all the flavors, one with at least 500 watts and a 62-ounce pitcher. You'll put all the ingredients into the blender on high until well blended (especially when using whole flaxseeds, make sure they grind up and disappear, or use a coffee grinder first). Then pour the smoothie into a large cup and sip slowly through a straw over twenty minutes. Straws help you avoid the dental issues that can come from the fruit sugar and acid interacting with the bacteria in your mouth and affecting your tooth enamel.[127] Consider glass, stainless steel, or silicone reusable straws to avoid BPA exposure and to lessen your environmental impact. Rinse your teeth with water after you're finished, and don't brush for an hour, because the enamel can't handle it. Sip any leftovers throughout the morning to keep the phytochemicals flowing. To mix things up, you can add vanilla, fresh mint leaves, fresh basil leaves, lime juice, lemon juice, fresh ginger root, cayenne pepper, or 1 to 2 drops of clove oil. (Warning: clove oil is extremely potent. Do test drops in a small portion of your smoothie to see what you can handle. The first time I tried it, my lips went numb for an hour, but then again, I used 20 drops!)

DR. FUNK'S ANTIOXIDANT SMOOTHIE

1 1/2 cups soy milk or almond milk

1 teaspoon *amla* (powdered Indian gooseberries)

1/4 teaspoon turmeric or 1/4 inch fresh turmeric root

1/4 teaspoon black pepper

1 tablespoon flaxseed

1/4 cup inner fillet aloe vera gel (gel, not juice or aloe water, and only
    inner fillet)

2 ounces brewed green tea, or 1 teaspoon matcha powder, or cut a
    green tea bag open and empty contents

1 dried date

1 teaspoon ground Ceylon cinnamon

1 custom Pink Lotus Green Pod or 2 packed cups of dark leafy greens like
    spinach, kale, collard greens (for a berry taste, use pods; for a green
    taste, use leaves)

2 cups berries (fiber listed in grams): raspberries (8), blackberries (8),
    boysenberries (7), blueberries (4), and/or strawberries (3). Use frozen

to make it frostier. Can use 1 cup berries and 1 cup other fruits like apples or oranges. Break the routine with new flavors such as mango, pear, and peach.

1 small banana (I freeze mine)

ALL IN A DAY'S DIET

I love lists. Nothing-oh-nothing can replace that satisfying, bold ✓ of accomplishment in the box next to a completed to-do item; I even like to double up on the achievement by checking the box followed by a decisive strikethrough of the whole item. Below is a master list that sums up all the powerful foods we've discussed and offers portion sizes to make your grocery shopping easier. You can download this list at pinklotus.com /eattobeat. Strive to consume the number of appointed servings from each of these food categories every single day. This goal is more achievable than it might appear after glancing at this seemingly long food inventory. For example, my antioxidant smoothie *alone* has you checking off ten of the twenty food and spice boxes!

DR. FUNK'S FAVORITE 14: EAT TO BEAT BREAST CANCER TODAY

SERVINGS	FOOD	PORTION	EXAMPLES
☐	Cruciferous vegetables	• $1/2$ cup chopped • $1/4$ cup sprouts • 1 tablespoon horseradish	Broccoli, broccoli sprouts, cauliflower, cabbage, brussels sprouts, turnip, radish, horseradish
☐☐	Leafy greens	• 1 cup raw	Kale, mesclun mix, spinach, arugula, romaine, watercress, bok choy, chard, collard greens, turnip greens, mustard greens

SERVINGS	FOOD	PORTION	EXAMPLES
☐☐	Other vegetables	• 1/2 cup cooked or raw • 1/4 cup dry mushroom • 1/2 cup veggie juice	Beets, artichokes, carrots, peppers, corn, zucchini, purple potatoes, sweet potatoes/yams, squash, tomatoes, seaweed, mushrooms, garlic, onions, leeks, shallots, chives
☐	Berries	• 1 cup fresh/frozen • 1/2 cup juice • 1/4 cup dried	Blueberry, blackberry, raspberry, cranberry, strawberry, cherry, acai, goji, boysenberry, kumquat, gooseberry
☐☐☐	Non-berry fruits	• 1 medium size whole • 3/4 cup chopped • 1/2 cup juice • 1/4 cup dried	Apple, orange, pear, peach, nectarine, plum, papaya, tangerine, watermelon, kiwi, passion fruit, kumquat, cantaloupe, honeydew, banana, grapes, guava, grapefruit, lychee, mango, apricot, lemon, pomegranate, pineapple, dates, figs, olives
☐☐☐	100 percent whole grains	• 1 bread slice • 1 cup dry cereal • 1/2 cup cooked cereal, rice, pasta	Brown rice, wild rice, oats, quinoa, whole rye, whole barley, whole wheat pasta, popcorn, buckwheat, whole wheat couscous, millet, bulgur, freekeh, amaranth, sorghum, teff
☐☐	Beans/ legumes	• 1/2 cup cooked • 1/4 cup hummus/dips • 1 cup fresh peas or sprouted lentils	Beans (kidney, garbanzo, lima, fava, black); peas (green, snow, snap, split, black-eyed); lentils
☐☐	Soy	• 1/2 cup tofu • 1/2 cup soy milk	Tofu, tempeh, miso, nattō, edamame, roasted soybeans, soy milk
☐	Nuts/seeds	• 1/4 cup raw • 2 tablespoons nut or seed butter	Walnut, cashew, almond, pistachio, peanut, macadamia, pecan, hazelnut; pumpkin, chia, sunflower, sesame, hemp seeds

SERVINGS	FOOD	PORTION	EXAMPLES
☐	Flaxseed	• 1 tablespoon	Golden or brown
☐	Turmeric	• $1/4$ teaspoon • $1/4$ inch	Turmeric or turmeric root
☐	Spices	• Per desire	Ceylon cinnamon, clove, cumin, curry, dill, fenugreek, bay leaves, chili powder, coriander, ginger, saffron, rosemary, sage, thyme, paprika, oregano, basil, allspice, pepper, parsley, cilantro, mint
☐☐☐ ☐☐☐ ☐☐☐	Water Green tea Other tea, coffee	• 12 ounces • 4 ounces • 4 ounces	Water, coffee, tea: green, matcha, hibiscus, black, white, rooibos, chai, chamomile
☐	Supplements: B_{12}, vitamin D, methylfolate, omega-3	• As needed	You know who you are

CHAPTER 4

Don't Eat That

If, after reading that last chapter, you have assumed that I've always been a normal weight, robust, cancer-slaying machine, I've got news for you: I grew up chubby in Southern California. Let's just say that when my family visited my cousins in Laguna Beach, and we'd drive past the Goodyear Blimp, my brothers would shout, "Hey Kristi, look! There you are, waiting for takeoff."

All together now: *awwwwwww*.

When I was young, most parents and even the medical community had a much different idea about what was considered nutritious than we do now. A healthy lunch during the school week included a sandwich on either Home Pride "wheat" bread or Wonder Bread with deli slices—my faves were bologna, salami, turkey, or liverwurst. I'd also get a piece of fresh fruit and a Twinkie, Ho Ho, or Ding Dong for a treat. When we'd go to McDonald's, the Happy Meal was too small for me. At eight years old, I remember eating a Big Mac, large fries, and *strawberry* milkshake (I thought it was healthier than what I really wanted, which was the chocolate milkshake). Similarly, at KFC, I'd order the sugar-drenched coleslaw, thinking mashed potatoes and gravy were too heavy. To my mom's credit, when she cooked, she made great dinners with tons of vegetables from our backyard. My father loved to garden, and eventually he dug up most of our small yard, transforming it into a veritable world of leafy greens. A few healthy dinners a week, lots of fruit, and unstoppable sports saved me from obesity, but it was a close call.

If it weren't for my older sister, Kim, I wouldn't have understood the basics of healthy eating for years to follow. When I was ten years old, she was twenty-two, and I did everything she did. She became a vegetarian, so I did too. She introduced me to kefir and acidophilus milk. She took me to places like Mrs. Gooch's health food store in West Los Angeles (acquired by Whole Foods in 1993), and to lunch in Topanga at the Inn of the Seventh Ray, known for its seasonal, organic ingredients. We even frequented a Hare Krishna restaurant in Westwood for the all-you-could-eat five-dollar brown rice, tofu, and veggies. When I was sixteen, Kim started to eat meat again, so just to prove my independence, I stayed vegetarian. Eventually, I added reintroduced fish, lean chicken, and turkey to my palate, and that's where I parked it for over thirty years (alongside a carbohydrate phobia avoiding all pasta, rice, potatoes, and bread)—until I learned all of the rock-solid evidence we discuss in this chapter.

In the last chapter, we learned how to build an arsenal of phytochemical weapons to fight cancer adversaries like inflammation, blood vessel formation, and free radicals. Not only does embracing the wisdom of chapter 3 ward off illness, it *reverses* illness—cancer, diabetes, heart disease, and more. In July 1990, Dr. Dean Ornish published picture-perfect proof (i.e., angiogram before-and-afters) of blocked heart arteries opening up again in response to a whole food, plant-based diet and other healthy lifestyle changes (like exercise and stress reduction) in patients with severe heart disease.[1] We're talking about *reversal of chronic illness*, *reversing* the number one killer of human beings on planet Earth, by eating broccoli and lentils (without medications, without surgery). In just *two weeks* of healthy eating, type 2 diabetics for over twenty years using over twenty units of insulin a day suddenly needed no medication at all.[2] Why don't all type 2 diabetics know that blindness, renal failure, and amputation don't have to threaten their futures? Dr. Ornish also documented that the same dietary and lifestyle principles *reverse* prostate cancer.[3] You now understand that the underlying common ground of all these disease processes involves oxidative stress, and *antioxidant* dietary interventions remarkably slow, stop, or reverse breast cancer progression. But hold on, where do all the *oxidants* come from? It's time to investigate what *not* to eat, and pay attention to where popular items like meat, dairy, eggs, alcohol, certain sweeteners, and organic foods rank in the carcinogenic scale. Can you eat red meat if it's grass-fed? Are certain types of cheeses better for you than others? Are eggs all they're cracked up to be? Hint: my childhood diet would never pass muster—and neither did my adult one.

GOT MEAT?

In the United States, 58 percent of all meat consumed is red meat (beef, pork, veal, mutton, lamb, sheep, goat, game); 32 percent is poultry (chicken and turkey); and 10 percent fish.[4] With all this muscle comes cautionary advice to carnivores: many compounds present in meats (natural and synthetic estrogens, heme iron, N-nitroso compounds, saturated fat) may promote the development of cancer by increasing insulin-like growth factor-1 (IGF-1), producing carcinogenic heterocyclic amines, and stimulating inflammation and oxidative stress.[5] More than one hundred studies from multiple countries look at high versus low consumption of red meat, white meat, total meat, or fish, and they generally find an unalarming zero to 6 percent increase in breast cancer in the high consumer group.[6] If meat is so bad for your breasts, why aren't the studies screaming about it? Well, possibly for two reasons. One, we lack well-designed nutrition studies lasting decades, which is the time frame required to spot a true division in health due to meat consumption. And two, the previous studies all compare meat-to-meat consumption, and overlook the possibility that *any degree of meat* consumption is just plain ol' bad for you—so damaging that comparing meat-to-meat will likely never show a decrease in cancer rates. It's like comparing people who smoke two packs a day to people who smoke one pack a day and concluding,

"Looky here. Smoking cigarettes doesn't increase lung cancer." Similarly, maybe we have been comparing the wrong diets. What would happen if we looked at studies that compare *any* meat at all to *no* meat whatsoever? Very few studies separate out vegetarians and look at breast cancer risk, but the ones that do might make you raise your eyebrows at the results. The UK Women's Cohort Study followed 35,372 women for eight years, with 1,850 subsequent breast cancers.[7] Compared to *no meat* consumers, *high intake* of the following meat had the corresponding spikes in risk: total meat 34 percent; red meat 41 percent; processed meat 39 percent; poultry 22 percent. The Adventist Health Study-2 followed 69,120 participants for 4.1 years, and categorized their eating as meat, vegan (no meat, dairy, eggs), lacto(milk)-vegetarian, pesco(fish)-vegetarian, and semi(sometimes meat)-vegetarian.[8] Vegans were the *only* subgroup to show a statistically significant 44 percent drop in breast and gyne-cologic cancers relative to meat-eaters. Based on this sneak-peek into a vegetarian/vegan world, it's plausible that avoidance of meat altogether translates into avoidance of cancer. We don't need any more inconclusive studies talking about fourteen versus three strips of bacon; if we want meaty answers, it's time for all-meat versus all-plant/no meat/no dairy comparisons to seize the spotlight. I am not only concerned about meat itself, but also *what's in the meat*—especially when it comes to additives.

Enter: Zeranol

As of this writing, nothing has changed since the following concern was published in the *International Journal of Health Services* in *1990* (that is not a typo): "In the absence of effective federal regulation, the meat industry uses hundreds of animal feed additives, including antibiotics, tranquilizers, pesticides, animal drugs, artificial flavors, industrial wastes, and growth-promoting hormones, with little or no concern about the carcinogenic and other toxic effects."[9] How can scientists study what we're eating if we don't know what we're eating?

This lack of transparency should sound alarms regarding breast and overall health. Because its use requires FDA approval, we know that a chemical named zeranol (brand name, Ralgro), a synthetic estrogen given to US and Canadian cattle to accelerate their growth and girth, exists in all conventional red meat we eat (not in organic, optional in grass-fed). Since a baby calf needs to become a seventeen-hundred-pound heifer or steer by slaughter time at eighteen months, it helps to give it some growth-promoting zeranol. Who cares? Does it matter if you ingest a little zeranol with your burger or milk? Well, in 1981 (yes, that long ago), the European Economic Community (the EEC, now the European Union) banned zeranol and other growth promoters in cattle farming after a group of Italian boys and girls ages three to ten suddenly began sprouting breasts, and all signs pointed to the zeranol used in beef.[10] Zeranol's estrogenic effects were apparently strong enough to accelerate the arrival of puberty in these young children, a condition called *precocious puberty*. Citing the potential to cause cancer in humans, in 1989, the EEC prohibited the import of beef products from the United States or Canada—*and North America still uses zeranol as a growth promoter to this day.*

Yup—to this day.

In terms of breast cancer risk specifically, zeranol is the most potent growth hormone found in human food, boasting 100,000 times the estrogen influence of bisphenol A (BPA) from plastics, which we'll talk about soon.[11] A hundred thousand times? Any beef-eater worried about the BPA in water bottles needs to know that stat. In fact, in the lab, zeranol turns benign human breast cells into cancer within twenty-one days and causes existing cancer cells to proliferate.[12] It gets in our bodies, as evidenced by 78.5 percent of 163 New Jersey nine-to-ten-year-old girls testing positive for zeranol in their urine.[13] Zeranol has been implicated in precocious puberty in Europe, as noted above, and in Puerto Rico.[14] Could it also be the reason that when the Nurses' Health Study II followed over 39,000 premenopausal women for seven years, they found a 34 percent increase in estrogen-positive premenopausal breast cancer for those who ate the most red meat during their high school years?[15] Among 88,804 women followed twenty years, animal fat (but not total fat) consumption between ages twenty-six and forty-five also independently increased premenopausal breast cancers by 18 percent.[16]

It gets worse. Zeranol potentiates leptin activity, a breast cancer–promoting hormone produced by fat cells; as you might predict, obese women have higher leptin levels.[17] Hence, there is a rising concern that obese beef consumers increase their cancer risk via this zeranol–leptin friendship.[18] In the largest study on human nutrition ever done, the European Prospective Investigation into Cancer and Nutrition (EPIC) study followed nearly 400,000 Europeans from ten countries.[19] EPIC revealed that those who ate red meat, poultry, and processed meat gained 4.4 pounds (2 kilograms) more weight than low meat consumers in just five years. So the more beef you eat, the fatter you are, the more leptin you make, and the more zeranol can transform cells from normal to abnormal.

Enter: Insulin-like Growth Factor-1 (IGF-1)

All meat, chicken, and fish (yes, including chicken and *fish*—patients often ask, "Fish is okay, though, right?") have another man-made cancer-promoting secret, but it doesn't come as a synthetic pellet. *You* make it everyday. Insulin-like growth factor-1 (IGF-1) has one mission in life—to tell everybody to grow, grow, grow! This critical growth promoter works the miracle of a child becoming an adult. But we only get so tall, and our hands only become so large, so what's IGF-1 doing for the rest of your adult life? Well, we turn over around fifty billion cells a day, and they need replacing, post-exercise muscles need repairing, and brain cells need protecting.[20] Once these tasks are complete, however, if there's excess IGF-1 screaming at cells to grow, then grow they will—into cancer, into metastases, into the lung and liver, into the brain and bone.[21] *Whoa.* Someone better settle that IGF-1 down.

It turns out, you're that someone. Your brain tells your liver to produce IGF-1 predominantly in response to eating animal protein (meat, dairy, eggs). A study followed 6,381 adults aged fifty and up for eighteen years; among those ages fifty to sixty-five, higher protein levels linked to a 430 percent higher chance of dying from cancer and a 7,300 percent increase in diabetes when compared to those in the low protein group.[22] IGF-1 emerged as an important moderator of the association between protein consumption and mortality, since wherever protein went, IGF-1 levels were sure to follow. (Just like Mary and her lamb.) Notably, no such elevations in risk happened with proteins derived from plants—only animals.

If you could not respond to IGF-1 at all, you would have Laron syndrome, and you would be very short, which makes sense, since you wouldn't have anyone yelling at you to grow.[23] But guess what else you wouldn't have? Drumroll, please . . . cancer. *Not one person with IGF-1 deficiency has ever gotten breast cancer.*[24] (In fact, only one person with Laron syndrome *ever* has gotten any type of cancer.) Okay, that's astounding. *No one with IGF-1 deficiency ever gets type 2 diabetes.* Astounding again. Clearly, IGF-1 contributes substantially to the causation of all cancer and diabetes. IGF-1 creates a microenviroment proven to be conducive to breast cancer, and increases breast cancer invasiveness.[25] Women with high circulating levels of IGF-1 have 38 percent more estrogen-driven cancers than those with low IGF-1.[26]

I can tell you how to lower IGF-1 and how to make more of an IGF-1 binding protein that acts like a body snatcher, retiring IGF-1 from circulation. As my son, Ethan, would say, easy peasy lemon squeezy. Just do what a group of obese women did following the Pritikin plan: eat a low-fat (10–15 percent of daily calories), high-fiber (30–40 grams per 1,000 calories per day) plant-based diet and attend daily exercise classes for two weeks.[27] On day 1, a blood sample from these ladies was dripped onto breast cancer cells in a petri dish, and a small number of cells died (apparently, everyone has a few cancer defenses in their veins). On day 12, researchers dripped the same women's blood on cells again, and, presto chango, *the majority of cancer cells* died. The researchers also measured blood hormone levels in these women. In just two weeks of healthy eating, IGF-1 and insulin went down, binding protein went up, and cancer cells went away. Although exercise alone also improves IGF-1 levels, it does so to only half the degree of plant-based eating.[28] The IGF-1/cancer connection is real—and reversible. I share the Pritikin experiment story of whole food plant-based eating whenever I hear people say "it's too late" to turn back time and undo the damage their diets have done; oh no, sister, you can absolutely transform your blood into a cancer-fighting machine.

NOT ALL PROTEIN IS CREATED EQUAL

While *animal* proteins cause IGF-1 levels to skyrocket, *plant* proteins make IGF-1 hit rock bottom and IGF-1 binding proteins soar.[29] Depending on your activity level, you should aim to consume 50 grams of protein a day—and not all protein comes from meat. Remember our 70/30 plate from chapter 3? A big chunk of meat protein wasn't the star of the dish. The protein macronutrient belongs in the "best supporting actor" section as a cup of lentils or small wedge of wild-caught fish. Or let it trickle into your day as a snack of nuts or edamame with a pinch of paprika and sea salt.

MEATLESS MONDAYS ALL WEEK LONG

Here are ten additional ways to get your fill of protein each day without eating meat:

- $1/3$ cup seitan = 21 grams protein (avoid in celiac disease or gluten intolerant)
- $1/2$ cup soy as tempeh/tofu/shelled edamame = 20 grams protein
- 1 cup cooked lentils = 18 grams protein
- 1 cup beans (kidney, pinto, black, white, green, garbanzo) = 15 grams protein
- $1/4$ cup nuts or nut butters (almond, walnut, cashew, pistachio, brazil); $1/4$ cup seeds (sunflower, sesame, flax, pumpkin, chia, hemp) = 7 to 10 grams protein
- 1 cup green peas = 8 grams protein
- $1/2$ cup cooked quinoa = 7 to 9 grams protein

- 1 cup cooked wild rice = 6.5 grams protein
- 1/4 cup dry steel-cut oats = 5 grams protein
- 1/2 cup cooked spinach, broccoli, brussels sprouts, organic corn, avocado = 2 grams protein

---

Enter: Meat-related Mutagens

If you're thinking, "Doc, I love myself a cheeseburger, and I won't stop eating meat," I get it. You don't have to swear off meat, and you're not alone—overall meat consumption continues to rise throughout the entire developed world, and averages 128 grams per day in the United States, which is three times higher than the global average. But before you order a crisp burger at the pub or nibble the skin off your roasted chicken, you must know that even if you eat organic or grass-fed beef, how you *prepare* your meat can make it even more carcinogenic.

Certain mutagens—polycyclic aromatic hydrocarbons (PAHs) and heterocyclic amines (HCAs), to be exact—are cancer-causing compounds that form on the surface of well-done and otherwise deliciously grilled, smoked, roasted, pan-fried, and barbecued meats.[30] HCAs form within minutes at high temperatures, but even baking chicken at lower temps for fifteen minutes leads to HCAs on the surface because of a chemical reaction between the heat and the creatinine in muscle tissue[31] (fried and grilled veggie burgers, on the other hand, don't have any measurable HCAs).[32] You'll want to avoid very well-done meat, then, since it has been linked to breast cancer: 54 percent higher for hamburger consumers, 64 percent higher for bacon eaters, and 121 percent higher for beefsteak lovers.[33] Women who eat all three of these meats well-done have a *362 percent higher* risk than women who choose rare or medium done meat. Note that we're not comparing well-done–meat eaters to vegetarians here; when comparing meat versus meat, burnt meat is bad. One culprit behind the cancer connection is PhIP, an HCA found in cooked meats that possesses a power equivalent to pure estrogen to fuel both the initiation and growth of breast cancers.[34] When the breast milk of nonsmoking women is tested for PhIP, it exists in meat eaters, but not vegetarians.[35] Within twenty-four hours of ending meat consumption, PhIP in urine samples disappears.[36] We've been given a forgiving body.

Is there any way to compensate for the risk? When you do eat meat, add a strategic side dish. Adding three cups of daily greens like broccoli and brussels sprouts drops HCA in urine by 23 percent, despite ingesting the same level of carcinogens.[37] Green, black, and white teas have all been shown to stop DNA mutations caused by PhIP.[38] Avoid broiling meats, and limit baking and roasting. It's best to use moist heat at low temperatures such as slow cooking in a crockpot, steaming, poaching, simmering, stewing, or *sous-vide* (a French method of boiling meat). Pressure cookers accelerate healthy moist heat cooking too. If you panfry or stir-fry, minimize the production of HCAs by using antioxidant-rich marinades and healthy fats like organic canola oil. Did someone just ask, "What about deep-frying?" In other words, surround your meat with batter and then immerse it into some kind of boiling saturated fat until it becomes a crispy golden cancer ball? I don't think you want me to answer that.

Enter: Nitrates

Of all the meats eaten in the United States, 22 percent include processed meat, the source of several known mutagens, including *N*-nitroso compounds. Processed meat means that smoking, curing, salting, fermenting, or adding preservatives has altered the meat. In a UK study of 35,372 women, those consuming the most processed meat exhibited 64 percent more breast cancer than those who ate *none* of the hotdogs and deli slices.[39] Recall the theory that comparing *more* meat to *less* meat needs to be revisited with a simple meat versus none comparison. When you look at studies on high versus low consumption of processed meat, increased risk surfaces, but it's 8 to 10 percent,[40] not 64 percent . . . so even just an occasional slice of salami or chorizo cuts a big slice out of life. You might call "processed" by friendly names like sausage, hot dog, ham, salami, pepperoni, deli meat, cold cuts, corned beef, beef jerky, and bacon, but the International Agency for Research on Cancer (IARC) calls them potentially deadly.

In 2015, twenty-two scientists from ten countries met at the IARC in Lyon, France, to answer the question, "Are red meat and processed meats bad for your health?"[41] The working group assessed over eight hundred epidemiological studies looking into cancer and red or processed meat consumption in countries from several continents, with diverse ethnicities and diets. Their conclusion? The IARC bestowed the highest warning level possible to the consumption of processed meat, labeling it flat-out "carcinogenic to humans" (on par with smoking and asbestos), and classified red meat as "probably carcinogenic to humans." Truth be told, after I read the IARC ruling, I cringed with remorse realizing that sending my sweet boys to school with "healthy" turkey slices amounted to throwing a cigarette or two into their lunchboxes. Sure enough, when the NIH-AARP Diet and Health Study followed an impressive 193,742 postmenopausal women over 9.4 years, they found 25 percent more breast cancer in red and processed meat consumers.[42]

In response to the IARC determinations, the World Cancer Research Fund International said to avoid all processed meat,[43] but the American Cancer Society only recommended limiting consumption of red and processed meat. And while my focus is on your breasts, it's worth noting that the human evidence linking meat intake to cancers of the colon, rectum, esophagus, lung, and liver is beyond compelling, as is the data implicating meat for all cancer mortality and cardiovascular disease.[44] So there's more than breast cancer to consider while making smart food choices at the grocery store.[45]

Besides fat and sodium, the real beef here comes from nitrates. They are harmless, but they have the ability to shape-shift—and that's where it gets tricky. Nitrates become nitrites, which are good when eaten in plant form, as they become nitric oxide (which improves blood flow). But nitrates become bad with the addition of an *amine* or *amide* when eaten in meat form, because they transform into carcinogenic *nitrosamines* or *nitrosamides*. I want you to understand this verbiage because your packaged meats that boast "No nitrates added" might have a disclaimer like "except for those naturally occurring in celery powder." That natural celery nitrate becomes an unnatural carcinogen thanks to the "meat plus amine," just the same as if they added nitrosamine directly without the veggie trap. Your best bet is to eliminate processed meat. This is where the whole "everything in moderation" mantra rubs me the wrong way. Why consume cancer-causing meats "in moderation" when all level of processed meat consumption has been deemed dangerous? So that maybe I can remove a *moderate* part of your breast instead of the whole gland?

GLOBAL MEAT CRISIS

Around the world, we've seen a rapid surge in all-meat consumption as countries such as Brazil, China, Latin America, and Asia pursue the diet of industrialized nations such as the United States, France, and Spain. According to the Food and Agriculture Organization of the United Nations (FAO), meat consumption per person per year increased between 1964 and 2015 as follows: East Asia nearly sextupled from 8.7 kilograms to 50.0 kilograms (110.2 pounds); developing countries tripled from 10.2 kilograms to 31.6 kilograms (69.6 pounds); Latin America more than doubled from 31.7 kilograms to 65.3 kilograms (143.9 pounds); and industrialized countries apparently still have room for more, increasing 36 percent from 61.5 kilograms to 95.7 kilograms (210.9 pounds). To satiate our carnivorous appetites, 19.6 billion chickens, 1.5 billion cows, 1 billion pigs, and 1.9 billion sheep and goats populate the planet alongside us (or somewhere hidden from us)—that's over three times the number of people.[46]

Global agriculture, dominated by livestock production and the grains grown to feed it, contributes to climate change and threatens planet sustainability and, ironically, exacerbates world hunger. Animal agriculture accounts for 30 percent of greenhouse gas emissions[47] (more than all transportation sources combined; cows produce 150 billion pounds of toxic methane farts a day[48]), uses 80 to 90 percent of US water consumption[49] (55 trillion gallons/year;[50] 1 pound of beef requires 5,000 gallons;[51] 1 gallon of milk takes 1,000 gallons[52]), occupies around 45 percent of the earth's land,[53] has caused 90 percent of Brazilian Amazon destruction,[54] intensifies world hunger[55] (82 percent of starving children live where livestock consume the food, and then Westerners consume the livestock), and paves the way for ocean dead zones,[56] habitat destruction,[57] and species extinction.[58] If humans really plan to escalate all their meat consumption as per the FAO, agriculture emissions will increase by 80 percent by 2050,[59] so we really should figure out that whole living-on-Mars thing sometime soon, where hopefully there'll be room for vegetables too.

Stay updated on the evolving global meat crisis. Learn how it affects your health and the health of those you love. Find out ways to help yourself and others at pinklotus.com/meatcrisis.

You Have My Attention, Now What?

Even if you're intrigued, going from all-to-none or simply consuming less total meat will be challenging for many people. Do damage control by consuming wild-caught fish, organic poultry, grass-fed beef (as opposed to grain-fed), and sustainably harvested canned fish (when fresh isn't an option) such as wild salmon, "pole-caught" tuna, sardines, and mackerel. I would suggest, however, limiting meat servings to three or less a week, and *eliminating* (no financial sponsors here) all processed meat.

DEAR DAIRY . . .

Dairy products come from milk from the mammary glands of mammals. Examples include the milk itself, all cheeses (cheddar, Swiss, mozzarella, jack, goat), cottage cheese, cream, cream cheese, sour cream, ice cream, gelato, butter, and yogurt. As mentioned in chapter 2, you'd think that the presence of hormones, growth factors (IGF-1), fat, and chemical contaminants (pesticide residues, antibiotics, aflatoxins, melamine) would lead to a proliferation of hormonally sensitive breast cancer cells.[60] However, research shows increases, decreases, and null effects of dairy consumption on breast cancer risk, so naturally, meta-analyses combining tons of studies conclude that dairy's fine.[61] The healthy connection between dairy products and breast tissue seems to involve the protective effects of calcium, vitamin D, butyrate, lactoferrin, and conjugated linoleic acid.[62]

Trim the Fat

Hold up, put that Häagen-Dazs down. When studies *do* show a causal connection, is there something there we should notice? While low-fat dairy doesn't seem to pose breast problems (and correlates with *less* breast cancer in some studies[63]), the saturated fat in full-fat dairy definitely raises eyebrows (think whole milk versus skim). In the Life After Cancer Epidemiology Study (LACE), breast cancer patients eating one or more daily servings of high-fat (not low-fat) dairy increased all-cause mortality by 49 percent compared to those consuming less than a half-serving per day.[64] Really, deadly dairy? Well, unlike their pasture-fed buddies from a hundred years ago, modern dairy cows are genetically modified organisms (GMO) that continually produce milk throughout pregnancy—and actually throughout their entire lifetimes because they are reinseminated shortly after birthing a calf and are basically constantly pregnant—a condition that significantly elevates estrogen in the milk.[65] These estrogens reside primarily in fat, so you ingest substantially more cancer-fueling estrogens from full-fat dairy (organic included[66]), which possibly helps explain the LACE study mortality bump.

Before you get your daily calcium from a dairy-delicious chunk of cheddar, we should talk more about foe fats. Foe fat directly contributes to our top killers: heart disease, cancer, stroke, obesity, Alzheimer's, and diabetes. We talked about friendly fats in chapter 3. Foe fats are another story. One unmistakable foe source is *trans* fats—fats that need to be immediately *trans*ferred out of your diet. We find them in foods such as cakes, donuts, margarine, shortening, fried chicken, microwave popcorn, and French fries. You might as well push Crisco straight into your arteries and watch blood flow come to a screeching halt. When Denmark banned trans fats, deaths from cardiovascular disease dropped by 50 percent.[67] These man-made fats appear in clever ways on the labels of processed food innocently noted as "partially hydrogenated oil" or "high stearate." Don't be fooled by "No Trans Fat" marketing on a box or container; read the ingredients label on the back to be sure you don't spy any covert trans fats. Trans fats affect breast cancer. In a study from Greece, where the MedDiet abounds, using margarine just once a week bumped breast cancer up by 5 percent.[68] Breast cancer patients who consume butter, margarine, or lard on a daily basis have a 67 percent increase in cancer recurrence, and a 212 percent increase in *death* for the highest third of fat consumers relative to the lowest third.[69] So trans fats might preserve food, but they expire *you*.

Avoiding junk food may not be enough. The *only* other source of trans fats occurs naturally in *meat* and *dairy*. Yes, I just said that. With the 2018 ban on trans fats in processed food, animal meat and dairy now account for the majority of the daily trans fat intake in America.[70] Animal trans fats from all meat and dairy sources, including non-cow animals, increase bad LDL cholesterol and lower good HDL cholesterol, just the same as the man-made variety.[71] Heart disease goes up 23 percent for every 2 percent of calories coming from trans fats.[72]

In addition to trans fats, saturated fats are also bad for your breasts. A Seattle research center followed over 4,400 breast cancer patients who had not yet recurred, and found that 3 percent died within seven years.[73] While the highest trans fat intake led to 78 percent more death, the highest *saturated fat* eaters had 41 percent more death than the lowest intake. Saturated fats are solid at room temp (butter) and come from animal sources: cheese, milk, butter, cream, meat, and eggs. When patients change toward healthier eating, what's the one food they say they miss the most? Hint: it's dusted with hormones, and packed with calories, cholesterol, salt, and saturated fat.

Cheese. What's that you said? Oh, it was a scream: "Nooooo!" I'm right with you. But after acknowledging the rock-solid evidence about the health dangers of saturated fat, I gave up my manchego. Do you want to know why cheese and pizza (a.k.a. cheese) rank numbers 1 and 2 for how Americans eat their fat? Besides the lip-smacking truth that cheese is salty, fatty, and gooey delicious, it's also addictive like a street drug. It takes ten pounds of milk to make one pound of cheese, so that little bite of solid cheddar boasts 73 percent fat, 25 percent protein, and 2 percent carbs. The protein, casein, breaks down into the addictive opioid caso-*morphin* in your stomach, which stimulates the same brain receptors as *morphine* with one-tenth the affinity—making you come back again and again for just one more slice of pizza.

After following 188,736 postmenopausal women for 4.4 years, those who derived 40 percent of their daily calories from fat had a 32 percent higher rate of invasive breast cancer than those with 20 percent of calories from fat.[74] So avoiding saturated fat-laden foods will reduce the creation, recurrence, and killer effects of breast cancer. It's never too soon to start healthy fat consumption. Eating more vegetable fat from avocados, olives, seed butters and nuts during youth (ten to fifteen years old) decreases postmenopausal breast cancer forty years down the road.[75]

FAT FACTS

The National Cancer Institute (NCI) surveyed Americans and ranked their favorite ways to eat saturated fat. The following made their top ten, listed from most to least calories coming from saturated fat consumption.[76] If any of these is part of your diet, your breasts politely request that you trim the fat. It's time to trade that TGIF pepperoni pizza for avocado whole grain toast.

- cheese
- pizza (a.k.a. more cheese)
- grain-based desserts (cake, cookies, pastry, and donuts)
- ice cream
- chicken (one skinless breast = 19 percent fat; with skin, 36 percent fat)

- sausage/hotdogs/bacon/ribs (oink oink)
- burgers
- Mexican dishes
- beef
- reduced fat milk*

* Thanks, milk labeling tricks: 2 percent fat by weight is still 30 percent fat by calories; for reference, whole milk is 3.25 percent fat.

In chapter 3, we talked about healthy PUFAs like the omega-3s found in oily fish such as salmon, herring, sardines, and mackerel; plus flaxseed, walnuts, and healthy oils, including unhydrogenated soybean oil, walnut, sesame, canola, almond, flaxseed, and borage oils. But there are also the unhealthy PUFAs—omega-6 polyunsaturated fatty acid vegetable oils—that include safflower, sunflower, hydrogenated soybean (versus good *un*hydrogenated), corn, coconut, palm, evening primrose, black currant, hempseed, and grape-seed oils. Just keep in mind that even though they are essential PUFAs, a Western diet has us consuming them at a ratio of 16:1 against omega-3 PUFAs, when what we want is 1:1, so go easy on them.[77] The imbalance works against all the omega-3 benefits and leads to a cascade of inflammation that feeds a host of chronic illnesses, with heart disease and cancer chief among them. This even includes the almighty coconut oil, which is about 90 percent saturated fat and outranks butter (64 percent saturated fat), beef (40 percent), and even lard (also 40 percent) in terms of its PUFA harm.

To sum this up and make it easy: throw away every bottle of oil in your home except for extra virgin olive oil and organic expeller-pressed canola. Reserve saturated and trans fats for special occasions only. Deep-fried anything, butter, lard, and oils like cottonseed, corn, safflower, and sunflower are bad for your breasts, heart, and basically every vital organ.

Since you want to limit your dairy intake, especially in its higher-fat versions, where do you get your calcium? You'll find plenty of easily absorbed calcium in dark leafy greens, such as bok choy, kale, mustard greens, collard greens, and turnip greens, as well as broccoli, beans, figs, almonds, calcium-fortified whole grain cereals, soy milk, and other nondairy milks. Bonus: these foods contain all the other cancer-fighting phytochemicals missing from dairy products, like fiber, iron, folate, and antioxidants.

It's the Milky Way

Besides fat and estrogens, is there anything else unhealthy in milk we should know about? Well, remember zeranol in beef cattle? Dairy cows can get a different artificial hormone that increases milk production by 10 to 15 percent; it's called recombinant Bovine Growth Hormone or rBGH. No safety studies have been done to evaluate rBGH, but due to concerns regarding animal and human health, and elevated IGF-1 levels,[78] other countries ban its use, including the European Union, Japan, Australia, New Zealand, and Canada. In a human study, plasma IGF-1 concentration increased by 10 percent when healthy subjects consumed cows' milk,[79] but as noted above, the detrimental effect seems to be counteracted by protective factors. As demand for rBGH-free milk has increased in the United States, its use has decreased to 17 percent of cows.[80] Also, in addition to IGF-1 that promotes cancer cell growth, milk products may contain carcinogenic contaminants such as pesticides (organochlorines).[81]

And then there's a virus called bovine leukemia virus (BLV) that infects the mammary glands of cows and gets into the milk supply we consume. How many cows are we talking about here? Exactly 100 percent of cows on farms with more than five hundred cattle.[82] BLV matters to your health, since 74 percent of tested humans show circulating antigens to BLV in their blood, proving a human immune response to a cow's breast infection.[83] What's more, when researchers at University of California–Berkeley in 2015 looked for BLV in the excised breast tissues of 239 noncancer and cancer patients, they found cancer patients were *twice* as likely to have BLV in their breasts (59 percent versus 29 percent), leading to the statistical conclusion that up to 37 percent of all breast cancers might be caused by BLV exposure.[84]

What about finding BLV in all those benign breasts? Since studies on cell biology show that it takes years to decades for cancer cells to form a detectable cancer, perhaps those BLV samples came from women who would *eventually* get breast cancer. This same study supports that theory. They found BLV in 38 percent of tissues harboring precancerous breast cells—a number perfectly in between the numbers of benign and cancerous breasts noted above, correlating to finding the most BLV with cancer, second-most with precancer, and the least BLV in normal tissues. Using similar techniques in 2017, an Australian team studied ninety-six women, finding BLV again in twice as many of the cancer samples: 80 percent versus 41 percent noncancer. What's equally interesting, forty-eight of the subjects also had breast tissue removed three to ten years earlier for benign reasons. In 74 percent of those with cancer now, the specimen from three to ten years ago contained BLV. This supports (but doesn't prove) the idea of a causal relationship between BLV infection and subsequent development of cancer.

What can we do about BLV if it really does cause breast cancer? Well, we could easily screen for BLV infection and prevent thousands of breast cancers every year simply by administering a BLV vaccine, not to mention mandating the elimination of its source in cow's milk. For those with a BLV-induced cancer, targeted antiviral therapies could possibly prevent recurrence (like HIV antivirals). Should we eradicate the infection from cattle now, just in case this all turns out to be true? More than twenty other countries have already managed to do so, but the effort and money it would take for the American milk industry to eliminate the transmission of BLV would likely preclude them from doing it unless forced. BLV is a retrovirus, so like HIV, it spreads from blood to blood contact, from the blood of one cow entering into another cow. *Ew.* This happens because ranchers don't disinfect the blood-contaminated instruments they use all day long, and so they introduce one cow's blood into another cow. Also, ranchers impregnate cows by pushing an arm up cows' rectums to insemi-nate them, bleeding occurs, and then they just move on to the next rectum. *Oof.* In other words, what happens on the farm doesn't stay on the farm.[85]

NOT SO EGGS-CELLENT

Chickens were purposefully fed arsenic until, after seventy-two years of doing so, the United States poultry industry was forced to stop using this additive in 2016.[86] Arsenic kills off internal and external chicken parasites (tapeworm, lice, mites, and so on) and makes the meat turn a pretty pink color. A 2012 study measuring exposure to toxins in 207 preschoolers ages two to four years old found that 100 percent of the children exceeded the arsenic-to-cancer risk ratio by a factor of over one hundred, and their number-one source of arsenic was poultry.[87] Even though arsenic has been eliminated from the feed, dumping two million pounds a year for seventy-two years into the environment has spiked our soil, such that even rice and plants can be arsenic-laced.[88]

What else is fed to the mama of our eggs? As noted earlier, it's hard to say since feed ingredients aren't disclosed, but grains fortified with pesticides and antibiotics exist legally. However, *illegal* antibiotics, like fluoroquinolones, showed up in a lab analysis of chicken feathers, which, by the way, farmers grind up and feed back to chickens as feather meal.[89] What else was in those feathers? Acetaminophen (like Tylenol), Prozac, antifungal medications, antihistamine, a sex hormone, and caffeine. Look, if chickens have a headache, or feel depressed and sleepy, I get it, but just tell us. We have to interrogate feathers in a lab to find this out because there are no labeling requirements for poultry and eggs.

So do eggs cause breast cancer? Individual studies land all over the place, showing no risk, increased risk, and even protective effects. When this happens, it's sometimes helpful to pool all the studies together to hopefully get enough "statistical power" with large numbers. The only meta-analysis to look solely at egg consumption and *breast* cancer risk took thirteen studies and concluded that consuming two to five eggs per week was associated with a small but definite 4 percent increased breast cancer risk and up to 9 percent risk among European, Japanese, and postmenopausal populations.[90] Another dietary meta-analysis with a fifteen-year follow-up of 351,041 women found no link between cancer and meat or dairy, but did find one positive correlation: for every two large eggs (100 grams) consumed daily, breast cancer rates went up 22 percent.[91]

Scientists have uncovered a number of possible explanatory carcinogenic pathways regarding egg consumption. Choline is a vitamin-like compound for which there is no Recommended Daily Allowance (RDA) because deficiencies don't exist, so you don't need to proactively seek out sources of choline, and too much can be a bad thing. Why? Gut bacteria feast on the high choline content in eggs, leading to a toxic metabolite called TMAO (trimethylamine *N*-oxide).[92] Harvard researchers linked the TMAO from just 2.5 eggs a week to an 81 percent increase in *lethal* prostate cancer, so it's possible that the same inflammatory cascade caused by TMAO could increase breast cancer as well.[93] Heterocyclic amines (HCAs), the carcinogenic compounds that we discussed as forming on cooked meat, also form in fried eggs, along with powerful carcinogens, PhIP and IQ[4,5-*b*].[94] Eggs are man's number one source of cholesterol with 425 milligrams per two large eggs (there's 79 milligrams in a Big Mac). Guess what cancer cells order for breakfast? Eggs! Breast cancer cells suck up LDL (bad cholesterol) to stimulate their own growth. In fact, the more LDL receptors found in breast cancer tissue, the shorter a woman's survival time.[95]

In summary, it seems safe from a cancer risk perspective to consume up to two eggs per week. However, never let your guard down against our number-one global killer, heart disease. Cholesterol is a major player in the growing worldwide cardiovascular health crisis. The American Heart Association (AHA) recommends consuming less than 300 milligrams per day, but you never need to eat cholesterol since your body can synthesize all it requires without your help.[96] Keeping your cholesterol level under 160 will drop breast cancer by 17 percent.[97] Eggs crack a double whammy to the chest: heart *and* breast.

I HATE TO BE A BUZZKILL . . .

Of all the controllable risk factors for breast cancer, none is more prevalent across diverse populations and cultures than alcohol. Why? Alcohol increases estrogen levels (a.k.a., cancer fuel), impairs immune function, creates toxic metabolites like acetaldehyde, and inactivates folic acid, which repairs DNA when it goes awry. All of these actions are like soldiers in the oxidative stress battle, turning the tide toward free radicals and cellular damage. I can hear your thoughtful protestations. "But wait a minute. Doesn't alcohol prevent heart attacks?" Yes, it does, and you are seven times more likely to die from a heart attack than from breast cancer. One drink a day significantly decreases mortality from heart disease largely by increasing good cholesterol (HDL).[98] So, my drinkers, be of good cheer. However, no abstainer should consider consuming alcohol for the sole reason of reducing heart disease.

Okay, now, what's a drink? The National Institute on Alcohol Abuse and Alcoholism, a branch of the NIH in the United States, defines one drink as fourteen grams of alcohol—that's a twelve-ounce can of beer, five ounces of wine, or 1.5 ounces of hard liquor (80-proof spirits: gin, vodka, whisky, and so forth).[99] So pick your poison, and read on. (You might actually need a drink after reading what comes next.) Relative to a nondrinker, studies show that one drink a day increases breast cancer 10 percent; two drinks a day increases your risk 30 percent; three drinks a day, 40 percent, and you can add 10 percent per drink thereafter.[100] So to balance the cardio-protective effects of alcohol with the carcinogenic effects on breast tissue, keep your weekly intake of alcohol to approximately seven drinks (fourteen for men). How's that for some educated justification for a weekend trip to Napa?

Let's take a closer look at what alcohol does to folate, a.k.a. folic acid, a.k.a. methylfolate in the active form. Methylfolate ensures that as your DNA replicates, it maintains its original structure without allowing mutations to occur and propagate. Methylfolate has an extra methyl group that it donates to DNA as new strands are synthesized. So you can imagine how a folate *deficiency* might increase the incidence of breast cancer when there isn't enough methylfolate around to babysit the dividing DNA. What would cause a folate deficiency (which, by the way, is the most common vitamin deficiency in the world)? Besides low dietary intake, it's good ol' alcohol, which decreases folate absorption from the intestines and increases its excretion in the kidneys and interferes with the necessary conversion of folic acid to its helpful form, methylfolate.[101] The enzyme that turns folic acid into its active form, methylenetetrahydrofolate reductase (MTHFR), contains "polymorphisms" (variations) in 30 to 50 percent of people (you can do a saliva test for this), but for the majority, their MTHFR works fine at reduced efficiency.[102] However, if MTHFR is compromised enough (genetically or from alcohol), then methylfolate levels are problematically low. In fact, women with certain MTHFR polymorphisms show a 37 to 66 percent increased risk for breast cancer, but high dietary folate should mitigate this risk.[103]

Does low dietary folate lead to higher breast cancer incidence? The Nurses' Health Study looked into folate levels, and all women ingesting at least 300 micrograms a day had 27 percent less breast cancer than those not getting folate. Among all those drinking at least one alcoholic drink a day, 600 micrograms a day of folate reduced breast cancer by 89 percent versus without folate.[104] In the Iowa Women's Health Study, over 34,000 women were followed for thirteen years. An increase in breast cancer correlated to low-folate/high-alcohol intake, and interestingly, the cancers were primarily estrogen receptor-negative tumors, so folate deficiency seems more important than the estrogen increase when it comes to alcohol.[105]

Two tips. One, you have to *consume* folate (human cells can't make it), and heat destroys it, so folate food sources, which contain some methylfolate, have to be eaten raw: broccoli, leafy greens like spinach, kale, and asparagus. Which leads me to the second tip. For moderate drinkers only (averaging at least one drink a day), folate would be one of those exceptions I mentioned regarding taking supplements—just go straight for the active form your DNA needs, methylfolate (not folic acid),

800 micrograms a day—see pinklotus.com/alcohol for more details. Take methylfolate once daily (more is *not* better) at any time. It does not need to be taken with your happy juice. On the flip side, you could drink less than a glass a day.

The Nurses' Health Study also reported their fourteen-year follow-up of over 83,000 participants and showed that in women who consumed at least one alcoholic drink a day, eating five or more servings per day of fruits and vegetables conferred a 47 percent drop in breast cancer as compared to drinkers having two or less servings per day.[106] What's the magic? Beta-carotene. So . . . (insert Bugs Bunny voice) what's up, doc? Eat carrots, sweet potatoes, kale, spinach, broccoli, yellow squash, apricots, cantaloupe, and sweet red peppers—that's what's up. When it comes to beta-carotene, supplements seem to work, but to a lesser degree than food sources, so eat those plants.

Although all types of alcohol can reduce cardiovascular disease, decades of research correctly blame that same alcohol for causing cancers of the mouth, esophagus, liver, colon, and breast.[107] However, one and only one exception to this rule has emerged from recent literature: women consuming 120 to 240 milliliters (4 to 8 ounces) a day of *red wine* as their sole alcohol of choice (FYI, a bottle has 750 milliliters or 25 ounces) actually show a *decrease* in all cancer relative to teetotalers.[108] Wait, what? How? Well, all other alcohol increases estrogen levels, but red wine actually behaves like an aromatase inhibitor (AI), which is a drug given to estrogen-positive breast cancer patients to stop the conversion of your body's steroids into estrogen. Naturally occurring AIs exist in grapes, grape juice, grape-seed extract, and red wine, but not white wine.[109] Can you believe that cancer cells use aromatase to actually create their *own* estrogen so they can fuel themselves? Sinister little beasts. So the AI compound in our red wine–caped hero inactivates the aromatase enzyme, taking away the cells' abilities to auto-fuel. Foiled!

Another kudo awarded to red wine is resveratrol. Resveratrol from red grapes inhibits all three requirements for cancer to form: initiation, promotion, and progression.[110] As such, a large number of human clinical trials are investigating its use as a possible agent against cancer. The resveratrol molecule and AI actions of red wine help explain why moderate red wine consumption (in contrast to all other alcohol choices) does not appear to elevate breast cancer risk. You can also get all these benefits minus the alcohol by eating red grapes, the kind with seeds.[111] The secret is in the skin.

That being said, the International Agency for Research on Cancer (IARC), the official World Health Organization division that decides what causes cancer, has concluded that *all* alcoholic beverages are "carcinogenic to humans."[112] If you want to implement every possible action to reduce breast cancer, the safest amount of alcohol to consume is zero. However, if you choose to consume alcohol, limit intake to 120 to 240 milliliters a day, favor red wine, supplement with methylfolate, and eat your veggies (beta-carotene).

DON'T TAKE MY WORD FOR IT

In 2007, the World Cancer Research Fund (WCRF) and the American Institute for Cancer Research (AICR) released their top recommendations aimed at preventing the most common cancers worldwide.[113] Guess which three, when adhered to in real life, led to a 62 percent drop in postmenopausal invasive breast cancer? Maintaining a healthy weight, limiting alcohol, and consuming plant foods. Sound familiar? That would prevent about ten million diagnoses of invasive breast cancer in the upcoming decade. Ten million!

TOO SWEET TO BE TRUE?

Artificial sweeteners, or synthetic sugar substitutes, allegedly help us decrease the intake of refined sugar and high-fructose corn syrup by providing zero-calorie sweetness in favorite standbys such as soda, ice cream, breakfast cereal, baked goods, and chewing gum. Five FDA-approved sugar substitutes exist in the United States, including aspartame (Equal, NutraSweet, Sugar Twin), sucralose (Splenda), saccharin (Sweet'N Low, Necta Sweet), neotame (Newtame), and acesulfame potassium (Sunett, Sweet One). The US banned cyclamate, but it's widely used in more than one hundred countries.

Bottom line for our main focus: no known link exists between artificial sweeteners and breast cancer. Despite reports to the contrary, no convincing evidence points to any of the artificial sweeteners causing any kind of cancer. You probably remember hearing that sweeteners cause bladder cancers in rats? Turns out that those rats had a bladder cancer–causing parasite (and now, a sugar addiction). At the end of the day, humans aren't rats. Primate studies also showed no malignancies, and neither did a number of studies in humans.[114] That's a relief, because 40 percent of adult Americans consume no-calorie sweeteners on a daily basis, and studies measuring sweeteners in blood and urine show that many who report not using artificial sweeteners do, in fact, consume them unwittingly in anything from baked goods to cough medicine. For completeness, one human study did show an increase in bladder cancer if you consume 1,680 milligrams of sweetener daily (approximately ten cans of diet soda).[115]

The initial hope behind the calorie-free hype was that if you can cut calories, you'll lose weight, leading to better control of blood sugar and possible avoidance of diabetes, heart disease, and obesity. Spoiler alert! You'll never guzzle Diet Pepsi with delight again. The scientifically reported negative associations between artificial sweeteners and health include *excessive weight gain*, obesity, metabolic syndrome, type 2 diabetes, high blood pressure, cardiovascular disease, headaches, migraines, and a deleterious reduction in healthy gut bacteria.[116] These rebound effects come from a tendency to overcompensate for thinking you have caloric room to spare, and therefore doing something like ordering extra fries because you had a Diet Pepsi;[117] also, that sweet taste boosts hunger, but without hunger-satiating calories coming, you just revved up your appetite.[118] *Oops.*

Are there any safe no-calorie or low-calorie sweeteners? Yes. Stevia, thought to be harmless given that it's derived from a South American plant, morphs into mutagenic compounds in your gut and gets absorbed into the bloodstream, but you can safely limit stevia to two sweetened beverages a day (per the World Health Organization, the limit is 4 milligrams of stevia per kilogram of body weight; 1.8 milligrams per pound).[119] Probably the safest sugar substitute in moderation is erythritol (you know it from sugarless gum). Erythritol is made commercially from yeast and contains antioxidant properties.[120]

Although artificial sweeteners don't cause cancer directly, they cause health problems linked to breast cancer like obesity and insulin resistance, and they ultimately reduce more healthful choices. Rather than nibbling on nutrient-dense sweet dates, for example, which are high in fiber and low in glycemic load, someone will choose a Splenda-sweetened muffin. Frequent use of sweeteners stimulates the same addiction-related and pleasure-center pathways in the brain as would shooting heroin (yes, I just said that).[121] Sweeteners decrease interest in consuming less intensely sweet foods, such as fruit, and might make the thought of eating vegetables downright disgusting.[122] Every day, think about trading in a few packets of sweetener for a spoonful of something packed with antioxidants, vitamins, and minerals, such as maple syrup, blackstrap molasses, date sugar or paste, balsamic glaze, brown rice syrup, or real fruit jam.

DO I HAVE TO SHOP ORGANIC?

Let's begin at the end: consuming as many fruits and vegetables as you can fit onto your plate and into your stomach supersedes any concern you should have regarding whether your purchases are organic or not. An inorganic strawberry reduces breast cancer risk more than an organic pizza. What does *organic* mean, anyway? Organic foods are grown without synthetic additives like pesticides, chemical fertilizers, and dyes and are not processed using industrial solvents, irradiation, or genetically modified organisms (GMO). Animals do not receive antibiotics or hormones, and they consume 100 percent organic, non-GMO feed. A "Certified Organic" seal on your food means 95 percent of the ingredients meet these criteria; the remaining 5 percent are additives on an approved list. A "100 Percent Organic" seal means all of the ingredients are organic, whereas "Made with Organic Ingredients" means that at least 70 percent of the food is organic. The claims "Natural" or "All Natural" do not mean organic and basically mean nothing at all, since no laws govern their use on packaging.

What's GMO feed? Seeds can be genetically modified to stay alive when crops are heavily sprayed with pesticides and glyphosate weed killers, and so the question becomes, "What happens if we ingest a small fraction of these toxic chemicals in our food?" One study showed that at the levels you would ingest from GMO soybeans, glyphosate activates estrogen receptors, causing human breast cancer cells to grow in a petri dish.[123] But we don't live in dishes, and no human studies have been done to prove harm (or safety) from eating GMO foods.

Does eating organic translate into health benefits and higher nutritional value? Not really. In a large study of over 623,000 UK women followed over nine years, no reduction in breast cancer was found in the group eating organic food (the only cancer reduced was non-Hodgkin's lymphoma).[124] Scientists at Stanford University compared the evidence in decades of studies regarding the health effects of organic versus conventional foods. They reported significantly lower pesticide levels in the urine of children consuming organic, but biomarker and nutrient levels in blood, urine, breast milk, and semen in adults did not identify any meaningful differences.[125] They did find more vitamin C and cancer-fighting phenols in organic produce, and as we know, those phenols can fight. Organic chicken and milk contained more healthy omega-3 fats. But in the end, researchers concluded that the body of published literature on this subject shows no significant increase in nutrition with organic over conventional foods.

Should we choose organic to avoid pesticide and bacterial exposures in the name of health? Probably. The Stanford review found that organic foods contained 30 percent fewer pesticide residues (all levels were below the danger zone) and no difference in bacterial contamination of *produce*, but watch out for the conventional, nonorganic chickens and pork—they were 33 percent more likely to harbor antibiotic-resistant bacteria (a deadly threat on the rise in our own hospitals, called *superbugs*). When the US Department of Agriculture (USDA) tested 10,187 conventionally grown produce items, they found that 85 percent were contaminated with a variety of 496 different pesticide residues. In contrast, organic produce will consistently have 30 to 50 percent less residues, and far less of a potpourri, than conventional.[126] Confused about how "organic" plus "pesticide" doesn't equal an oxymoron? Organic farming still uses pesticides, but they are derived from natural sources on a USDA-approved list.[127]

Residues often persist after washing and, in some cases, peeling. Remember, consuming as many fruits and vegetables as your plate can hold trumps any concern you should ever have regarding risks from pesticide residue. Fancy products meant to wash off residues better than water don't pass the test, so don't waste your money.[128] To rinse off pesticides as effectively as special washes in cute spray bottles, mix one part table salt to nine parts water, rinse and rub produce, then wash again with only water to get rid of the salt.[129] Chemicals in animal products, however, can't be washed off; they build up in the fats, and cooking can make them worse, not better.[130] You'll just have to eat it (or don't). Tip: boiling eggs reduces more pesticides than scrambling.[131]

Besides avoiding contaminants, when eating organic you also support local agriculture, a healthier work environment for farmers who are exposed to less toxic crops, and environmental sustainability with improved biodiversity due to the earth-friendly farming and livestock practices that shun harsh additives. On average, buying organic costs more—especially for milk, eggs, and meat—but these foods might be the most important ones to prioritize as we strive to limit breast cancer risk. In addition to the chemicals we just mentioned being stored in animal fat, all the approved estrogen-mimicking hormonal additives pumped into animals could interfere with the natural pathways of cell function in the human body. Back in 1981, what's now the European Union became concerned about this harmful estrogen-mimicking in humans and banned the use of all six FDA-*approved* hormone additives: estradiol, progesterone, testosterone, trenbolone acetate, zeranol, and melengestrol acetate (MGA). As we discussed, the literature regarding meat consumption and cancer risk remains inconsistent, but at the very least, consider this: these additives quickly and purposefully fatten a calf with less feed; why wouldn't they do the same to you?

Despite similar nutrient values between organic and conventional foods, it seems wise to avoid unhealthful additives such as harsh pesticides, chemical fertilizers, growth hormones, and antibiotics. I suggest eating organic whenever financially feasible, and prioritize having children, pregnant women, and immune-compromised people eat organic. Strive to purchase organic for animal products (meat, milk, cheese, eggs) and the most heavily contaminated foods, which the USDA updates annually. Visit the Environmental Working Group's (EWG.org) posting of these fruits and veggies for a fun way to review the latest "Dirty Dozen"—the produce most likely to be contaminated with pesticides and pesticide residue. Frequent flyers include strawberries, spinach, nectarines, apples, peaches, celery, grapes, pears, cherries, tomatoes, sweet bell peppers, and potatoes. On the other hand, save your dollars when purchasing from the "Clean Fifteen"—produce least likely to contain pesticide residues: sweet corn, avocados, pineapples, cabbage, onions, frozen sweet peas, papayas, asparagus, mangoes, eggplant, honeydew melon, kiwis, cantaloupe, cauliflower, and grapefruit. An easy way to remember the difference is that most of the clean ones have an outside skin you do *not* eat, whereas all of the dirty ones have edible skin.

A final word (okay, two words) about organic: junk food. You can readily find organic cookies, crackers, chips, ice cream, cheese puffs, donuts, soda, French fries, pizza, jelly beans, and lollipops, to name a few delicious-not-nutritious fake-outs. I recently picked up my son Justin from my parents' house and found him eating an organic double chocolate chip multigrain granola bar. When I asked my mom why he had it, she looked all innocent and wide-eyed at me, and exclaimed, "It's good for him; it's *organic*!" The first ingredient was cane juice with 16 grams of sugar in a 1.3-ounce bar. Inviting labels like "organic" and "multigrain" could trick anyone. It's called a "health halo"—foods considered healthy are consumed in higher quantities, ascribed more nutritional value, and thought to contain fewer calories than they actually do.[132] It's a trap!

FAST FACTS ON FOOD LABELS

Ready for a crash course in how to read food labels to boost not just your breast, but overall health? Nourishment that leaves the bad stuff on the supermarket shelf and only lets you bring the best ingredients into your home and body? For starters, know that *unlabeled* foods get all the gold stars here—apples, fresh kale, frozen berries, nuts, wild rice, and the like. But we can also eat lightly processed and packaged foods while arming our cells with anticancer fuel. Here's how.

1. Ignore front-of-box claims. Phrases like "Excellent Source of Calcium," "Wholesome," "Low-fat," and "No added sugar" are largely unregulated by the FDA. They exist only to get your attention because marketers know you're interested in making healthy choices. Head, instead, to the list of ingredients on the back of all packages. Ideally, an ingredient list reads like a recipe you'd whip together in your own kitchen.

2. Ingredients always get listed in order from the highest quantity to least, so the first three better be good for you and include what you'd expect to see—i.e., whole wheat bread should list "whole wheat" *first*. The shorter the list, the better.

3. Sugar hides behind many sneaky names and shouldn't be one of the item's first three ingredients (I'm looking at you, ketchup). Sugar doesn't directly cause cancer, but your liver turns excess sugar into fat, which leads to weight gain, and being overweight or obese elevates breast cancer risk. By the way, sugar feeds cancer in the *exact same way* that blood glucose (sugar) feeds *all* cells, so don't think that eating more or less sugar can speed or slow

cancer like a game of Red Light/Green Light. When the ingredients contain more than two sugar sources, consider that so-called food a dessert. Any sugar or sweetener, high-fructose corn syrup, honey, molasses, any sugar ending in "ose" (dextrose, fructose, glucose, lactose, maltose, sucrose) and the words *cane, nectar, syrup,* and *juice* are nothing but fat makers, usually with no essential nutrients. Low-cal or calorie-free sugar substitutes from sugar alcohols like mannitol, sorbitol, and xylitol can accompany both good-for-you and not-so-hot foods.

4. Avoid words straight out of a chemistry lesson like butylated hydroxyanisole and ammonium sulfate. These preserve the shelf life of foods, but not *your* life.

5. When it comes to fiber-rich foods, a grain must be the first ingredient listed, and you must see the word *whole* before it, as in whole wheat and whole oats. Put back the fake-outs like multigrain, stone-ground, bran, or even 100 percent wheat. The word *enriched* before a grain means it has been stripped of the germ, bran, nutrients, and fiber, which leaves only a refined plop of a simple carbohydrate sugar that's devoid of nutrition, rapidly enters the bloodstream, spikes insulin levels, and turns to fat. Ever hear the saying, "The whiter the bread, the sooner you're dead"? Sadly, it's true, and it applies to white rice too (e.g., sticky, sushi, basmati, jasmine, and arborio white rices).

6. Don't overconsume GMO soy protein isolate, textured soy, hydrolyzed or textured vegetable protein, soy flour, or soybean oil until we have more scientific data about how these affect human health. Soy by-products are ubiquitous, added to everything from candy bars to beef as emulsifiers, meat extenders, meat analogues, cheap flour, and cheap oil. Per the National Academies of Sciences, Engineering, and Medicine, there's no proven harm from any of these GMO soy products in humans.[133] While we don't have to put this package back every time, favor non-GMO products containing these additives in order to avoid glyphosate, hexane (a chemical solvent used to extract soybean oil from raw soybeans), and high pesticide residues (the USDA reported fourteen different ones in soybean grain alone).[134] By the way, soy by-products don't provide the breast benefits we discussed as coming from non-GMO whole food soy in chapter 3.

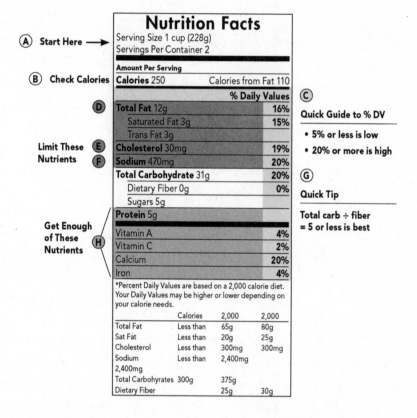

Nutrition Facts

Serving Size 1 cup (228g)
Servings Per Container 2

Amount Per Serving

Calories 250   Calories from Fat 110

	% Daily Values
Total Fat 12g	16%
Saturated Fat 3g	15%
Trans Fat 3g	
Cholesterol 30mg	19%
Sodium 470mg	20%
Total Carbohydrate 31g	20%
Dietary Fiber 0g	0%
Sugars 5g	
Protein 5g	
Vitamin A	4%
Vitamin C	2%
Calcium	20%
Iron	4%

*Percent Daily Values are based on a 2,000 calorie diet. Your Daily Values may be higher or lower depending on your calorie needs.

	Calories	2,000	2,000
Total Fat	Less than	65g	80g
Sat Fat	Less than	20g	25g
Cholesterol	Less than	300mg	300mg
Sodium	Less than	2,400mg	
2,400mg			
Total Carbohyrates	300g	375g	
Dietary Fiber		25g	30g

(A) Start Here →

(B) Check Calories

(D)

Limit These Nutrients (E) (F)

Get Enough of These Nutrients (H)

(C)

Quick Guide to % DV

• 5% or less is low
• 20% or more is high

(G)

Quick Tip

Total carb ÷ fiber
= 5 or less is best

7. If the ingredients pass your test, then take a good look at the charted numbers on the package's "Nutrition Facts" label as well. The letters below reference the label above.

A. Servings Per Container: All of this info pertains to one serving, not the whole box, so know thy serving size—and how many servings are in the entire box (and how many you plan to consume).

B. "Calories" listed are also per serving, so multiply that number by how many servings you're about to chow down. Tell me I'm not alone here. I found the most delicious 35-calorie-per-serving popcorn and devoured the whole bag while watching a show, only to flip the bag over to discover I gobbled fifteen servings and 525 calories! When it comes to "Calories from Fat," consume 20 percent or less of your daily calories from healthy fats, and saturated fats should be no more than 5 percent of your daily calories. Fat is the only dietary percentage I pay any attention to when it comes to my daily intake. Divide the calories from fat by the calories per serving and make sure it's 0.20 or less (above, 110 ÷ 250 = 44 percent fat calories). Or allow 2 grams fat per 100 calories. Or if you splurge with one food, be done with fat for the day.

C. The "% Daily Value" column tells you what percent of the recommended daily total is in one serving, assuming 2,000 calories per day. Tip: Peek at these percentages and just note extremes, less than 5 percent and more than 20 percent, to make sure nothing surprises you, like getting 80 percent of your daily fat from one cookie. And then move on.

D. Minimize saturated fat and avoid trans fat completely. Do you see how saturated plus trans equals less than the total fat, accounting for 6 grams out of 12 grams? Labels do not have to tell you the polyunsaturated fat and monounsaturated fat breakdown, but PUFA and MUFA make up the missing 6 grams here. Tip: If the package dazzled you with the claim "Reduced Fat," immediately check the sugars. Gram for gram, fat has nine calories, but sugar only has four. So I can turn a healthy 100 calories (like peanut butter) into a sugar nut bomb with 100 calories (reduced-fat peanut butter) by saying: give me one fat, and I'll give you more than two sugars back. Sometimes, the full fat version is actually healthier.

E. Our cells can make all the cholesterol they need to function, so don't purposefully consume extra LDL to hand over to cancer cells. If this number isn't "0," there's an animal product in there somewhere; plants are naturally cholesterol-free.

F. According to the American Heart Association, the average American eats 3,400 milligrams of sodium a day, but the ideal limit is 1,500 milligrams per day or less (3/4 teaspoon). Tip: sodium content shouldn't exceed the calories per serving. If it does and you still eat it, guzzle a couple glasses of water. Also, "reduced sodium" doesn't mean "low." Kikkoman's "37 percent Less Sodium" Soy Sauce has 575 milligrams of sodium per tablespoon, so it's basically 37 percent less than a salt lick.

G. The majority of your food calories should come from complex carbohydrates and fiber, as these burst with all the phytonutrients that fight cancer: whole grains, fruits, vegetables, and beans. To find nutritious bread and cracker products, divide the total carbohydrates by the grams of fiber; the number should be less than five. In 2021, labels will specify refined added sugars here. Unrefined sugars like fructose from eating apples and beets come packed with the food's fiber, which slows sugar absorption, avoids insulin spikes, evens out energy levels, works against weight gain, and lowers estrogen levels. Therefore, if the product has sugar, look for an even number of fiber grams to balance out the sugar grams. You can currently identify added sugars by scanning the ingredients list for additives like high-fructose corn syrup. According to the American Heart Association, women should limit sugar to 25 grams (6 teaspoons) per day, but we average 76.7 grams (19 teaspoons). One can of Coke has 39 grams of sugar. Mary Poppins should switch to water to help her blood pressure medicine go down.

H. Excellent plant sources of protein like lentils, soy, and beans comingle with healthy carbs and good fats in such an elegant fashion that you don't need to count calories or pay attention to the rest of this label—you're good to go (eat).

HOW DO YOUR FAVORITE FOODS ADD UP?

So now that you're practically an expert on what to nosh and not nosh to maintain breast health, aren't you curious about how their cancer-fighting abilities compare? In my favorite food study, researchers recorded the total antioxidant content of 3,139 foods, beverages, spices, herbs, and supplements used worldwide—everything from Coca-Cola to coconuts.[135]

At the very tippity-top of the scale sits the Indian gooseberry (it's in my Antioxidant Smoothie as *amla* powder), scoffing at the blueberry 124 times beneath it. Plants, on average, carry *64 times* the antioxidant power of meat, fish, eggs, and dairy. Let that sink in. So that means, gram per gram, in order to ingest the antioxidant content in one cup of blueberries (100 grams, 57 calories, 0.3 grams fat), you would need to eat 27.5 slices of cheese pizza (2,750 grams, 7,590 calories, 323 grams fat).[136] Cancer only needs one of the more than fifty trillion cells in our bodies to make a mistake while dividing and a window of opportunity opens. Let's hope you just poured a bunch of free radical–scavenging antioxidants in the way of that window. If the only thing defending your cells is a chicken wing and white rice, that cancer cell will fly much faster than the bird you sent after it.

So as you decide what to eat for dinner tonight, remember that the preponderance of scientific evidence points to the irrefutable, lifesaving power of whole food, plant-based eating. Anything particularly healthful gained by consuming meat, dairy, and eggs might very well be offset by the contaminants, additives, cholesterol, and fats that ignite a cascade of oxidative stress and angiogenesis. You don't have to abandon your favorite foods, but make choices that shift the balance of health on your plate into Camp Antioxidant for most of the meals of your life. There are twenty-one meals a week, and Americans eat out four to five times a week, on average. Seize these opportunities to find plant-based restaurants or new items at your favorite places that offer fresher fare. At home, try my Antioxidant Smoothie for breakfast a few times a week. Trade out the animal products within your standby faves. For example, we tweaked our family burrito bar to eliminate meat and dairy: black beans, refried beans, cilantro, kale, guacamole, pico de gallo, olives, dairy-free cheese and sour cream (cashew based), and meatless ground turkey (soy-based). *Delicioso.* To inspire your culinary curiosity, I offer these trusted sources for you to find hundreds of free recipes, cookbooks, kick-start plans, online cooking classes, meal planners, smartphone apps, articles, and educational resources in the hopes that you will discover your healthiest self in evidence-based nutritious eating:

- NutritionFacts.org (Dr. Michael Greger); and his books: *How Not to Die: Discover the Foods Scientifically Proven to Prevent and Reverse Disease* and *The How Not to Die Cookbook*
- Forks Over Knives: forksoverknives.com

- Physicians Committee for Responsible Medicine: pcrm.org
- Center for Nutrition Studies (Dr. T. Colin Campbell): NutritionStudies.org

Get your loved ones involved and transform your whole family's health for the better.

COME TO THE TABLE!

Transitioning to whole food, plant-based eating? What has helped you the most? Found any rock-star recipes? Beloved brands? I want to hear about it. Log onto pinklotus.com/myexperience to share your tips and tricks!

CHAPTER 5

Beyond Food: What You Should Do

What in the world? An estimated 1.67 million new breast cancer cases were diagnosed worldwide in 2012, but I've seen the math, and guess what that number will be in 2050?

You might want to sit down for this.

The predicted international incidence of female breast cancer will be a shocking 3.2 million cases *per year* by 2050.[1] *That's double the rate in less than forty years.*

Ladies, we have *got* to get this under control. Strategically improving your diet is a huge step, but there's still more you can do to reverse this killer trend.

As you read this chapter, I'm not insisting that if you don't cut all the risk factors here out of your life, your breasts are doomed. All known breast cancer risk factors are *contributory* causes, meaning the exposures *add to* risk, but alone and by themselves, they do not possess the power to independently cause breast cancer. This applies to everything from nutrition and obesity to alcohol and the air we breathe. Think about the proverbial straw that breaks a camel's back: the camel plods along appearing healthy and strong, carrying a seemingly manageable load, until one more little strand of straw atop his back sends him crashing to the ground under the weight of it all. Any and every straw we can avoid will lessen the total burden we have to carry. If we can avoid or remove enough elective straws, our backs and breasts will never break.

ADDRESSING A WORLDWIDE CATASTROPHE

Around the world, breast cancer already ranks as the most frequent cause of cancer death annually in women in less developed regions (324,000 deaths, 14.3 percent of total), and it is the second cause of cancer death after lung cancer in women in more developed regions (198,000 deaths, 15.4 percent).[2] A few telling trends emerge when comparing breast cancer incidence from eighteen selected cancer registries and ethnic/racial groups in East Asia, Europe, and the United States between 1973 and 1997.[3]

First of all, these decades witnessed an explosion in worldwide breast cancer with all the numbers and figures moving up, up, and away with no downturn in sight. Second, it's clear that cancer rates in Europe and the United States far exceed the levels in Asia. But what about Asians in the US—are rates lower like back home, or do they mirror their new home? Japanese immigrants in Los Angeles and Hawaii show a sharp breast cancer increase after 1982, and then Chinese in Hawaii do the same hockey-stick shaped spike after 1992 *at rates over 100 percent higher than Japanese and Chinese still in their homeland.* What happened when they left home? And while we're talking about home, those in urban areas of China (Hong Kong), Singapore, and Japan had a 50 to 100 percent increase in cancer, so what happened when they stayed home?

Since only 5 to 10 percent of all breast cancers come from inherited mutations, and deleterious DNA mutations don't suddenly affect an entire planet of women all at once—doubling breast cancer rates in twenty-five years—another very significant factor must be marching this disease forward at such a rapid pace. Also, the short time frame in which the worldwide cancer rates have risen makes a purely genetic explanation impossible. So what can we blame? Well, what grows worse every year in America? What was happening in Asia in the 1970s and

1980s that incubates trouble for ten to thirty years before you notice it? What dramatically accelerated the breast cancer mortality rate in Japan by 55 percent between 1990 and 2000?[4]

I'll tell you what: the American lifestyle. From our habits, to our food, our weight, our inactivity, our delayed childbearing, our hormones, and our whole way of life.[5] Asians started chasing our culture, and as a result, they caught our cancer. Sadly, our contagious lifestyle has infected the entire world.[6] Ironically, the antidote is to revert to the dietary and lifestyle behaviors that the world possessed *before* it successfully emulated the behavior of the affluent United States.

Beginning in the 1970s, the growing economics and increased prosperity in Japan, Singapore, and urban China sparked westernized changes in how people went about their days. Data even shows that migration from a low-risk country to the United States increases breast cancer risk in proportion to (1) the length of time lived in the US, (2) the number of preceding generations that are American-born, and (3) the degree to which an American lifestyle is adopted.[7] We shouldn't be surprised, then, that the international trends from the next decade, 1998 to 2008, look even worse, displaying increased breast cancer rates in all eight Asian American populations evaluated (Indians/Pakistanis, Chinese, Filipinos, Japanese, Kampucheans, Koreans, Laotians, and Vietnamese), with incidence hikes ranging from 20 percent in Filipinos to 370 percent in Koreans.[8]

The problem looks the same in the East and West: instead of laboring all day in the home, tending to children, and preparing fresh meals, women in the United States and around the world now enter the work force in droves, leading stressful and sedentary lives, delaying childbearing until later years (if at all), eating leftover pizza for lunch while sending off that e-mail ASAP, and then dashing home just in time to put takeout on the table, pour a glass of wine, and catch a favorite TV show before bed. We're not healthy. I've spent some time in this club—how about you?

Perhaps we shouldn't be surprised that the same unhealthy lack of balance that increases our risk of breast cancer is seven times more likely to permanently stop our hearts. Heart disease is twenty-one times more likely to exist and seven times more likely to kill you than breast cancer. You don't need to be a statistician to be floored by the numbers of American women diagnosed and killed annually:[9]

ILLNESS	NEW CASES	DEATHS
Heart disease	6,600,000	289,758
Invasive breast cancer	252,710	40,610

We need to rediscover balance: a way of life where physical, emotional, relational, intellectual, and spiritual needs receive daily nourishment to keep our souls—and our cells—rejuvenated. "How bad is it?" you ask. Oh, sister, it's bad. But just as I proposed in the food chapters, you can control this, too, so come on, give me a biceps flex and let's exert some power.

LOSE THE LOVE HANDLES

I'm just going to be blunt here: if you're too chubby, your extra pounds can kill you. When an obese cancer patient looks at me and asks, "How did this happen?" I'd never blame or shame her, but *shame on me* if I pass by a critical opportunity to help this woman make healthy changes that might save her life. The truth is, I don't know for a fact that her fatness made a difference, but with or without other identifiable risk factors, odds remain that the fat mattered. Being overweight or obese is the single most preventable contribution to the causation of breast cancer worldwide, with 25 percent of all cases being due to the deadly combination of obesity and a sedentary lifestyle.[10] In the United States, up to 50 percent of postmenopausal breast cancer *deaths* can be attributed to obesity.[11] Are you one of the 2.1 billion people in the world (nearly 30 percent of the planet) or one of the 68.8 percent of American adults who is overweight or obese?[12] To find out, calculate your body mass index (BMI).

CALCULATE YOUR BODY MASS INDEX (BMI)

BMI = [Weight in pounds ÷ Height in inches^2] x 703

BMI metric = Weight in kilograms ÷ Height in meters^2

Calculate your BMI at pinklotus.com/bmi.

How do you look? Underweight = <18.5; Normal weight = 18.5–24.9; Overweight = 25–29.9; Obese = 30–39.9; Morbidly obese = >40

Every other breast article I read seems to highlight yet another study proving that overweight and obese women have more (1) postmenopausal breast cancer, (2) breast cancer recurrence, and (3) breast cancer-related death than non-obese women. No question. No controversy. Curiously, being overweight in youth exerts a protective effect against getting breast cancer prior to age fifty, except for those with a family history of the disease,[13] but overweight and obese adult women have a 50 to 250 percent greater risk for postmenopausal breast cancer than normal weight women.[14] If you were plump as a child, it's unlikely you lost that weight by age eighteen, but if you did, you get the best of both the overweight and normal-weight worlds. Once breast cancer happens, women with a BMI of 30 or more suffer a 57 percent increase in breast cancer recurrence.[15] The American Cancer Society studied 495,477 women for sixteen years and stratified the groups according to BMI. They compared breast cancer mortality among the BMI groups and found that the following increases in *death* correlated to increased weight:

BMI = 18.5 to 24.9, baseline risk
BMI = 25 to 29.9, 34 percent
BMI = 30 to 34.9, 63 percent
BMI = 35 to 39.9, 70 percent
BMI at or over 40 = 112 percent increase in breast cancer *death*[16]

We could literally stop around 14,500 postmenopausal breast cancer deaths per year if American women maintained a BMI of less than 25 throughout their adult lives.[17] Wouldn't that be incredible?

Obesity and breast cancer risk go hand-in-hand thanks, in part, to estrogen receptors that sit like little antennas on some normal breast cells and about 80 percent of cancer cells.[18] Whenever estrogen lands in the receptor, it sends signals inside the cell that make cancer multiply and divide. It stands to reason, then, that excess estrogen is a risk factor for estrogen-positive breast cancer.

High estrogen levels *after* menopause increase your breast cancer risk. How is this possible if your ovaries have already shut down? Well, before menopause, most estrogen comes from your ovaries, but after, it's from adipose—a.k.a. fat. Wherever fat hangs out, it has an enzyme called *aromatase*, which it uses to convert other steroids in your body into estrogen. Your adrenal glands produce these steroids, and your postmenopausal ovaries still secrete testosterone, and *fat* converts it all to active estrogen. So we still make estrogen after menopause (though apparently not enough to stop a hot flash).

All that estrogen-creating fat explains why blood tests confirm that obese women have 130 percent higher estradiol levels (the main cancer-fueling estrogen) than lean women.[19] By the way, premenopausal obese and lean women have similar estradiol levels, so the fat factor really kicks in after menopause.[20] The fat inside your breast also contains aromatase, and so does that sinister tumor itself. In fact, with enough breast fat, estrogen levels inside tumors can be tenfold higher than blood estrogen levels.[21] In addition, fat cells (adipocytes) secrete a number of inflammatory mediators that all promote tumor growth, with fancy letters like TNFα, IL-6, VEGF, HGF, IGF-1, and leptin. These increase aromatase, stimulate angiogenesis, cause hyperinsulinemia, and create inflammation—all requirements for carcinogenesis, which we discussed in chapter 3.[22] So we make estrogen forever, and obese women have more estrogen, more aromatase, more angiogenesis, and more hyperinsulinemia, but *do obese women have more cancer?*

To answer this, we turn to postmenopausal women with cancer who never took hormone replacement therapy (HRT), because HRT would be an external estrogen source not attributable to the adrenal gland/fat

115

connection. When we do this, we find that, relative to the weight women were at age eighteen, the amount of weight gain corresponds linearly to a gain in risk (the heavier you are, the higher the cancer chances). As I said, childhood chubbiness seems to be protective, but those days are long gone for most of us, and now the risk is real. So what was your weight in high school? Got that number? Now subtract that from your current weight. Got that number? All right, here we go.

If you have lost weight, wow, good for you and your skinny jeans. If you gained less than 8 pounds, there is 0 percent increased risk (hooray); an 8-to-13.9-pound gain yields a 25 percent increase in risk; a 14-to-29-pound gain, 60 percent; and over 21 pounds gained nearly doubles your risk with a 90 percent increase in breast cancer.[23] *Gulp.* Your chances of getting a postmenopausal breast cancer go up as fast as the dial on your scale. As you would expect from this discussion, the cancers obese women get are usually estrogen-positive.[24]

Cue the good news. If you are overweight and lose that fat, you will lose your risk—and it doesn't take years to take effect. Seriously, it's that simple. Weight loss through either caloric restriction or gastric bypass surgery leads to a reduction in circulating estrogens.[25] And, as hoped, this leads to less cancer. A recent study showed an incredible 85 percent reduction in breast cancer after gastric bypass surgery.[26] Another study followed 33,660 women over fifteen years, and 1,987 got cancer. The highest rates were in women who steadily gained weight throughout life, but for women who maintained or lost weight, their chances of getting breast cancer dropped 64 percent for premenopausal weight loss, 52 percent for postmenopausal weight loss, and 34 percent for weight maintenance.[27] It pays to be a loser, and the younger the better.

Not to scare you, but to incentivize you, if you have already been diagnosed with cancer, gaining more than 5 percent of your initial weight during or after treatment—irrespective of baseline BMI—increases the risk of recurrence and reduces survival fivefold, that's 400 percent.[28] So let's at least not *gain* weight, okay? To lower or maintain body weight poses a challenge for many women, but remember, it's always simple math: burn more calories than you eat.

SKINNY TIPS FOR HEALTHY BREASTS

As a former chubster still wanting to knock off the final five, weight loss tips are my jam. My number-one rule to maintaining a healthy BMI is to know thy portion size. Use your hand as a rough guide for how much of a given food you should eat at any meal or snack:

Palm of your hand: Protein from seitan, tofu, beans, lentils, peas.

Fist: Whole grain rice, pasta, cereal, fruit, or vegetables.

Two open handfuls: Soup or salad.

One open handful: Dried fruit and nut snack.

Thumb: Peanut butter or cheese.

Other favorite tricks?

1. Drink a glass of water twenty minutes before a meal so you consume fewer calories.

2. When you feel like eating something, ask yourself, "Am I hungry?" We eat for so many different reasons, it's hard to find a reason *not* to eat. But you should eat because you're hungry.

3. Don't have food in the house that you should ban from your lips, like chips.

4. Keep healthy snacks at the ready: carrots and hummus, a handful of nuts, a piece of fruit.

5. Drink three 4-ounce cups of green tea a day to boost metabolism.

6. Use small plates, chew solid food thirty times before swallowing, take at least twenty minutes to eat a meal, and stop eating when you feel three-quarters full.

7. Read food labels and cut out the refined sugar and high-fructose corn syrup.

8. Don't diet. Create a healthy eating style you can maintain lifelong. See chapters 3 and 4.

BUST A MOVE

If your idea of exercise is twisting the cap off a peanut butter jar, we've got some room to improve. A study compared 17,171 postmenopausal women who briskly walked for 1.25 to 2.5 hours per week to those who didn't. The walkers reduced their breast cancer risk by 18 percent.[29] Life saving benefits from *eleven minutes a day*. What would happen if you put some pep in your step, carried a five-pound weight, or bumped it up to thirty minutes? Women who exercise for three to four hours per week at moderate to vigorous levels (breaking a sweat and impossible to carry on a conversation) have 30 to 40 percent less breast cancer than sedentary women.[30] More than four hours? A 58 percent decrease.[31]

So exercise helps you avoid breast cancer, but what if you already have breast cancer, can exercise save the day? Apparently so. A study revealed that, *even when obese*, the combination of merely walking thirty minutes six days a week with consuming five or more servings of daily vegetables conferred a 44 percent survival advantage over those who adhered to one or neither of these lifestyles.[32] And compared with those who were basically totally lazy, doing no exercise whatsoever both before and after diagnosis, women who increased physical activity after diagnosis had a 45 percent lower risk of death, while women who decreased physical activity after diagnosis had a 300 percent increase in death.[33] Seriously, if you have breast cancer, it's time to feel empowered by facts and do some joyful jumping jacks.

How, exactly, does physical activity decrease our number-one cancer risk or the threat of its recurrence? First and foremost, it causes estrogen levels to drop; even among women who are all obese according to their BMI, we find fewer cancer-fueling estrogens in the more active ladies.[34] In addition to reducing body weight and circulating levels of sex hormones, exercise reduces insulin resistance, and all the other letter-factories in the above obesity section like $TNF\alpha$, IGF-1, and leptin that adversely affect the immune system and stoke the cancer cell microenvironment.[35] Other advantages of exercise for all women with or without breast cancer include: decreased heart disease, lower blood pressure, less type 2 diabetes, happier mood, sounder sleep, improved bone health with less osteoporosis, decreased fatigue, increased endurance, reduced stress, and less lymphedema (arm swelling after lymph node surgery).[36] The only downside is that you'll soon need smaller clothes.

How much activity gets you the cancer risk reduction you want? The latest guidelines from the National Institutes of Health (NIH) state that for the most overall health benefit, we should do 300 minutes (5 hours) of moderate intensity aerobic activity (like power walking) or 150 minutes (2.5 hours, that's 22 minutes a day) of vigorous supersweaty activity each week.[37] The more active you are, the more you will benefit. Add moderate to vigorous muscle-strengthening activities two or more days a week. These should work all the major muscle groups (legs, hips, back, chest, abdomen, shoulders, and arms). Examples include lifting weights, working with resistance bands, doing sit-ups and push-ups, and yoga. Unfortunately, less than 13 percent of patients with breast cancer attain *half* the time stated in these goals.[38]

Here's the simple and unglamorous key to exercise: make a plan and just do it—alone, with a friend, or with a trainer. Don't make exercise a choice. Mark it on the calendar, and make it happen. If five minutes makes you pant, that's awesome. Shower and move on. Don't get discouraged, and show up again tomorrow. A slow or short walk/run is always better than no movement at all. Stick with it and amaze yourself at how a mere two weeks ago you could not make it half the distance you achieve today. Work up to the time goals as best you can.

Just shy of forty years old, I delivered my triplet boys, and time was not on my side. Three months earlier, Andy and I had also just birthed our first baby, the Pink Lotus Breast Center, at the absolute nadir of worldwide financial collapse, so post-babies, I went straight back to work and had no time for gyms or spin classes. I got into home DVD workouts, specifically *Beachbody* with Tony Horton's P90X. I occasionally used the boys, then a very convenient ten, twelve, and fifteen pounds, as swaddled dumbbells (I'm kidding, but I did like to do bicep curls with them in my arms just to make them giggle). Like I said, ladies, the key to exercise is to *just do it* (right, Nike?).

DO OLDER MOMS GET MORE CANCER?

Speaking of forty, the age at which a woman delivers her first child impacts the risk of breast cancer. While you and I can control this to a certain degree, no one would advocate multiple pregnancies in your teenage years for the sake of breast cancer reduction. Nevertheless, women who deliver children prior to age twenty show a 50 percent reduction in breast cancer relative to women who never have children.[39] And those of us who wait until after age thirty-five for a first full-term pregnancy receive a baby and a 40 percent increase in breast cancer compared to women without kids. Yikes. The good news, however, is that this elevated risk only lasts for ten to fifteen years and then drops *below* that of the never-pregnant woman. It turns out that pregnancy exerts opposing influences on the risk of breast cancer: a short-term detrimental effect caused by pregnancy hormones grows existing cancer cells (present pre-pregnancy but undetected), and a long-term protective effect enables some breast cells to resist carcinogenic stimuli.[40] This protective effect doesn't really kick in until ten years after the last delivery, and in the interim, older childbearing women demonstrate a slight increase in breast cancer relative to their never-pregnant peers.[41]

Harkening back to my brief statistics lesson on relative and absolute risk in chapter 3, if you deliver your first child at age thirty-eight, this changes your absolute risk from 1.9 percent to 2.7 percent by age fifty. Most moms would agree that's a risk worth taking. Women having their first child when they are eighteen years or younger have about one-third the lifetime breast cancer risk of those who delay their first birth until they are thirty-five or older.[42] Are you wondering why your calculated decision to delay childbearing in pursuit of a meaningful career or the right partner has this unfair payback? Well, the most plausible explanation for the age factor, pregnancy, and breast cancer risk is this: your first pregnancy creates permanent changes to the cells that line your breast ducts and lobules, which are the cells that form the vast majority of breast cancers. These cells become "locked" into their DNA at the time and spend the rest of their lives in growth and division phases. When you lock in the cell DNA at a young age, cells tend to be healthy, but DNA mutations come along with aging, so a first-time pregnancy after age thirty has a greater chance of locking in a mutated cell.[43] This mutated cell usually takes years to repeatedly multiply and divide until it finally manifests as a cancerous lump.

Although studies differ on the matter of breastfeeding and cancer reduction, the majority demonstrate protective effects, and insofar as you are able or interested, nursing can only lead to health benefits and no detriments for you and your baby. A 2015 meta-analysis of twenty-seven studies concluded that women who breastfeed decrease their lifetime breast cancer risk by an average of 39 percent.[44] Some studies show even higher benefits with a lifetime total of twenty-four or more cumulative months of breastfeeding and with earlier age at first lactation.[45] Three studies looked at receptor status of tumors and concluded that if you've ever breastfed, you reduce aggressive triple-negative breast cancer (TNBC) rates by 22 percent but do not affect estrogen-positive tumors.[46] This report goes hand-in-hand with another that found a 32 percent reduction from breastfeeding for one year and 49 percent reduction for two years or more in BRCA-1 mutation carriers (high TNBC risk); in contrast, BRCA-2 mutation carriers (low TNBC risk) only showed a 17 percent reduction.[47] Other studies from southern Europe, Italy, and the United States present counterpoint data, concluding that no cancer protection exists from breastfeeding.[48]

HANDLE MENOPAUSE WISELY

Menopausal symptoms come in three flavors: vasomotor (hot flashes and night sweats), central (insomnia, mood changes, brain fog, lost libido, memory loss), and urogenital (frequent urinary tract infections, urinary urgency, vaginal dryness with painful intercourse). Each symptom can adversely affect your quality of life on multiple levels. Hopefully, you weren't dealt the entire constellation of craziness, but whatever you do have, you may have considered taking hormone replacement therapy (HRT) to alleviate the unwelcome changes. HRT ameliorates some or all of these symptoms and protects against osteoporosis (accelerated bone loss). But as with any medicine, risks exist. Given alone, estrogen can increase endometrial cancer, and that's why you protect your uterus (if you have one) by taking progesterone with the estrogen. Anything else? Oh, yes, HRT can also cause breast cancer.

How did estrogen become the bad guy here? As I've touched on already, breast cancer cells often have receptors that bind estrogen and progesterone, and when hormones fit into their little receptor, they launch cell growth and division events that culminate in a cancerous cell turning into a detectable lump. You know how I occasionally mention lab experiments using petri dishes filled with human breast cancer cells? Guess how scientists make those cells in the first place? They drip *estrogen* (specifically, 17-beta-estradiol) onto normal breast cells to transform them into cancer.[49] Hormones both initiate breast cancer and promote its growth, and those receptors don't care if the hormones came from your own ovary or horse's urine (from which the HRT drug Prempro is made). Estrogen metabolites also yield by-products that can directly cause DNA damage and mutation, so HRT enters into the battle of oxidative stress, which we have discussed as the key fight in all of this cancer business.[50] For these reasons, I feel it's important to permanently shy away from HRT if you have already had breast cancer, but that issue is controversial.

What if you've never had breast cancer and aren't considered high risk to get it; isn't it safe to take HRT? Studies show that HRT increases breast density in 75 percent of users (more so from the progesterone component), and denser breasts create more cancers (see the next chapter), so that's one strike against HRT.[51] And then there are studies—two biggies. The Women's Health Initiative (WHI) randomized 16,000 postmenopausal women to either Prempro (estrogen plus progesterone) or placebo.[52] After 5.2 years, they called it quits for ethical reasons, since 26 percent more breast cancers had accrued in HRT users (along with heart attacks, strokes, blood clots, and dementia, but fewer colon cancers and hip fractures). In response, a whopping 33 million women abruptly stopped their HRT and leapt into the ring for Menopause Round Two: Woman Versus Hot Flashes/Night Sweats/Insomnia/Mood Swings. Guess what got knocked out the very next year? Breast cancer. Rates plummeted an unprecedented 6.7 percent in 2003. Also in 2003, researchers in the UK published their observation in over 1.1 million women that HRT causes a 66 percent increase in breast cancer.[53] The results were in: HRT fuels breast cancer; stopping HRT reduces breast cancer.

Those conclusions pertain to estrogen *plus* progesterone. What if you don't have a uterus and therefore only need estrogen? Studies confirm the following regarding estrogen-only use: estrogen yields 23 percent less breast cancer after ten years' use,[54] but poses a 57 percent *increase* in cancer risk if that use occurs within five years of menopause,[55] *or* if taken for more than ten years total.[56] Therefore, it seems safest to wait five years into menopause before initiating estrogen-only HRT (which probably doesn't help you when you really need it and is not possible if you have a uterus), and you should discontinue its use within a decade.

I'm not telling you to tough it out in drenched sweats, but I always advise a little education. Balance personal risk versus benefit from HRT. With your doctor, look at your risk profile for getting breast cancer, uterine cancer, colorectal cancer, heart disease, dementia, strokes, blood clots, and bone fractures. Then tell your doctor why you want HRT. Is it because you heard that taking HRT in your fifties decreases heart disease and strokes, and your father died from a heart attack at age forty-eight?[57] You should eat more salads, jump on the treadmill, and stay far away from HRT until more studies prove it's cardio-protective. Did Mom have a horrible hip fracture at eighty, and you never want to suffer like she did? We can offer bisphosphonates, calcium, vitamin D, and a weight-bearing exercise routine. By the way, if you barely notice menopause symptoms, you don't need to do anything regarding this entirely normal and expected phase of life.

On the other hand, if you're low-risk for adverse outcomes, and high-risk for breaking the menopause misery meter, then we have some good options. Again, what do you want to eliminate? Vaginal dryness could be treated with a topical vaginal estrogen, which gives 80 to 100 percent relief, and has very little absorption into your bloodstream. We also have an array of new laser treatments that stimulate collagen and moisture "down there" like MonaLisa Touch and ThermiVa. Be encouraged that 90 percent of women have no hot flashes after four to five years, and symptoms can often be relieved by an increase in fiber, fruit, and vegetable consumption and exercise. Always consider nonhormonal options first that don't elevate cancer risk.[58] Menopause Miracle is an estrogen-free herbal supplement that dramatically improved menopause symptoms in three double-blind, randomized, placebo-controlled, peer-reviewed human studies.[59] Be sure to work with an appropriate practitioner to dispense the right doses and monitor your progress.

ALTERNATIVES TO HRT FOR HOT FLASHES

- Complementary medicine: acupuncture, Chinese herbs
- Herbal remedies: black cohosh (*Actaea racemosa*, plant extract); *dong quai* (*Angelica sinensis*, a medicinal root); evening primrose oil (*Oenothera biennis*, wildflower seeds, an omega-6 essential fatty acid); ginseng (a medicinal root); melatonin (a brain hormone that regulates the sleep/wake cycle); Menopause Miracle (a proprietary blend of Korean and Chinese roots: *Cynanchum wilfordii, Phlomis umbrosa,* and *Angelica gigas*); vitamin E (an antioxidant)
- Prescription medications that change nerve impulses and blood flow: Bellergal (ergotamine), Catapres (clonidine), Neurontin (gabapentin)
- Prescription medications that block brain chemicals like serotonin and norepinephrine—you know them as antidepressant and antianxiety meds: Effexor (venlafaxine), Paxil (paroxetine), Prozac (fluoxetine)
- Body movement: biofeedback (a technique that teaches voluntary control of muscle tension, temperature, heart rate, and brain activity), focused breathing, exercise, stretching, *tai chi* (stress reduction through gentle, flowing movements), yoga

- Phytoestrogens/isoflavones act preferentially on beta estrogen receptors (alpha receptors are the ones associated with breast cancer): red clover extract (*Trifolium pratense*, an herb); soy (consumed in whole foods: tempeh, sprouted tofu, edamame)

You might also consider bioidentical HRT (BHRT) that chemically matches our naturally occurring steroids, including progesterone, estradiol, estrone, estriol, pregnenolone, testosterone, and dehydroepiandrosterone (DHEA). Drug companies make them from animal or plant sources, with FDA regulation to ensure uniform dosing and purity, while compounding pharmacies also make them by creating personalized non-FDA approved hormonal blends suited to your needs. They sound fancy, but do they work, and are they safe? I sure hope so, because US doctors write an estimated 26 to 33 million prescriptions annually for unregulated compounded BHRT.[60]

BHRT products often come from some of my favorite food sources, such as soybeans and yams, which sounds so beneficial and friendly, but lab alterations morph those phytoestrogens from their natural state. How do we know if they remain as protective as they once were, or maybe they have become harmful? BHRT still needs to be tested in large-volume, high-quality clinical trials for efficacy and safety. Without studies, we don't know if they reduce or surpass the problems we saw in the WHI group with Prempro, such as breast cancer, heart attack, and stroke. Whether compounded or FDA-approved, BHRT is available in various dosages, combinations, preparations, and routes of delivery that may have differing effects on risk to an individual patient.[61] Given the molecular match to our own hormones, one would guess that BHRT effects are lower than synthetic versions, but when it comes to breast cancer and other critical health issues, guessing isn't good enough. If you do decide to use either HRT or BHRT, I advise doing so at the lowest dose that controls your symptoms and for the shortest amount of time needed to carry you through a rough patch.

TRASH YOUR CIGARETTES

Did you know that lung cancer is the number-one cancer killer of women? In 2017, 105,510 women were diagnosed with lung cancer, and 71,280 died from it—because we can't cure them.[62] Since smoking causes 87 percent of all lung cancers, if smokers would stop smoking, then they (and secondhand smokers) would stop dying. Smoking damages nearly every organ in your body. Besides lung cancer, tobacco use also causes cancer of the mouth, nasal cavities, larynx, pharynx, esophagus, stomach, liver, pancreas, kidney, bladder, and uterine cervix, plus myeloid leukemia.[63] It causes infertility and, *egads*, unsightly pucker wrinkles around your mouth. So not only does smoking kill you, it makes you look ugly at your own funeral.

But does smoking cause breast cancer? Over one hundred studies have investigated this issue, and smoking seems to be a compelling cause if you are young, have yet to get pregnant, smoked more than forty years, or already have breast cancer. There are a number of smokers who don't land on that short list. How can smoking be so carcinogenic and toxic everywhere else in the body, and yet maybe not in the breast? Smoking causes genetic mutations in breast tissue and carcinogens build up in breast fluid,[64] but smoking also increases the breakdown of estradiol.[65] By now, you recognize estrogen's name as a major driving force in the causation of most breast cancers, so clearly, less estrogen protects you. The net effect on breast tissue might be that the antiestrogen and pro-cancer components of smoking cancel each other out.

Before you rush out to buy a pack of Virginia Slims, many studies repeatedly point to certain subgroups of women smokers who have an increase in breast cancer. Smoking during adolescence or early adulthood exposes breast cells to chemical carcinogens before the breasts finish developing, which helps explain why smoking has more consistent links with premenopausal breast cancer.[66] Young women who smoke the equivalent of a pack a day for twenty years before their first pregnancy have a 73 percent breast cancer increase.[67] Women who smoke ciga-rettes for forty or more years have a 50 percent increase in breast cancer relative to nonsmokers.[68] The California Teachers Study followed over 116,000 women and found that active smokers of any duration had a 32 percent higher chance of breast cancer versus never-smokers or those who had quit.[69]

What about those who get diagnosed with breast cancer and then quit smoking? Is it too late to do any good? In a recent prospective obser-vational study involving 20,691 women with breast cancer, the 10 percent who continued to smoke after diagnosis were 72 percent more likely to die from breast cancer than those who never smoked.[70] Among the smokers, those who quit smoking dropped their death rates by 33 percent compared to those who continued to smoke after diagnosis, and the quitters were 61 percent less likely to die from lung cancer. With respect to weight, I asked you to be a loser, and now I want you to be a quitter. I love losers and quitters. Don't smoke.

STAMP OUT AS MANY ENVIRONMENTAL RISKS AS YOU CAN

Environmental risk factors vary in magnitude, and all are challenging to measure (how much pesticide did *you* consume from fruits before puberty?). Each threat can affect a woman differently, depending on her cumulative risks, the dose and timing of exposures, how factors interface with one another and with genes and genetic susceptibilities, and the body's hormonal milieu. The complexity of these interactions, the diffi-culty of quantifying exposures, and our incomplete understanding of the intricate pathways of carcinogenesis, all make singling out environmental contributions to the breast cancer conundrum very difficult. There are three broad factors, however, that carry a lot of weight—radiation, endo-crine disruptors, and stress. Let's control what we can.

Radioactive Risk Factors

In 1979, my parents bought a nifty device that made cold food turn hot, called a microwave. As a kid, I'd stand on a chair to look through the glass window, fascinated to see a hot dog bubble out in patches or spaghetti sauce splatter all over the inside of the box. My dad would caution, "Don't do that! You will get brain cancer or your head will explode." He made up a rule about being three feet away at all times. To this day, whenever I use the microwave, I duck down and slither away from its nonionizing (not harmful) rays until I can't wait for my food anymore, and then I go back and hit stop, usually with one second left on the timer.

All of us in the industrialized world coexist with an unmonitored barrage of environmental exposures such as radiation, industrial emissions, pollutants, pesticides, and countless synthetic compounds. The earlier exposures occur in our lives, the worse our future cancer risk. Breast cells are more susceptible to the carcinogenic effects of hormones, chemicals, and radiation during early stages of development—and I'm talking *early*, as in, our prenatal days hanging out in mother's womb—and then small, chronic exposures accumulate throughout early life, puberty and adolescence, until the first full-term pregnancy.[71] A New York study measured air levels of PAHs (polycyclic aromatic hydrocarbons) in residential areas from 1959 to 1997 and followed 3,200 women into their postmenopausal years.[72] Those exposed to high levels of PAHs at the time of birth were 142 percent more likely to get breast cancer than those with lower exposure levels. International regulatory agencies have implicated at least 216 chemicals and radiation sources for their part in causing breast cancer.[73]

What is our greatest environmental enemy? Ionizing gamma radiation, which mostly comes from medical treatments and X-rays, but unfortunately, we also have a few tragedies that prove the point. Survivors of the atomic bomb explosions in Hiroshima and Nagasaki and thousands living near the 1986 Chernobyl nuclear power plant disaster in the former Soviet Union (Belarus and Ukraine) received massive amounts of radiation; the *doubling* of breast cancer has been observed in women, and the younger they were at the time of the explosions, the higher their risk.[74]

We have startling data regarding early life exposures to medical X-rays resulting in shockingly high breast cancer rates as well. Reasons for X-rays that zapped developing young breast tissue range from important therapies for other diseases, like Hodgkin's lymphoma and tuberculosis, to rather ridiculous indications (now that research has revealed the risks) for things like acne, postpartum mastitis, enlarged thymus glands, and skin hemangiomas. Even just one measly spine X-ray to monitor scoliosis, a curvature of the spine, at age ten causes a 170 percent increase in breast cancer.[75] Thirty years after getting thymic radiation in infancy, women are 3.6 times more likely than their non-irradiated sisters to have breast cancer.[76]

My fifty-seven-year-old patient Linda came in to see me because her left nipple would intermittently discharge bloody fluid. Diagnosed with stage IV lymphoma at age thirteen, she endured tons of radiation and chemo and had been in remission for decades. No one had ever told her that she was basically guaranteed to get breast cancer. In fact, she didn't even have routine mammograms, because by her own admission she considered herself immune to future cancers—as if she had already had her fair share for one lifetime. With this history in her chart, I knew before I walked in the room to meet her that I had a cancer to find. How could I be so sure without even doing a breast exam? Chest irradiation used to treat Hodgkin's lymphoma prior to age fifteen causes an astounding increase in invasive breast cancer risk to 136 times the general population (that's *13,500 percent*; I am not sure that even makes mathematical sense). Radiation between ages fifteen and twenty-four carries a nineteenfold increase; ages twenty-five to thirty, a sevenfold increase; and women treated after age thirty have no increased risk of breast cancer due to radiation exposure.[77] As compared to the general population, these cancers occur at a younger age (forty-one versus sixty-two years old), are more often in both breasts (10 to 22 percent versus 3 percent), and are located in the inner breast (toward the sternum), as opposed to the upper outer breast, where 50 percent of most sporadic cancers occur.[78] If you had chest wall radiation for any reason prior to age thirty, begin a breast screening program eight years after radiation, or at age twenty-five, whichever comes first.[79] By the way, Linda had five different subtypes of cancer in both breasts.

Regarding routine medical X-rays, I limit whole-body staging with PET, CT, and/or bone scans to later-stage breast cancer patients or those with aggressive tumor subtypes. Save your exposures for when you really need them. Mammograms have much less radiation than these scans, and benefits outweigh the risks. No evidence implicates nonionizing radiation and electromagnetic fields from cell phones, power lines, microwaves, or televisions in breast cancer, which we explored in chapter 2.

Evil Endocrine Disruptors

You know when medical ionizing radiation waves penetrate you, because *you've given consent*. On the other hand, over 90 percent of the estimated 100,000 synthetic chemicals used in the United States have never been tested for their effects on human health,[80] and nobody has asked for my permission—have they asked yours? A substantial number of these compounds behave as xenoestrogens (chemicals that mimic the actions of estrogen in our bodies), and yet no regulatory body has mandated that we test products for xenoestrogen levels or their effects. *Xeno* means "foreign" in Greek, so these foreign estrogens behave as endocrine disrupting compounds (EDCs), a term applied to mimickers of not only estrogen, but of any naturally circulating hormone: insulin (from the pancreas), DHEA and testosterone (adrenal gland), PTH (parathyroid), oxytocin and growth hormone (pituitary gland), melatonin (pineal gland), and calcitonin and thyroxine (thyroid). EDCs exist in many pesticides, plastics, tobacco smoke, prescription drugs, food additives, fuels, detergents, industrial solvents, and personal care products.[81] They attach to the same receptors as our natural hormones, but can cause a stronger downstream reaction than normal hormones, a weaker one, or a totally different one. Your guess is as good as mine. We wouldn't know, because nobody has tested most of them.

In 1998, the Environmental Protection Agency (EPA) formed

the Endocrine Disruptor Screening Program. Their first update came seventeen years later in August 2015 when they published their initial review of fifty-two pesticides. Fifty-two? At that rate, we can expect them to report on the remaining 99,948 chemicals in 32,674 years. Talk about a slow clap. In the meantime, EDCs can affect gene expression, thereby potentially adding to the burden of breast cancer. Many EDCs are super stable. Stable is good for things like marriage and a job, but no one wants EDCs parking themselves in fat cells for decades.[82] They are everywhere. The sunscreen you put on this morning? EDC. The gas pump you handled at the station? EDC. The plastic fork and water bottle from lunch? EDC. The detergent you used to wash the pillow you're sleeping on? That too.

We can't become obsessed with invisible toxicities that individually contribute rather minimally to the threat of breast cancer. Remember the seed and soil discussion from chapter 3? EDCs add to cancer cell *initiation*, but all of the food and lifestyle behaviors we have investigated determine cancer cell *promotion*, and promotion has the final say when it comes to controlling cancer. Limit your exposures as best you can, and then just live . . . but live *well*. The following EDCs have been shown in human or animal studies to definitely affect the risk for breast cancer,[83] and at the end of this chapter, we'll explore ways to minimize their influence.

ALKYLPHENOLS: Industrial chemicals in laundry detergents and cleaning products.

BISPHENOL A (BPA): A ubiquitous chemical in modern life, BPA is used to make polycarbonate plastic, the global production of which reached 288 million metric tons in 2012, a 620 percent increase since 1975.[84] The main product is disposable packaging. Once thrown away, plastic goes to the landfill, and BPA enters the soil and groundwater, so be sure to *recycle* all plastics. The older plastic is, the more EDCs it releases. By 2012, Canada, the EU, China, Costa Rica, Malaysia, and the United States banned BPA from baby bottles, sippy cups, and infant formula cans.[85] You commonly find BPA in food packaging, the lining of canned food and beverages (beer and soda), epoxy resins, dental sealants, some sports water bottles (often marked with a #7 or "PC"), receipt paper, and paper money.

DIOXINS: The body fat of every human being, including newborns, contains dioxins. They form after the incineration of products containing polyvinyl chloride (PVC), polychlorinated biphenyl (PCB), and other chlorinated compounds; due to this and the combustion of diesel and gasoline, dioxins contaminate crops that livestock eat. Primary exposure is via consuming meat, dairy, and human breast milk.

FLAME RETARDANTS: Polybrominated diphenyl ethers (PBDE) and tetrabromobisphenol A (TBBPA) are used in plastics, paint, furniture, electronics, and food to make them flame-resistant. Top food sources include meat, fish, dairy, and eggs. Toxins accumulate in organs over time, including the breast, and then infants get PBDE from breast milk. Breast milk levels in the United States are ten to twenty times higher than in Europe, but I don't think this makes us fireproof.[86]

FOOD ADDITIVES: Recombinant bovine somatotropin (rBST) and zeranol replaced banned diethylstilbestrol (DES) to enhance the rapid growth of cattle and sheep.

METALS: Copper, cobalt, nickel, lead, mercury, cadmium, and chromium hang out in batteries, thermometers, paint, fish, dental fillings.

PESTICIDES: Now banned, the insecticides dichlorodiphenyltrichloroethane (DDT), dieldrin, aldrin, and heptachlor were used pervasively until the 1980s, so cancer risk persists for those exposed back then, and toxins also remain in today's soil. Currently, legal pesticides exist abundantly in food, soil, and water. An association between the herbicide atrazine and breast cancer was first reported in 1997. The EU banned atrazine in 2005 after it demonstrated harmful effects on wildlife *and* was found abundantly in human drinking water. However, approximately seventy million pounds of atrazine are still applied annually in the United States, primarily to control weeds in corn and sorghum crops.[87] At levels *lower* than considered "safe" in your drinking water, atrazine transforms male frogs into females, complete with lady parts like eggs.[88] Whoa.

Atrazine also turns on aromatase, which by now you know is an enzyme that converts other steroids into estrogen. Double whoa.

PHTHALATES: Phthalates make plastics more flexible and are used in food packaging, vinyl shower curtains, car seats, cleaning agents, and cosmetics. If a product has a fragrance or perfume, it probably has phthalates, which promote fat cell growth and alter IGF-1 levels. The fifty billion–dollar cosmetics industry can put anything they want into items like cosmetics, shampoo, and lotion. The EU banned the use of over 1,100 chemicals in cosmetics; by contrast, the United States has banned ten chemicals.

POLYCYCLIC AROMATIC HYDROCARBONS (PAHS): Burning meat, coal, oil, gasoline, trash, tobacco (active and passive users), or wood releases over one hundred different PAHs.

Until studies reveal EDC potency and mechanisms of action, we won't know which are safe and which cause irreparable harm. For instance, the widely used cardiac medication digoxin resembles estrogen chemically so much so that current users of the drug have a 39 percent elevated risk of invasive breast cancer; stopping the medication reverses the risk.[89] And while medications have consistent dosing and known metabolites, chemicals are difficult to understand because exposures are ubiquitous and levels in the body aren't easy to track. No one should question, however, that some of these compounds behave like an evil estrogen, hiding under a black mask with guns blazing. Take the tragic tale of diethylstilbestrol (DES). Prior to the 1971 DES ban in people and cattle, doctors prescribed the estrogen look-alike for millions of pregnant women to prevent miscarriages. Suspicion arose when the children of these women kept dying from an extremely rare vaginal cancer compared to those who were not exposed to DES in the womb.[90] Both the mothers and their DES daughters manifested a threefold increase in breast cancer risk after age fifty.[91] Now that cattle can't get fed with DES, the meat industry switched to zeranol (see chapter 4).

You know what story sounds like DES in the making? Bisphenol A (BPA). In 2007, international EDC experts analyzed all available evidence about BPA and concluded that the wide range of adverse effects of low doses of BPA in laboratory animals seem to be manifesting in humans as well: breast cancer, precocious puberty, obesity, type 2 diabetes, to name a few.[92] Globally in 2015, the annual output of BPA reached 6.8 million tons;[93] in 2009, BPA generated about 3.3 million dollars *a day* in revenue for each of the five corporations that produce it: Bayer, Dow, Hexion Specialty Chemicals, SABIC Innovative Plastics (formerly GE Plastics), and Sunoco.[94] Cue the pushback, as if we wouldn't notice: of 115 government-funded studies exploring the health effects of BPA, ninety-four (82 percent) of them from labs all over the world confirmed adverse effects at low-dose exposure; however, exactly zero of the studies funded by Big Plastics reported adverse effects, fueling their argument that evidence for low-dose effects of BPA is "very weak" and nothing needs to change.[95] Those researchers, from the Harvard Center for Risk Analysis, should receive a *plastic* golden statue for their performance, which was funded by the American Plastics Council.[96]

Not all chemicals exert their carcinogenic potential by being EDCs; they can just directly damage breast cell DNA or change that cell's ability to protect itself from oxidative stress. The International Agency for Research on Cancer (IARC) and the National Toxicology Program (NTP) have classified each of the following compounds as "definitely" or "probably" causing breast cancer:

- Benzene: inhaled from gasoline fumes, car exhaust, tobacco smoke
- Polyvinyl chloride: PVCs used in medical products, food packaging, appliances, toys, water pipes
- Organic solvents like carbon tetrachloride and formaldehyde: found in fabricated metal, lumber, furniture, and in the printing, chemical, textile and clothing industries
- 1,3-butadiene: a by-product of petroleum refining, vehicle exhaust, synthetic rubber
- Ethylene oxide: in cosmetics
- Aromatic amines: by-products of plastics, pesticides, dyes, and polyurethane foams, grilling of meats and fish

DOES YOUR JOB HURT YOUR BREASTS?

Certain occupations chronically expose women to radiation, EDCs, and other toxic chemicals that increase their risk of breast cancer. Any office exudes this stuff all day long from sources like carpet fibers, copiers, printers, and toner cartridges. Evidence shows the following jobs pose a threat. I'm on the list; are you? Aircraft and automotive workers; barbers and hairdressers; chemists and chemical industry workers; clinical laboratory technologists; computer operators; crop farmers; dental hygienists; dentists; dry cleaning workers; flight attendants; food, clothing, and transportation workers; fruit and vegetable packers; furniture and woodworking workers; homemakers; journalists; librarians; chemotherapy nurses; paper mill workers; physicians; publishing and printing industry workers; meat wrappers and cutters; microelectronics workers; radiologic technologists; rubber and plastics industry workers; social workers; telephone workers.[97]

EIGHT SIMPLE WAYS TO LOWER TOXIC EXPOSURE

The good news about carcinogens and EDCs is that you can minimize your breast cancer risk by exposing yourself to them less. There are better ways to do this than others, so here are the biggies that I encourage everyone to implement:

1. **Wash your hands:** Frequently. Always before you eat. Avoid triclosan-laden antibacterial soaps and just use soap and water. The World Health Organization calls antibiotic resistance a major threat to global health security (antibiotic resistant superbugs), so don't help a bug out.

2. **Dust and vacuum:** Chemicals fly off flame-retardant electronics and couches and collect in dust. Zip it up.

3. **Ban plastics:** Use glass, steel, or ceramic for storing, preparing, and serving food and drink; use glass not plastic baby bottles and wooden

not plastic toys; never microwave food in plastic containers or cover them in plastic wrap; when food comes in a "microwavable bag" or TV dinner tray, unwrap it and heat in glass or ceramic; don't heat Styrofoam; do not leave water bottles or plastic containers in the sun because the heat makes BPA and dioxins leach into your water and food; do not freeze plastic bottles; avoid plastic baggies and plastic wrap.

PLASTICS RECALL!

The 500 billion plastic bags we throw away annually take 450 to 1,000 years to degrade, releasing chemicals all the while. And that's just bags. By choosing plastic alternatives of all kinds, you not only reduce your endocrine disrupting compound (EDC) exposures but also stop adding to the 22 billion plastic bottles a year sinking into landfills,[98] the 5 to 12 million pieces of plastic dumped into the ocean annually,[99] and the 1 million seabirds killed by plastic each year.[100] These substitutes for plastic can help save your breasts *and* the planet:

- **Storage:** Tempered glass containers with steel lids or stainless-steel storage containers come in many sizes and can go straight from fridge to oven; mason jars hold stews and soups with style.
- **Wrapping food:** Use parchment or soy-derived wax paper; kitchen dishcloths or paper towels wrap lettuce and veggies and trap moisture; mesh bags with drawstrings work for veggies; and remember—not all food needs to be wrapped up.
- **Reusable bags:** Zippered cloth sandwich bags and silicone storage bags stash food for home or travel use; keep a few bags made from canvas, denim, jute, water hyacinth, or paper in your car for groceries or shopping trips.
- **Kids' dishware:** Stainless steel dishes, cups, bowls, and latch lunch boxes provide non-plastic, shatterproof options.

Six suggestions:

- Repurpose the wrap around super-sized packs of toilet paper into your next recyclable trash can liner.

- Bring your own mug to the coffee shop: plastic coats the inside of to-go cups that also sport a plastic lid and plastic stirrer.
- Buy water bottled in glass, not plastic.
- Say no to plastic straws (use reusable stainless, silicone, or glass ones).
- Pick the boxed pasta over bagged.
- Stop chewing gum (a synthetic rubber, a.k.a. plastic).

---

4. Eat wisely: Choose organic or locally grown foods whenever possible to avoid consuming hormones and pesticides as best you can. Splurge for organic when consuming the skin (like berries, not bananas); wash fruits and veggies with a 10 percent salt solution (see chapter 4); peel nonorganic fruits and vegetables; go fresh (say "no can do" to cans lined with BPA, but not all cans are); limit exposure to carcinogenic dioxin by eating less meat, fish, milk, eggs, and butter; if you eat fish, choose wild salmon, mackerel, and sardines.

5. Make better choices for household products: Filter your drinking water, and all household water sources if possible, so even your shower water is filtered; trade nonstick Teflon pans for cast iron or stainless steel; choose chemical-free, biodegradable laundry and household cleaning products (or make your own: 1 cup white distilled vinegar with 1 cup water); find chlorine-free products and unbleached paper products (think tampons, toilet paper, coffee filters); ditch your vinyl shower curtain and hang one made of fabric; use metal or bamboo cooking utensils, strainers, and cutting boards (not plastic); put a high efficiency particulate air (HEPA) filter in rooms where you spend the most time; as you replace big items like couches and mattresses, select those that contain naturally less flammable material like leather, wool, and cotton to avoid flame-retardant chemicals; get rid of things with crumbling, old lead paint; don't kill ants or cockroaches with chemical pesticides; don't use weed killers and artificial fertilizers on your lawn; open windows and allow fresh air to circulate through your home.

6. Grow houseplants: Carpets, couches, ovens, cleaning solutions, and synthetic materials all constantly emit chemicals, but in 1989, NASA discovered that houseplants absorb harmful toxins from the air (specifically, benzene, formaldehyde, and trichloroethylene).[101] Choose any of these low-maintenance potted air purifiers to detoxify your home and double as décor: philodendrons (heartleaf, elephant ear, spider plant, golden pothos), mother-in-law's tongue, peace lilies, dracaenas (marginata, mass cane, Warneckei, Janet Craig), aloe vera, areca palms, and potted mums (mildly poisonous; beware of toddlers and pets). For greener thumbs, bamboo palms, English ivy, rubber plants, Chinese evergreen, gerbera daisy, and weeping fig decontaminate the air, but need more attention.

7. **Make better choices for cosmetic products**: Turn up your nose to fragrances or use essential oils to avoid phthalates; find chemical-free soaps and toothpaste; avoid lotion and cosmetics that have toxic chemicals and estrogenic ingredients; avoid nail polish and polish removers; avoid shampoos, conditioners, body washes, and moisturizers with phthalates or parabens on the label; sunscreens (UV filters) also contain chemicals like padimate O, so use appropriately but sparingly. To find out what you are putting on your skin, nails, and hair (70 percent of which gets absorbed into the body), visit the Environmental Working Group's database of chemicals at ewg.org.

8. **Exercise**: Many toxins are excreted through sweat, separately from stool and urine.[102] Get moving!

FIND YOUR HAPPY

When I ask a newly diagnosed patient if she faced a stressful or heartbreaking situation five to ten years ago, she all too often responds, "Yes, how did you know?" Loss, disappointment, emotional pain, regret, illness, suffering—life happens, and every person passes through difficult times. But it's particularly tragic when that "something" occurred during the five-to-ten-year window when cancer cells were too few to detect, but plenty enough to gain momentum. Not all stress announces itself like a massive earthquake; chronic stress results from the cumulative effect of tiny shocks. I believe that how we handle life's struggles, large and little, directly impacts our physical well-being.

Does science agree? It sure does. Your mind exerts tremendous power over your body. Has a scary movie ever caused sweaty palms and a racing heart? You're just sitting in a chair! Healthy doses of stress can lead to a successful presentation or victorious tennis match. You need your heart rate up, faster breathing, and energy coursing through your veins if you plan to close an important deal or outrun a bear, but many of us spend our days trapped in a fight-or-flight phenomenon. We respond to life as if we are about to get eaten. What happens when deadlines, traffic, work, childcare, bills, and relationships cause psychological stress? It becomes *physiologic* stress that wreaks havoc on your body. It sets off a chain reaction with a series of chemical messengers running around preparing for battle. What starts with epinephrine ends up elevating levels of estrogen, testosterone, cortisol, dopamine, and serotonin. Inflammatory cytokines such as Interleukin 1 (IL-1), Interleukin 6 (IL-6), and tumor necrosis factor alpha (TNFα) rise up, and natural killer (NK) cells diminish. Aptly named, natural killer cells bind and destroy tumor cells. Chronic stress induces oxidative stress as the immune system starts to shut down. Indeed, a meta-analysis of three hundred independent studies confirms that stress alters immunity.[103] Our stress decorates the scene with inflammation and immunosuppression, just as illness wanders on stage.

Stressful life events and/or chronic stress have been linked in human studies to cardiovascular disease and death,[104] major depression,[105] asthma,[106] obesity,[107] diabetes,[108] progression of HIV to AIDS,[109] headaches,[110] Alzheimer's,[111] and gastrointestinal disease.[112] Scientists have clearly associated acute and chronic stress with a number of biological changes and other diseases known to commonly coexist with breast cancer, but studies do not prove stress to be a stand-alone cause. Breast cancer is never caused by *one thing* anyway, such as a virus or fat; the cause is always multifactorial. A perfect storm of predisposing factors dwells within your body for a long enough time to initiate cancerous change, and then to promote its growth and spread. Stress, therefore, is but another one of those storm factors. But contrary to how you might feel when you are particularly stressed out, you can reduce stress. Mind over matter.

For one, your outlook and attitude matter in everything you do. Canadian researchers found that a positive outlook—feeling happiness, joy, contentment, enthusiasm—decreases heart attacks by 22 percent for each attribute people express that's positive.[113] Literally choose to smile, and make it a point to forgive those who hurt and upset you. Do it for your health. Forgiveness improves both mental and physical health; it lessens anxiety, anger, and depression; reduces stress; relaxes facial muscles; and decreases cortisol levels and blood pressure.[114] Forgiveness even links to less alcohol and cigarette use.[115] Also, don't forget to breathe. Deep breathing activates the *para*sympathetic nervous system, opposing the functions of the sympathetic stress system. Finally, say no to people whose anger, jealousy, or negativity brings you down. And the more you say no to activities that don't matter to you right now (even good ones like that fund-raiser), the easier it becomes to own your choices and to fill your time with joy.

Gratitude stops stress before it starts. When I jump out of bed in the morning and my feet hit the floor, I say "Thank" with the left foot, and "You" with the right. Try it! For me, no matter what challenges the day holds, my first utterance reminds me to be grateful to God that I am alive to face them. Since I am not talking to *myself*, saying these words also reinforces that today comes with divine help and ever-present company. Next time you're stressed out, regroup for a second and remember what you're grateful for—like eyes that see, or a car that starts, or friends who love you. Count your blessings—it really works.

There's also a lot to gain from joining a faith-based or spiritual community. Finding a community that supports your beliefs provides social support and connectedness, as well as the opportunity to be altruistic toward others, and can be a boon to sustained health. Both giving and receiving friendship lead to feeling well; in fact, studies show that those involved in a religion were 29 percent more likely to be alive at any point during the study follow-up than those who were not in a faith-based community.[116] Spiritual families also reinforce a common belief system, and remind you that you are not meant to carry the weight of the world alone but to be part of a whole, and together you can accomplish more than you can alone. Finally, faith attaches *meaning* to events; when events lack purpose, stress shows up. Faith gives you reasons and hope. Nothing reduces stress better than hope!

Also, get your sleep, so your body can rest and repair. According the American Psychological Association, stress keeps 40 percent of adults lying awake at night. Limit caffeine at night, no TV or computer screens in the bedroom, and keep a routine. Get seven to eight hours of sleep a night. And if you work the night shift, you need to recreate natural darkness when you sleep in the day. Working at night increases breast cancer by 40 percent, with the highest rates found in long-term employment for jobs like nurses, flight attendants, and janitors.[117] Even the International Agency for Research on Cancer (IARC) classifies the night shift as "probably carcinogenic."[118] Melatonin peaks between 2:00 AM and 5:00 AM; your brain's pineal gland secretes this hormone when it's dark and stops when it's light. In this way, melatonin controls your internal clock, your circadian rhythm. It knocks you out at night and wakes you up in the morning, but it also suppresses breast tumor cell growth.[119] This is actually why blind women have lots of melatonin and less breast cancer—57 percent less if totally blind.[120] Guess what happens when it's light all day, and then artificially light all night (night shift) too? No melatonin. Your organs rely on melatonin to coordinate hormone production. "Oh, it's daytime! Let's make estrogen," say your ovaries, so now the night shift not only has more estrogen running around, they also lost the melatonin signal that keeps tumor cells from growing.[121] About 20 percent of women in the United States and Europe work at night. Exposure to light at night in industrialized countries might also increase breast cancer rates by the same low melatonin mechanism.[122] If you're a natural night owl, try exercising during the day to help induce sleep. It also lowers blood pressure, improves mood, and reduces stress.

Finally, in your pursuit of stress-free, joyful living, ask for help when you need it. Maybe you feel overwhelmed and strapped for time, and you could use some assistance with cooking, driving, childcare, cleaning, or caring for an elderly loved one. Do everything you can to get it. Or it might be enough to unload on a licensed mental health professional who can offer guidance about the situations and behaviors that add stress to your life.

REMEMBER, YOU HAVE THE UPPER HAND

Part of why I want you to reign in as many controllable risk factors for breast cancer as you can is because, as you'll read next in part 3, some risks aren't up to you.

LEARN YOUR PERSONAL RISK FACTORS AND CONTROL WHAT YOU CAN

CHAPTER 6

Uncontrollable Risk Factors: Do You Have Them?

You now understand the latest science about how food and other lifestyle choices can help reduce your risk of developing breast cancer, so it's time to move on to other less malleable risk factors that might affect you personally. I love working with every patient to develop the right path for her—and for many, the strategies in parts 1 and 2 are enough to create confidence and maximize breast health. When researchers in Mexico developed a healthy lifestyle checklist, a combined strategy emerged that reliably drops breast cancer risk: when women (1) exercise; (2) don't drink alcohol; (3) don't smoke; (4) shift diet away from meat and dairy toward whole food, plant-based eating, breast cancer rates plummet. For my premenopausal friends, your odds of getting breast cancer drop in half, and older women, you're protected by 80 percent![1]

All women carry a degree of cancer risk over which they have no control—some, more than others. Yet despite these inherent uncertainties, those who make healthy lifestyle choices still dramatically reduce their chances of a cancer diagnosis. In part 3, I'll walk you through all the factors that gently nudge, or in some cases rudely shove you toward the need for more intense risk reduction choices. That's how we control even the uncontrollable. In this chapter, we'll explore the uncontrollable risk factors that you cannot will, wish, or warp into any other shape than the way they came. And the way they came might increase your risk for breast cancer.

145

YOU'RE A WOMAN

That's right, having XX chromosomes instead of XY—i.e., being female— is the number one risk factor for getting breast cancer, but honestly, sister, who would want to change *that*? According to the International Agency for Research on Cancer (IARC), breast cancer is by far the most frequent cancer among women with an estimated 1.67 million *new cancer cases* diagnosed globally each year (25 percent of all cancers). Breast cancer ranks supreme as the most frequent cause of cancer death in women in less developed regions, and lands second to lung cancer death in more developed areas. Incidence rates vary fourfold across the globe, ranging from 27 per 100,000 in Middle Africa and Eastern Asia to 93 in the United States to 112 in Belgium.

ESTIMATED AGE-STANDARDIZED
RATES (WORLD) PER 100,000

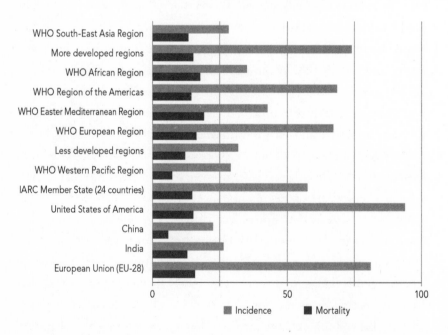

M. Ervik, F. Lam, J. Ferlay, L. Mery, I. Soerjomataram, F. Bray (2016). Cancer Today. Lyon, France: International Agency for Research on Cancer. Cancer Today. Available from http://gco.iarc.fr/today/data/pdf/fact-sheets/cancers/cancer-fact-sheets-15.pdf.

As one would expect, developed regions have higher survival rates. Have a look at the previous page to see where ladies across the globe rank, relative to your homeland.

As I mentioned earlier, though it bears repeating here, men do get breast cancer because they also have breast tissue, accounting for 0.8 percent of all breast cancer cases in the United States, which is about 2,470 men annually. This means women are 120 times more likely to get this disease. The following factors are significantly associated with male breast cancer: BRCA-1, BRCA-2, PTEN, and TP53 gene mutations; radiation; diabetes; never having had children; a history of fractures; and conditions that elevate the estrogen/androgen ratio, such as obesity, tall height, cryptorchidism (absence of one or both testicles), orchitis (inflammation of one or both testicles), Klinefelter syndrome (a genetic abnormality in which men have *two* female chromosomes and one male chromosome: XXY instead of the usual XY), and gynecomastia (excess growth of breast tissue in men).[2] Male breast cancer has been on a slow rise since 1975, but death rates have decreased 1.8 percent per year since 2000.

YOUR AGE

The older you become, the higher your risk. I see premenopausal women under fifty every week with cancer, so I will not minimize how devastating and real that risk can be. However, statistics don't lie, and what I am about to share should help you relax a little.

You've surely heard that an American woman's lifetime risk of getting breast cancer is 1 in 8, but your risk right now, today, this minute, is *not* 1 in 8. That is the lifetime roll of the dice to a newborn. Risk stretches itself out across your years on Earth, so you have escaped some of it already, and another amount looms ahead. Let's put the risk of age into perspective. Below is a chart that details the age-specific probability of developing breast cancer, extrapolated by decades of life.

BY THE DECADE: LIKELIHOOD OF US WOMEN DEVELOPING INVASIVE BREAST CANCER (BASED ON CASES DIAGNOSED 2012–2014)[3]

IF YOU ARE THIS OLD	CHANCES OF GETTING BREAST CANCER IN THE NEXT TEN YEARS ARE	IN OTHER WORDS, 1 IN
20	0.1%	1,567
30	0.5%	220
40	1.5%	68
50	2.3%	43
60	3.4%	29
70	3.9%	25
Lifetime risk	12.4%	8

Note: Numbers may not be numerically equivalent due to rounding.

Pretend your current age is forty. For the entire period of time between forty and fifty years old, 1 in 68 women (1.5 percent) will get breast cancer while in her forties. But in any given year—say, age forty-two—the risk of a diagnosis *at the age of forty-two* is actually one-tenth of the risk for the whole period, so the chance is 1 in 680 (0.15 percent). That's a far cry from 1 in 8, now, isn't it? And for some reason, all of our data seems to have us women dead at seventy to eighty. The average life expectancy for women in the United States is 81.2 (I want you *above* average), with Japan winning the longevity race at 86.8, and Sierra Leone having the shortest life expectancy, 50.8 years.[4]

YOUR FIRST VISIT FROM AUNT FLO

Menarche refers to your very first menstrual period, which unceremoniously marked the beginning of armpit hair, monthly cramps, and maniacal mood swings for years to come. On the bright side, it was time for a real bra with cup sizes. The average age of menarche in the United States is 12.5 years old, with ages ranging from nine to sixteen. It wasn't always this way. The mean age of puberty in girls in Western populations has been falling for the last 150 years.[5] In 1997, a landmark US study thrust precocious puberty (blossoming at an earlier age than expected) into the spotlight when it reported on over 17,000 girls, finding that 27.2 percent of black and 6.7 percent of white girls had started to develop breasts or pubic hair by age seven.[6] Just one year later, by age eight, these numbers rose to 48.3 percent and 14.7 percent of black and white girls, respectively. Here's a concerning fact: early puberty increases breast cancer. Young girls whose breasts begin to grow prior to age ten have a 23 percent increase in breast cancer over those whose breasts develop at or after age ten. Conversely, girls starting periods at or after age sixteen have 50 percent less breast cancer than those with menarche before age twelve, which highlights the protective effect of later puberty.[7] In addition to breast cancer, early puberty in girls has also been associated with increased risk of ovarian cancer,[8] obesity,[9] diabetes,[10] psychosocial disorders,[11] and raised triglycerides (think heart attack) in later life.[12]

Since estrogen fuels the majority of breast cancers, it makes sense that early puberty begins estrogen exposures sooner, thereby expanding the window of vulnerability for breast cancer development between first menstruation and first pregnancy. Recent evidence implicates a rise in obesity and endocrine disrupters (EDCs) in precocious puberty.[13] We mothers of young children must encourage maintenance of a normal weight in our kids and avoidance of EDCs in our food and homes. As we learned in the previous chapter, peripheral fat elevates estrogen levels, so there's nothing cherubic about chubby. And estrogen-mimickers found in meat, dairy, pesticides, hair and cosmetic products, laundry detergents, cleaning products, and plastics (polychlorinated biphenyls, bisphenol A, and phthalates) need to be minimized in the home environment. While chopping away at these root causes that prematurely elevate estrogen and promote early breast growth in preadolescent girls, don't forget that this is a critical window to avoid smoking and to pile on the vegetables and soy.

GOOD OL' MENOPAUSE

Menopause refers to the cessation of menstruation—to be specific, twelve consecutive months of quiet (which, of course, you only know in hindsight). The average age in the United States is fifty-one years old, but a recent study placed the median age in Europe at fifty-four years old.[14] Menopause can occur prior to the natural timeline secondary to chemotherapy or anti-estrogen therapy (both of which turn off ovarian function, thus stopping periods), surgical removal of the ovaries, or certain illnesses. Usually several years of "the change before the change," called *perimenopause*, precede natural menopause. You might notice that everyone around you has an attitude problem, your spouse suddenly agrees with everything you say, and your inner child seems to have found a stack of matches. Perimenopause generally involves some unwelcome combo of irregular periods, mood swings, hot flashes, night sweats, insomnia, poor memory, weight gain (including back fat, *really?*), breast pain, joint aches, vaginal dryness, painful intercourse, decreased libido, dry skin, and/or thinning hair. On the bright side, that monthly visit from Aunt Flo goes away.[15]

Now for a pop quiz. Which one increases your breast cancer risk: *early* (younger) or *late* (older) menopause? Answer: late menopause. For the same postulated reason as with menarche, the longer your breast cells are subjected to monthly estrogen surges, the higher your incidence of breast cancer. Women who go through menopause for any reason prior to age forty-four have 34 percent less breast cancer than those whose monthly curse waits until fifty-four years or older to call it quits. This protective effect of an early age at menopause is actually 44 percent for women with a BMI equal to or lower than 27 but drops to 24 percent in women with a BMI greater than 27, so being lean confers more protection. In fact, researchers found that when matched age-for-age between forty five and fifty-four years old (say, two forty-eight-year-olds), the woman without periods for a year (i.e., menopausal) had 43 percent less breast cancer than one still menstruating (premenopausal).[16] If you had a hysterectomy but kept your ovaries, you're not in menopause until your ovaries say so (you just don't have the monthly reminders). So starting periods older and stopping them younger protects the breast.

YOUR RACE

White women get more breast cancer than any other race, including African American, American Indian/Alaska Native, Asian/Pacific Islander, or Hispanic. The following graph shows the US breast cancer incidence and death rates according to race (numbers are per 100,000 women):[17]

BREAST CANCER INCIDENCE AND MORTALITY RATES PER 100,000 PEOPLE IN US WOMEN BY RACE/ETHNICITY[18]

RACE/ETHNICITY	BREAST CANCER INCIDENCE (2010–2014)	BREAST CANCER MORTALITY (2011–2015)
Non-Hispanic White	128.7	20.8
Non-Hispanic Black	125.5	29.5
American Indian/Alaska Native*	100.7	14.3
Hispanic/Latina	91.9	14.2
Asian/Pacific Islander	90.7	11.3

*Statistics based on data from Contract Health Service Delivery Area (CHSDA) counties. Note: Rates are age adjusted to the 2000 US standard population.

As you can see, although white women have the highest incidence of breast cancer, African Americans are 30 percent more likely to die from it. All other racial and ethnic groups have at least 22 percent less cancer than white women and 52 percent less death than black women. The clearly visible and encouraging news, however, is that the incidence bars *tower* over the mortality bars, which means a lot more living than dying happens in all races. In fact, compared to 1975, earlier detection and improved treatment for breast cancers have lowered the mortality rates in *all* races. Chinese and Japanese women have the highest breast cancer survival rates of all races.

A number of factors largely explain the increased death rate in women of color as compared to whites.[19] From SEER (Surveillance, Epidemiology and End Results) cancer databases, we find that, compared to whites, African Americans are more often diagnosed at later stages of disease (44 percent versus 33 percent); at a younger median age (fifty-eight versus sixty-two); and with more aggressive triple-negative cancer subtypes (22 percent versus 12 percent).[20] Investigating beyond subtypes, scientists have identified inherent biological differences in the invasive breast cancers from patients of African versus European ancestry that may adversely affect how genes and proteins and cellular mutations interact.[21] Multiple other factors, including earlier menarche, less mammography use, higher breast density, poorer access to health care, regional variations in quality of care, lack of health insurance, underuse of cancer treatments, obesity (50 percent more common), diabetes (60 percent more common), certain cultural beliefs, and communication barriers, especially in immigrants and refugees, all contribute to the differences in incidence and mortality between the non-Hispanic black and white races.[22]

Clearly, it will take leaders at the patient, provider, insurance payor, community, and national levels to drive system change if we plan to close the racial mortality gap in America.

SOCIOECONOMIC STATUS

Higher socioeconomic status (SES) correlates to higher breast cancer rates than lower SES. But this isn't what you may think. SES and risk do not directly connect to money or education, fancy homes, or Ivy League degrees, but higher SES women (higher income, education, and skilled occupation) tend to display *behaviors* known to elevate risk: white race, no or fewer children, older age at first full-term birth, fewer months breastfeeding, hormone use, alcohol use, increased childhood nutrition with taller height and increased weight,[23] and life in urban communities.[24] Additionally, women with higher SES tend to get their annual screening mammograms, thereby having their cancers diagnosed. Women with an income greater than $50,000 and those who are college graduates, married, or have health insurance are all more likely to have had a mammogram within the last two years than a woman who earns less than $35,000, did not graduate high school, was never married, or has no health insurance.[25]

On the other hand, higher SES women tend to be diagnosed with breast cancer at an earlier and more curable stage than lower SES—and owing to better access to medical care and superior treatment options, fewer high SES women die from breast cancer when compared to low SES women.[26] Those without insurance or with Medicaid more often present with later stages III and IV cancer and die 36 percent more often than privately insured women.[27] Even within the same race, we find that high SES African American women have a better survival rate than low SES African American women.[28] The high SES group can deescalate their risk by adhering to diet and lifestyle changes, and the low SES ladies would benefit from better access to timely, affordable health care and breast screening.

YOUR HEIGHT

Believe it or not, the taller you are, the higher your risk of breast cancer. In a study of 108,829 women followed twelve years with 1,041 developing cancers, women 5 feet 7 inches (1.75 meters) tall or taller were 57 percent more likely to get breast cancer than women shorter than 5 feet 2 inches (1.60 meters) tall; every 2 inches (5 centimeters) added 11 percent risk.[29] Breast cancer mortality also increases with increasing height. After fourteen years of following 424,168 postmenopausal women, 2,852 breast cancer deaths were observed.[30] Women 5 feet 5 inches (1.68 meters) tall or taller had a 64 percent increase in death from breast cancer compared to those shorter than 5 feet 0 inches (1.52 meters). Now the "vertically challenged" taunts don't sound so bad, do they?

This has nothing to do with the universe favoring petite women. The functions of estrogen, progesterone, androgens, growth hormone, insulin, insulin-like growth factor (IGF-1), and dietary factors during childhood, puberty, and adolescence together determine adult height.[31] These hormonal messengers interact with genetic factors, biological pathways, environmental exposures, and lifestyle factors like diet and exercise in complicated and poorly understood ways. How low can you go to dodge breast cancer altogether? Well, remember Laron syndrome from our discussion in chapter 4? Dwarfism due to vastly diminished IGF-1 levels and receptor insensitivity to growth hormone not only results in a short stature—those with Laron syndrome *never* get breast cancer. You read that right. Why? IGF-1 promotes carcinogenesis and inhibits cancer cell death (apoptosis). An analysis of seventeen prospective studies confirmed *higher IGF-1* levels among taller compared with shorter women, with a 38 percent increase in *estrogen-positive* breast cancer, again suggesting that IGF-1 and estrogens are at play.[32] So, short sisters, the next time an eight-year-old girl says to you, "Hey, I'm almost as tall as you!" just give a kind, knowing smile.

BONE DENSITY

Right about now, you're probably thinking, "If it's not one thing, it's another." Well, here's another thing. Strong bones correlate to *more* breast cancer. Bones actually contain estrogen receptors, and estrogen keeps your bones strong by inhibiting cytokines, which act to destroy your bones. While we're glad estrogen does a body good in the skeletal department by increasing bone mineral density (BMD), it does so by ramping up the production of IGF-1 and growth hormone, which build and protect your bones while simultaneously fueling carcinogenic breast changes.[33] In fact, two large studies comparing postmenopausal women in the highest to lowest bone mineral density show breast cancer risks 3.5 to 6.0 times higher for the top quartile BMD group.[34] It's not that a healthy BMD causes breast cancer, but it's a sign that other well-established risk factors are flying around, namely, higher lifelong estrogen, IGF-1, and growth hormone exposures.

As for Miss Wimpy Bones who has a low bone mineral density (BMD) due to less estrogen for reasons such as early menopause and low postmenopausal body weight, these things actually protect her against breast cancer. But it's not a total win since low BMD puts you at risk for osteoporosis, a condition in which brittle bones can fracture. Accordingly, we see *less* breast cancer in women with hip and forearm fractures.[35] Becoming prone to fractures probably isn't the most desirable way to reduce breast cancer risk. A dual-energy X-ray absorptiometry scan (DXA) is a fast, low-dose radiation way to diagnose osteoporosis—if you have it, try to reverse it, and if you don't have it, act as if you do. What do I mean? The same behaviors that improve osteoporosis in low BMD women help offset the breast cancer risk in high BMD women: avoid alcohol and cigarettes, exercise (include weight-bearing exercises twice a week where you work against gravity like lifting weights, hiking, or climbing stairs), and consume calcium and vitamin D. Sound familiar? I love it when the universe makes sense.

BREAST DENSITY

When you get a mammogram, a radiologist determines your breast density by visually comparing your actual breast and stroma (white/bright gray) to the fat (black/dark gray) in your breast on the image. The whiter the mammogram, the denser the breast; the denser the breast, the higher the risk of getting breast cancer—and the harder it is for a breast imager to detect it.

Dense breasts genetically have more breast lobules, ducts, stroma, and connective tissue in them than fatty tissue. Since ducts and lobules can form cancer, and the stroma provides regulatory functions that promote carcinogenesis, it makes sense that denser breasts have a higher risk of breast cancer than fatty breasts.[36] Fat carries no risk of developing breast cancer, and it also looks dark on mammograms, making fatty breasts easier to image because cancer looks white, and stands out like a bright star against the dark fatty sky. In contrast, white cancer in a white, dense breast looks like a snowball in a snowstorm on mammograms (and that's why cancer can get missed); in fact, breast imagers miss up to 50 percent of cancers in dense breasts.[37]

Are you dense? Four breast density classes exist. These exact words appear in all mammogram reports, like "code talk" describing how dense— and therefore how reliable—a mammogram might be: *entirely fatty* or *fatty* (Class A), *scattered fibroglandular densities* (Class B), *heterogeneously dense* (Class C), or *extremely dense* (Class D). When comparing classes D to A, the densest breasts to the fattiest, dense Ds carry four to six times the cancer risk of fatty breasts.[38] But don't panic; that's only 10 percent of us. Most women fall into the middle two groups, with the distribution as follows: 10 percent Class A, 40 percent Class B, 40 percent Class C, 10 percent Class D. In the United States, many states mandate that all women with Classes C and D be informed that they have dense breasts in writing. While this helps us individualize surveillance options regarding density, the letter you receive basically says, "Hi, your mammogram is normal, but it's dense. Good luck with that, see you next year." Half of women over forty have no idea their "normal" mammogram might not be normal at all. If you're in class C or D, talk to your doctor about additional screening exams such as whole breast screening ultrasound or breast MRI.

Once dense, always dense? Not necessarily. Breast density decreases with increasing age (you call it sagging), postmenopausal status, a higher number of births, and reduced body weight, all of which indicate that hormones influence breast density.[39] Women with denser breasts have increased levels of estrogen,[40] and hormone replacement therapy (HRT) increases breast density in postmenopausal women too.[41] One solution for high-risk women who are also dense-breasted is to take the antiestrogen tamoxifen, which reduces breast density in premenopausal and postmenopausal women within months, plus reduces the incidence of breast cancer up to 63 percent.[42] Two other density-reducers include losing weight if obese and avoiding HRT. Lose your breast density, and lose the associated risk.

MARKER LESIONS

There's a category of altered breast tissue referred to as *marker lesions* that in and of themselves are not cancer, but their mere presence within your breast signifies that you are at higher risk for developing breast cancer— anywhere in either breast, not necessarily at the site of the marker lesion. Why? Well, if your breast makes a marker lesion, this means your cells are "busy" getting stimulated by all of the free radicals, growth factors, and estrogen molecules we've been talking about. In other words, the same microenvironment that makes marker lesions can make cancer too.

Marker lesions result from cell proliferation, meaning breast cells multiply and divide and eventually can create targets that catch your doctor's attention and makes her want to biopsy them—targets like calcifications on a mammogram, palpable lumps, or solid masses on ultrasound. The concern with marker lesions is that they often keep close company with cancer. When it comes to marker lesions, you don't want an upgrade. An upgrade means that what we thought was just a cluster of busy cells turns out to be cancer once we take a bigger bite. For example, when the marker lesion, atypical ductal hyperplasia (ADH), gets surgically removed, the final pathology reveals the presence of preinvasive or invasive carcinoma more than 20 percent of the time.[43] So we remove ADH whenever we find it. On the other hand, atypical *lobular* hyperplasia (ALH) upgrades 5 percent or less, so we leave most ALH alone.

Wouldn't it be great to have a cheat sheet so if you ever get a breast biopsy, you can know what gets removed and what can be safely followed? I thought so. Peruse the box below if you'd like to know.

TO REMOVE OR TO FOLLOW

In 2016, the American Society of Breast Surgeons (ASBS) research committee performed a comprehensive review of the modern literature on the subject of marker lesions and recommended what to do about them.[44] Marker lesions require action (either removal or follow-up), and if your breast makes one, now you can reference this tidy little list to help you know what to do about it.

These high-risk marker lesions should be removed:

- atypical ductal hyperplasia (ADH)
- some atypical lobular hyperplasia (ALH)
- pleomorphic lobular carcinoma *in situ* (PLCIS)
- nonclassical LCIS variants
- atypical or palpable papillary lesions
- radial scars
- complex sclerosing lesions
- some fibroepithelial lesions
- mucocele-like lesions
- desmoid tumors
- spindle cell lesions

These marker lesions are commonly followed rather than removed:

- most atypical lobular hyperplasia (ALH)
- classic lobular carcinoma *in situ* (LCIS)
- flat epithelial atypia (FEA)
- incidental papillary lesions without atypia
- columnar cell lesions (CCL)
- fibroadenomas (FA)
- pseudoangiomatous stromal hyperplasia (PASH)

In addition to deciding whether a marker lesion will be removed or observed, you also need to learn what this little intruder has to say about your future cancer risk. Markers affect your risk to variable degrees, depending on what they are, so here's another list for you to reference whenever an intruder surprises you.[45] Let's start with the good news.

These *nonproliferative lesions* have no or negligible impact on future breast cancer risk:

- benign phyllodes tumor
- epithelial-related calcifications
- simple cysts
- ductal ectasia
- fat necrosis
- fibrocystic changes
- fibrosis
- mild hyperplasia without atypia
- non-sclerosing adenosis
- solitary papilloma without atypia
- periductal fibrosis
- squamous and apocrine metaplasia
- mastitis
- benign tumors including hemangioma, hamartoma, lipoma, neurofibroma

Next up, proliferative lesions *without* atypia increase future breast cancer risk anywhere in either breast between 1.3 to 1.9 (30 to 90 percent increase) and, depending on what other risk factors you have going on, you may or may not do anything extra because of these:

- moderate or florid ductal hyperplasia without atypia
- fibroadenoma
- sclerosing adenosis

- multiple papillomas (papillomatosis)
- radial scar

And finally, proliferative lesions *with* atypia invite you to take a more assertive stance on surveillance and risk reduction because they increase future cancer risk 3.9 to 13.0 (up to 1,200 percent increase):

- atypical ductal hyperplasia (ADH)
- atypical lobular hyperplasia (ALH)
- all types of lobular carcinoma in situ (LCIS)

We address increased screening and risk reduction options in the next chapter.

PERSONAL HISTORY OF BREAST CANCER

A personal history of breast cancer means whatever circumstances co-mingled in your breast DNA to create that first cancer just might continue to exert carcinogenic effects on the remaining breast tissue. Keep in mind that the treatments of your first cancer often have the side benefit of limiting the possibility of a second cancer; this especially applies to endocrine therapy like tamoxifen, which reduces a brand-new cancer in the opposite breast—called a *contralateral breast cancer* (CBC)—by 50 percent.[46] In general, a cancer recurrence within ten years near the area where it first happened, termed a local recurrence, happens in 4 to 6 percent of women.[47] Among breast cancer survivors, a CBC is the most likely second cancer they will get, as opposed to ovarian cancer or melanoma, for example.[48] CBC chances hover around 7 percent as long as you adhere to your recommended cancer treatment.[49] Women often mistake CBCs as a cancer *recurrence*, but this isn't the old cancer coming back again in the other breast; it is its own original thing and could very well have a totally different set of hormone receptors than your first cancer did.

CBC carries its own prognosis without affecting the cure rates of the first cancer you had.

YOUR FAMILY HISTORY

My son Sebastian and husband, Andy, are mirror images of each other; Ethan is my mini-me; and Justin, well, I remember for a few days after his birth I thought maybe we took the wrong baby home. He didn't look like either of us. And then I noticed the edge of his upper lip, called the vermilion border. A tiny sliver of the border appeared pale due to missing pigment—just like Andy's lip! Wow, the things we can inherit from our parents.

Inherited *traits* like lip pigmentation and eye color are one thing; inherited genetic *mutations* are another (discussed next), but does anything else get passed along that leaves us vulnerable to breast cancer? Even with a strong family history, odds might not be as high as you think. From the largest review to date looking at how family history affects your risk, this is what emerged: with *one* first-degree female relative (sister, mother, daughter) diagnosed with breast cancer, your baseline risk of 12.4 percent increases to 17.8 percent; if *two* first-degree relatives have been diagnosed, your risk jumps to 25.6 percent.[50] Risk goes a tad higher when it's your sister as opposed to mother who has cancer, and higher still when the cancer occurs prior to age fifty; second-degree relatives with cancer elevate your risk about half as high as first-degree (so if a mother bumps your risk by 5 percent, a maternal aunt will raise it 2.5 percent).[51] It's not clear to what degree male breast cancers in a father, brother, or son affect risk. So moms with breast cancer, I hope you can relax a little. Your daughter has an 82 percent probability of *not* getting breast cancer, your situation has contributed only a little to her risk (if at all), and once you finish this book, you and she will start sharing all the cancer-kicking behaviors that we discuss. Good as gold.

The habits you'll adopt from the first half of this book could fully eliminate whatever contribution one or two family members make to your risk. Why? Because odds are 90 to 95 percent that your relative does not have a genetic mutation that could be passed down to you. You share a lot more than genes, like "inherited" eating habits, cooking styles, exercise routines, religious beliefs, and environmental exposures. Change all that for the better, and watch those numbers drop.

What about really extensive cancer histories in multiple relatives at young ages? Women who test negative for BRCA mutations with a significant family history of two or more breast cancers under the age of fifty, or three or more breast cancers at any age, have approximately a fourfold risk of breast cancer (12.4 percent becomes 36.9 percent lifetime risk).[52] If multiple cancers exist in your family tree, seek out a genetic counselor who will use sophisticated risk calculators to personalize these numbers even further. When risk elevates to a percent that really feels risky to you, then it's time for you and your breast doctor to dive into the options that we discuss in the next chapter.

BRCA GENE MUTATIONS

This four-letter acronym gets a lot of attention though most people don't know what it stands for, what it is, or if it applies to them. Well, then, let's change that. BRCA refers to two genes that we all have called BRCA-1 and BRCA-2 (the acronym stands for BReast CAncer). Healthy BRCA genes suppress the growth of tumor cells by repairing or removing faulty cells before they can form a mass. But some families carry *broken* BRCA genes that get passed down from one generation to the next. Less than 10 percent of all breast cancers and 14 percent of ovarian cancers occur from a BRCA or other genetic mutation, inherited from *either* parent.[53] Remember, your father's history may hold the key to recognizing gene mutations and elevated risk. You are half your father's DNA, and half of all BRCA carriers are men. The general population carries BRCA mutations at a rate of 1 in 450, but Ashkenazi Jewish individuals (those from Germany, Poland, Lithuania, Ukraine, and Russia, as opposed to the Sephardic Jewish population primarily from Spain, France, Italy, and North Africa) carry them at a rate of 1 in 40.[54] With these odds, certainly all Ashkenazi Jews with breast or ovarian cancer in the family should consider genetic testing; we'll review all the red flags that trigger testing in the section below.

What makes BRCA such a big deal? When you carry one of these mutations, breast cancer rates skyrocket to twenty-five times the general population risk for breast cancer by age fifty, and to thirty times the general population lifetime risk for ovarian cancer. Women carrying BRCA-1 have up to an 87 percent lifetime chance of breast cancer and 54 percent chance of ovarian cancer.[55] Different populations have different types of BRCA mutations (there are over 1,000), each of which has a unique propensity toward causing cancer—that's called *penetrance*, and it's why we see a range of cancer predictions related to gene mutations. A recent meta-analysis reported slightly less startling numbers with lifetime risk to age seventy (they always aim low for longevity, don't they?) for BRCA-1 breast cancer = 57 percent, and BRCA-2 = 49 percent; and ovarian cancer BRCA-1 risk = 40 percent, BRCA-2 = 18 percent.[56] That's better, but still disconcertingly high. I worry a bit more about the breasts in my BRCA-1 carriers because 70 percent of their cancers will be a more aggressive triple-negative subtype that almost always requires chemotherapy, even at stage I.[57] Since both breasts have BRCA problems, once you get cancer, there's a 40 to 65 percent chance the other breast will eventually get cancer too.[58] As you can imagine, with odds like these, many BRCA carriers with cancer in one breast will choose to have a double mastectomy.

We dig into all your choices about what to do about BRCA mutations in the next section. Since the average age at diagnosis of breast cancer for BRCA-1 is forty-four years, and BRCA-2 is forty-seven years, the younger you find out about this gene, the more proactive you can be.[59] As if the breasts and ovaries weren't enough to worry about, female BRCA patients also have to screen for pancreatic cancer (2 to 5 percent chance)[60] and BRCA-2 carriers need to watch out for melanoma (2 to 5 percent).[61] By comparison, in the non-BRCA population, cancer rates are 12.4 percent breast, 1.4 percent ovarian, less than 1 percent pancreatic, and 2 percent melanoma.

Male BRCA carriers have cancer risks too. Male breast cancer is more common in the BRCA-2 carriers than BRCA-1 (8 percent versus 1.8 percent). Similarly, BRCA-2 elevates prostate cancer risk much more than BRCA-1 (16 to 25 percent versus minimal elevation, respectively).[62] Just like the ladies, male BRCA-1 and -2 have pancreatic cancer risk (3 to 6 percent), and male BRCA-2 carriers need melanoma screening (2 to 6 percent).[63] These rates compare to 0.001 percent breast, 14 percent prostate, 1.1 percent pancreatic, and 2.5 percent melanoma in the non-BRCA male population.

OTHER GENETIC MUTATIONS

Other genetic mutations can also lead to inherited breast cancers. This area of research is bursting with new information, which excites us because as genetic testing becomes widespread, we will have larger populations with known mutations that we can then follow and more precisely come to understand the risks each mutation carries. As you know by now, less than 10 percent of all breast cancers come from inherited genes; among those with mutations, about 50 percent are BRCA carriers, 10 percent are in the list I'm about to detail for you, and the remaining 40 percent are a work-in-progress via *next generation sequencing*, which is the catchall term given to fancy ways to look at your DNA.[64] Most mutations carry less cancer risk than BRCA does.

The following genetic mutations elevate breast cancer risk to the degree indicated. Whenever you see a range in incidence, know that having family members with breast cancer pushes your risk toward the higher end of that range. Everyone with any of these gene mutations should consider upping the ante with surveillance well beyond annual mammography and might even take special medications or remove organs at risk (all of which we discuss on the next page and in chapter 7). Mutations known to elevate breast cancer risk include PTEN (Cowden syndrome), 80 percent; TP53 (Li-Fraumeni Syndrome), 31 percent with average age at diagnosis being thirty-two years old;[65] PALB2, 35 to 58 percent; STK11 (Peutz-Jeghers syndrome), 32 to 54 percent with a young onset; CDH1, 39 to 42 percent, invasive lobular subtype;[66] CHEK2, 20 to 44 percent[67] (breast cancer survival rates are 40 percent worse than noncarriers);[68] NBN, 20 to 36 percent;[69] NF1, 26 to 39 percent;[70] ATM, 16 to 26 percent[71] (probable sensitivity to ionizing radiation, such as used to treat breast cancer, which leads to a higher chance of new breast cancers);[72] and BARD1, "elevated risk."[73] Visit pinklotus .com/genemutations to learn about other cancers and physical signs that cluster with these mutations.

GENETIC MUTATIONS: TO TEST OR NOT TO TEST

Patients often say, "I don't want to know if I carry a mutation. What would I do differently?" The answer is, *a lot*! First of all, you most likely do *not* carry a mutation, and finding that out could relieve you of much anxiety. Second, if positive for a mutation, insurance should pay for more intense surveillance (like breast MRIs), and you could benefit from the extra vigilance in that we're more likely to find cancer early with better imaging. Third, your doctors could screen you for non–breast cancers associated with whichever mutation you have. Fourth, your breast doctors can offer effective medications and operations to reduce your risk of getting cancer. Fifth, other family members benefit from knowing your status. Sixth, you might become more motivated to seize control of contributory risks like nutrition and weight, which translates into overall health benefits for you. And finally, if you are planning to start a family, you have the option of not passing along the mutation (see chapter 7). On the flip side, if knowing about a mutation would merely increase anxiety because these reasons all seem irrelevant to you, and you would decline all interventions, then perhaps it's better not to know.

Privacy and Protection

Patients also express concern regarding discrimination against known genetic mutation carriers, but laws exist to protect you. The Health Insurance Portability and Accountability Act of 1996 (HIPAA) made it illegal in the United States for insurers to consider gene mutations a preexisting condition and to deny or limit coverage. In 2008, the Genetic Information Nondiscrimination Act (GINA) became another law that protects you from health insurance discrimination (but not life insurance) and makes it illegal for employers to use genetic information in workplace employment decisions. If you're still concerned, reputable testing kits are available for under $250, so if that's affordable, you can always circumvent insurance and test under an alias (here's your chance to be legitimately called Wonder Woman).

Who Should Consider Genetic Testing?

Given the high likelihood of getting breast, ovarian, or other cancers with all these different mutations, a family history peppered with numerous or uncommon cancers usually raises red flags that trigger the suggestion to get genetic testing. To evaluate this, first do your homework. Find out about your first-, second-, and third-degree relatives from maternal and paternal sides. Do you know why your dad's mom's brother died? (I don't even know if my dad's mom had a brother.) Who had what cancers? Based on what you learn, if you have any *one* of the following nine red flags in yourself or on the same side of the family tree, your gene mutation risk exceeds 10 percent, and you should consider genetic testing (you or the genetic testing company can first check to see if your insurance pays for it):

1. Two of the following: breast cancer before age fifty or ovarian cancer at any age

2. Ashkenazi Jewish heritage plus *one* breast cancer before age fifty or ovarian cancer at any age
3. Any male relative with breast cancer
4. A known BRCA mutation carrier (first degree relatives of a carrier have a 50 percent chance of carrying the mutation)
5. Breast cancer in self prior to age fifty
6. Two breast cancers in self, any age (not a recurrence)
7. Triple-negative breast cancer in self prior to age sixty
8. Ashkenazi Jewish and breast cancer in self, any age
9. Just a whole lot of cancer going on: two or more family members on the same side with breast, ovarian, pancreatic, prostate, melanoma, uterine, colon, and/or stomach cancers

A physician skilled in genetics or a genetics counselor will discuss the implications of testing and help you interpret how having *or not having* a gene mutation impacts your future cancer risks and reduction options. Pink Lotus offers an anonymous, free, less than five-minute online quiz to assess whether your level of risk meets testing criteria at pinklotus.com /genetictest. Testing involves spit or a simple blood draw, and you can choose to evaluate the entire spectrum of cancer-causing genes or hone in on genes of interest. Pink Lotus also offers a spit kit that gets mailed to your home and includes genetic counseling regarding your results at pinklotus.com/elements.

HAVE A GENE MUTATION?
MAKE AN ACTION PLAN!

If doctors have a heads-up that you carry a gene mutation, then there's a whole host of weapons to unleash. Take Sarah, for example, a newly engaged twenty-six-year-old second grade teacher with a BRCA-1 mutation whose mother passed away from ovarian cancer at age forty-four (when Sarah was fourteen), and whose maternal aunt died from breast cancer at age fifty-one. Sarah had seen several doctors already, but she felt overwhelmed and confused and came to me expecting to leave feeling just as helpless as when she arrived. I quickly discovered that Sarah has been looking forward to having two biological children of her own for as long as she can remember, and breastfeeding matters to her. Although her breasts are a favorite part of her body, she feels that once their life-sustaining purpose of nursing children has ended, she will worry too much about cancer to want to keep them. Together with her supportive fiancé, Doug, we reviewed Sarah's *actual* risks of getting breast and ovarian cancer stratified by decade of life over her next sixty-five years (because I expect her to live until at least ninety). Based on that new information to her, the urgency she felt in all of this melted away into something manageable. We outlined a strategy that suddenly made perfect sense to both of them, involving staggered breast exams and imaging. They would try to get pregnant right away, and once childbearing is over, her ovaries will be removed. We will keep the dialogue about breast surgery open, but for now, she has targeted age thirty-five for a bilateral prophylactic mastectomy. Sarah and Doug exhaled deeply, and her eyes welled with tears. They left with a proactive plan suited to their situation.

Getting to Know You

If you carried a gene mutation and I were meeting you for the first time, I would learn as much about your preconceptions and personality as possible. How has the cancer experience of others colored your perception of treatments and side effects? Are you in a stable relationship, married, or single? Have you completed childbearing? Do you desire children? Is breastfeeding a strong priority? How much do your breasts mean to you in terms of body image, sexual pleasure, and femininity? Can you tolerate living with risk, or do you feel anxious about it? Which at-risk organ concerns you more: breasts or ovaries, and why? What is your occupation, and how would the plans we are making interfere with work or travel? The answers to all of these questions, and other issues unique to you alone, not only enlighten your doctor, but they often surprise you with some self-discovery.

Two Roads to Travel

Two main strategies exist for gene-mutation carriers: surveillance and surgery. Just because you have elevated risk doesn't mean you follow a one-size-fits-all protocol. Doctors must uniquely tailor plans to each woman they advise. The strategy depends as much on your current priorities and future hopes as it depends on test results. Some patients choose prophylactic surgery. Others don't want to go anywhere near the knife, preferring preventive medications. And some decide to focus on the lifestyle factors we discussed in chapters 3 to 5, combined with the aggressive screening regimen I outline below. I want to help women find a path that leaves them feeling confident and comfortable with their choices. We investigate options that actively drop cancer risk associated with inherited mutations in chapter 7.

Remember, surveillance is not prevention; it's just hoping to find cancer early. The surveillance path involves a combination of imaging and exams, as well as possibly taking risk-reducing medications and using traditional Chinese medicine. Below is the surveillance plan I use for women at elevated risk, and it's a little more intense than the National Comprehensive Cancer Network (NCCN) advises.[74] Yet even with a rigorous protocol, 16 percent of the cancers that get diagnosed will already have involved lymph nodes—a stark reminder that surveillance is not prevention or treatment.[75]

- At age eighteen, breast awareness and monthly breast self-exam (BSE) begin and continue forever.
- Also at age eighteen, I start doing clinical breast exams (CBE) every six months.
- At age twenty-five, we introduce annual breast MRI with macrocyclic gadolinium contrast and annual whole-breast screening ultrasound spaced six months from the MRI. In this way, you have breast imaging and an exam every six months.

- At age thirty, annual mammography enters into the mix, the drawbacks of which are discussed in chapter 8.
- BRCA-positive men need BSE and annual CBE at age thirty-five and prostate screening at forty-five.

When it comes to ovarian cancer, our inability to detect it at an early stage is disappointing and unsettling. I suggest discussing with your gynecologist if pelvic exams, transvaginal ultrasounds, and CA-125 tumor marker testing are worthwhile for you to pursue. Oral contraceptive pills (OCPs), a.k.a. birth control pills, reduce the risk of ovarian cancer by 50 percent and do not increase breast cancer risks enough to overrule their protection for ovaries.[76] All premenopausal BRCA patients with ovaries who are not trying to conceive should go on OCPs (unless contraindicated) even if they have breasts. I can monitor breasts; those ovaries hide from view, and once they harbor cancer, survival rates are dismal.

My deepest hope is that a solid surveillance plan replaces anxiety with answers, and fear with confidence. Sometimes we have to get a little more intense with the risk reduction, and so the next chapter displays all the tools in our chest. Have a look! As always, the goal is to save lives.

FACTORS THAT INCREASE THE RELATIVE RISK FOR BREAST CANCER IN WOMEN

This simple chart categorizes the different risk factors we have reviewed and groups them according to how heavily they impact your risk of getting breast cancer relative to someone who doesn't have that factor. Anyone who falls into categories with a relative risk at or above 2.1 should not only read the next two chapters, but also discuss a rigorous breast-screening plan with her physician.

THE BOTTOM LINE: WHAT INCREASES BREAST CANCER[77]

RELATIVE RISK	FACTOR
>4.0	• Inherited genetic mutations for breast cancer (BRCA-1, BRCA-2, PTEN, TP53, PALB2, STK11) • Age over 50 versus under 50 years • Biopsy in self showing LCIS or atypical hyperplasia (ADH/ALH) • Mammographically extremely dense breasts as compared to fatty breasts • High-dose radiation to chest prior to age 30
2.1–4.0	• Inherited genetic mutations for breast cancer (CDH1, CHEK2, NBN, NF1, ATM, BARD1) • Personal history of ER(-) breast cancer prior to age 35 • Family history: two or more first-degree relatives with breast cancer prior to age 50 • Family history: three or more relatives on the same parent's side with breast cancer at any age • High postmenopausal levels of naturally occurring estrogen or testosterone • Morbid obesity: BMI at or over 40
1.1–2.0	• Personal history of ER(-) breast cancer after age 35 or ER(+) breast cancer prior to age 30 • Proliferative breast lesions without atypia (usual ductal hyperplasia, fibroadenoma, radial scar) • Family history: one or two first- or second-degree relatives with breast cancer after age 50 • Height at or over 5 feet 7 inches • High socioeconomic status • High bone mineral density • Non-Hispanic white and black races versus other races • No full-term pregnancies • First full-term pregnancy after 35 years • Never breastfed a child • Menopause at or after 54 years • Menarche prior to 12 years • Diethylstilbestrol (DES) exposure • Night shift work • Obesity: BMI 25 to 39.9 • Adult weight gain exceeding 8 pounds • Sedentary lifestyle

RELATIVE RISK	FACTOR
1.1–2.0 (cont.)	• HRT (estrogen plus progesterone) within 5 years • HRT (estrogen only) within 5 years of menopause or for longer than 10 years • Recent oral contraceptive pill use • Smoking cigarettes for 20 years prior to first pregnancy or for more than 40 years • Alcohol consumption • Low fiber consumption • Low phytoestrogen consumption • Low green tea consumption • Vitamin and mineral deficiencies (A, B_6, B_{12}, C, D, beta-carotene, folate, calcium) • Regular red meat consumption • Regular high-fat dairy consumption

CHAPTER 7

Medications and Operations to Consider

For many of you, the threat of breast cancer looms as an ever-present anxiety that constantly disrupts your life by injecting fear where there could be peace. But you have power, you can exert control—you, and you alone, own your body and are responsible for managing the wellness and illness that exists within it. And when you're armed with the latest information on how to dramatically reduce your risk, for both first-time breast cancer and cancer recurrences, that information can change your life. If it seems from the prior chapter that you have more risk than your comfort zone allows, consider talking to your doctor about taking steps beyond diet and lifestyle modifications to manage your health.

The decision to intervene more aggressively with medications or operations should begin with a discussion between you and your doctor about how you can stomach surveillance alone. When I have these conversations, I quickly notice that one of three personality types emerges. There's what I call "The Sailboat," who tolerates risk and feels confident with imaging, breast self-exam (BSE), and clinical breast exam (CBE). Sometimes, this woman isn't so much easy breezy, but premenopausal or single and just doesn't want to rock the boat with menopause-inducing medications or breast removal. Then there's "The Cruise Ship," who craves more stability and predictability than a small vessel offers; we therefore add a risk-reducing pill to the screening plan. Finally, there's the woman I consider "The Speedboat." She has no interest in breast imaging, exams, or meds. She might even say, "These breasts are trying to kill me! I don't want them anymore." So we review surgical options and head straight to dry land.

Here, we'll tackle medications first and then move on to operations.

PREVENTIVE THERAPIES

There's a scary term called *chemoprevention* that gets its name from the word *chemo*, which means "chemical" in Latin; chemoprevention describes a number of chemicals (medications) intended for the purpose of preventing breast cancer. I use it here so that you can recognize it in other cancer literature, but for our purposes, let's join those who simply call it preventive therapy.[1] All preventive therapy is taken orally in pill or liquid form, and works by limiting the effects of your naturally circulating estrogens, which attach to estrogen receptors sitting on cancer cells and then fuel their growth and division. If any of the following three factors applies to you, I advise having a discussion with your doctor regarding preventive therapy:

- Atypical ductal hyperplasia (ADH), atypical lobular hyperplasia (ALH), or lobular carcinoma *in situ* (LCIS) on any previous biopsy
- Thirty-five years or older with a 1.66 percent or greater chance of developing breast cancer in the next five years (you can calculate this at pinklotus.com/gail)
- An inherited genetic mutation like BRCA

Aromatase Inhibitors (AIs)

Since 80 percent of all cancer happens after age fifty, something's up as you age—and it's estrogen. As I've mentioned before, you make estrogen forever because an enzyme called *aromatase* hangs out in adrenal glands, ovaries, fat, and brain tissue and converts androgens like testosterone into estradiol. Also, if you recall, breast cancer cells hijack the aromatase in breast fat and use it to make their very own estradiol supply. I'm reminding you of this because medications currently on the market named exemestane (brand name Aromasin), anastrozole (Arimidex), and letrozole (Femara) behave as "aromatase inhibitors" (AIs). They *inactivate* aromatase, thereby decreasing the amount of estrogen circulating in your body. So after your ovaries shut down, these antiestrogens will work by messing with the only other pathway that creates estrogen.

Trials prove that preventive therapies do a decent job of living up to the "prevent" part of their name. One trial put 4,560 high-risk postmenopausal women on exemestane versus a placebo every day for five years, and the AI cut invasive breast cancer by 65 percent compared to placebo.[2] Importantly, enrollees tolerated the side effects well, and adverse events were equal between groups. So taking exemestane is full of upside if you can handle the commonly experienced downsides of menopausal symptoms, joint pain, and bone density loss. A second big study looked at anastrozole versus placebo and reported that the AI cut breast cancer by 50 percent, dropping the cancer rate from 4 percent with placebo to 2 percent with anastrozole.[3] This might not sound dramatic, but that's over 4,600 US women every single year who don't have to deal with breast cancer. Pretty great!

Selective Estrogen Receptor Modulators (SERMs)

There's a second class of drugs available called *selective estrogen receptor modulators* (SERMs), taken in pill form. These currently include tamoxifen and raloxifene (brand name Evista). They chemically look like estrogen, and like a key fitting into a lock, they slide into the same estrogen-receptors as estrogen. But they outcompete estradiol, beat it to the receptor, and jam the lock. Brilliant! So instead of turning cancer cells into replicating machines, SERMs gum up the lock so the real deal estradiol can't do its cancer thing.

Tamoxifen

Several studies in the 1980s noted a surprise observation from the use of tamoxifen in cancer patients—not only did it reduce the recurrence of cancer in the affected breast, it significantly reduced contralateral breast cancers (CBC) in the opposite breast.[4] Hmm . . . so if high-risk women who have never had breast cancer took tamoxifen, would we *prevent* breast cancer? After following 13,388 high-risk women for almost six years, a tamoxifen versus placebo trial showed that tamoxifen slashes future estrogen receptor-positive [ER(+)] breast cancers and cancer death in *half*; if a prior breast biopsy showing *atypical* cells were your reason for taking it, risk dropped by 86 percent.[5] There are additional perks too: bone density increases (fewer fractures), cholesterol improves, and breast density goes down.[6] Wow, why don't we all just sprinkle a little powdered tam onto our whole-oats oatmeal every morning? I'll give you two reasons: side effects (hot flashes, vaginal discharge) and complications (blood clots, stroke, uterine cancer), but most women tolerate the side effects well, and complications are very rare.

Hey, BRCA friends, this tamoxifen trial also found a 62 percent drop in BRCA-2 carriers, which takes that roughly 80 percent lifetime risk of yours way down to 30 percent.[7] The problem is, there were only nineteen women in that subset, but there's another study that corroborates this tamoxifen effect. Guess what happens to the *opposite breast's* cancer risk when BRCA carriers get cancer, keep their breasts, and take tamoxifen? Data from 2,464 such patients revealed a 62 percent drop in BRCA-1 and 67 percent for BRCA-2.[8] If tamoxifen can knock second cancers down like that, it probably also reduces a *first-time* cancer for both BRCA-1 and -2. There's something bizarre hidden in this data; let me explain it to you. Tamoxifen dramatically reduced estrogen receptor-*negative* [ER(–)] cancers in BRCA-1 carriers, but all tamoxifen does is occupy estrogen receptors, so how does *that* make sense? Also, tamoxifen never stopped ER(–) cancers in *any* of the other trials. So what I'm saying is, tamoxifen can stop ER(–) cancers, but only when someone has a BRCA mutation. So . . . does that mean tamoxifen can undo the mutation? Well, yes, sort of, but it needs help. This help might come in the form of single-nucleotide polymorphisms—or SNPs, "snips"—which are basically typos when cells copy themselves (remember, you make around fifty billion new cells a day), so the new cell contains a misspelled word. Apparently, we're bad at typing, because you have around ten million of these SNPs, most of which mean nothing. However, scientists have identified more than ninety SNPs that elevate breast cancer risk.[9] Sometimes when SNPs occur in an area that controls a nearby gene, they directly affect that gene's function. Scientists found that BRCA-1 carriers have SNPs near estrogen receptors, so it's plausible that tamoxifen plus SNPs together alter a BRCA-1 carrier's inability to repair mutated DNA.[10] So both BRCA-1 and -2 women should consider tamoxifen for preventive therapy.

Raloxifene (Evista)

If you're in search of a sexier SERM with fewer hassles, the Study of Tamoxifen and Raloxifene (STAR) trial had these two drugs duke it out in 19,747 postmenopausal women at increased risk for breast cancer.[11] Both drugs equally and effectively lowered the risk of invasive breast cancer. Raloxifene, however, showed the following benefits over tamoxifen: less vaginal discharge, fewer blood clots, fewer cataracts, and less uterine cancer. Tamoxifen reduced stage 0 cancers (ductal carcinoma *in situ*, or DCIS) by 50 percent more than raloxifene and didn't cause insomnia. If you can't take tamoxifen because of say, a history of blood clots, then raloxifene's for you. But apples for apples, I like the fact that tamoxifen also knocks down DCIS risk, so that's my preference.

Who Takes What?

If you're considering any of these preventive therapies for risk reduction, remember that raloxifene and aromatase inhibitors are only used in postmenopausal women, not premenopausal women. Tamoxifen can be used in all women, and it's the only choice for premenopausal women. These drugs are usually taken for five years, but the SERMs (tamoxifen and raloxifene) continue to cut cancer risk for at least five years after stopping therapy.[12] Even though all of these meds offer more benefit than harm, most women perceive the opposite to be true and don't choose preventive therapy. Only exemestane, tamoxifen, and raloxifene are FDA-approved for preventive therapy. Together with your doctor, weigh the risks and benefits of these medications to decide which, if any, makes sense for you.

MORE PREVENTIVE THERAPIES AND RISK REDUCERS

Every once in a while, when people take medications to treat one illness, we accidentally discover that an unrelated ailment also improves on the same drug. The following medications have happily surprised us in that they seem to reduce breast cancer risk in addition to completing their original mission.

Bisphosphonates

First up is a class of drugs successfully used to treat osteoporosis called *bisphosphonates* (alendronate is the most popular one). They have the proven effects of managing breast cancer metastases to bone and bone loss induced by AIs or chemo, but bisphosphonates also might save you a trip down Cancer Lane. Within the large Women's Health Initiative study we reviewed regarding HRT risks, over 2,800 postmenopausal women used oral bisphosphonates for osteoporosis. After nearly eight years follow-up, the bisphosphonate users had fewer bone fractures (of course, since that's what the drug prevents) but also 32 percent less invasive breast cancer than women not taking the medication.[13] Echoing these findings, an Israeli study of 4,039 patients also found 28 percent less breast cancer in bisphosphonate users.[14] Other studies point to direct antitumor effects involving anti-angiogenesis (new blood vessel formation), antiproliferation (cell growth), and proapoptosis (cell death) to explain the benefit.[15]

Metformin

Metformin, another drug that's been around for ages, controls blood sugar in type 2 diabetics, but also has antiproliferative and anti-inflammatory effects, which you know favorably alter that tumor micro-environment I keep mentioning. In fact, a UK study evaluated 22,621 female users of oral antidiabetes drugs and found a 56 percent reduction in breast cancer for long-term metformin use of more than five years' duration, as compared to diabetics on any other medication.[16] Thiazolidinediones, drugs that work like metformin, have shown a 33 percent preventive effect on breast cancer too.[17]

Sugar and carbs do not cause diabetes (although they can exacerbate it); saturated fat—fat from a diet heavily focused on meat, dairy, and eggs—clogs the insulin receptors on your muscle cells. When that happens, insulin can't tell your muscle to open the glucose gates so that sugar can enter into the muscle for storage as glycogen, so glucose flies around your bloodstream making everyone think that sugar is the problem; we call this *insulin resistance*, because the cells resist what insulin tells them to do. In response, your body sends more insulin—known as hyperinsulinemia—as if it's saying, "Hey, receptor, what's your problem? Open the glucose gate!" It can't hear you, because it's stuffed with fat. Studies demonstrate that insulin resistance and hyperinsulinemia increase the risk of both getting and dying from breast cancer.[18] So it makes sense that normalizing the way insulin and sugar behave in your body with metformin proves to be an effective preventive strategy, but not all studies show a benefit, and other antidiabetic drugs, including insulin, don't offer cancer protection.[19]

On the other hand, type 2 diabetes can be entirely *reversed* in twenty-two weeks—I mean, off insulin forever, reversed—by exclusively eating a whole food, plant-based diet, so you could also try fixing your diabetes *and* saving your breasts with plants.[20] Dr. Neal Barnard and his colleagues have successfully treated thousands of diabetics with nutrition alone. Find tips and more information from the Physicians Committee for Responsible Medicine at pcrm.org.

Retinoic Acid

Emerging science on retinoic acid holds promise for lowering breast cancer risk. A derivative of vitamin A that's found abundantly in sweet potato and carrots, this metabolite plays a critical role in the way cells grow, divide, and die. All-trans retinoic acid (ATRA) turns precancerous cells *back to normal* in laboratory studies and in limited human clinical trials. Imagine three petri dishes with either (1) normal breast cells, (2) precancerous or noninvasive cancer cells (atypical or *in situ* cancer cells), and then (3) invasive cancer cells. Now let's drip different concentrations of ATRA onto each of them and see what happens. Incredibly, the precancerous atypical and noninvasive *in situ* cells reverted back to normal in terms of cell shape; not only that, but the way they communicated through 443 distinct genes also returned back to normal.[21] Thus even genetic pathways can change from good to bad and back to good again. The invasive cells did not revert to normal, which helps explain why dietary interventions alone once you reach the invasive stage of cancer progression are largely ineffective at curing breast cancer.

In human studies, when breast cancer patients were given a synthetic ATRA called *fenretinide* for five years after diagnosis, we see a remarkable 50 percent reduction in second breast cancers in women under forty, with a 38 percent reduction in all premenopausal ages, and these benefits persisted for several years after treatment cessation.[22] No benefit emerged in those over fifty-five years old. The explanation seems to involve an old frenemy of ours: IGF-1. Fenretinide makes IGF-1 go down while its main binding protein, IGFBP-3, goes up. We await the results of clinical trials in both the preventive therapy and treatment settings.[23]

NSAIDs

Here's an easy suggestion that I'll bet you already have in your medicine cabinet: aspirin and nonsteroidal anti-inflammatory drugs (NSAIDs). There's actually a side benefit to all that Advil popped for headaches and menstrual cramps. Preventive therapy from these anti-inflammatories makes sense because both acetylsalicylic acid (ASA; e.g., Bayer, Bufferin, Excedrin, generic aspirin) and NSAIDs (e.g., Advil, Motrin, Aleve, generic ibuprofen) obstruct an enzyme called *COX-2* that increases estrogen production, estrogen-mediated gene expression, and, thus, cancer growth. After analyzing the ASA and NSAID use in 80,741 postmenopausal women, researchers found that taking two or more tablets per week for five to nine years yields a 21 percent reduction in breast cancer; doing so for ten or more years provides a 28 percent reduction.[24] Many other studies confirm this effect, with breast cancer reductions consistently around 25 percent.[25] Regular use of acetaminophen (e.g., Tylenol) or low-dose aspirin (less than 100 milligrams) has little anti-inflammatory activity and no preventive effect. Recommended doses are NSAIDs 200 mg/tablet and ASA 325 mg/tablet. Unless you have had bleeding ulcers, a stroke, or another reason to completely avoid these meds, take two or three a week. By the way, they also protect against heart disease and colon cancer.

SURGICAL INTERVENTION:
BREASTS AND OVARIES

Angelina Jolie's op-ed piece in the *New York Times* called "My Medical Choice" awakened the world on May 14, 2013, to the existence of something called *BRCA*. When you hear that anyone would willingly remove two totally healthy external parts of her body that symbolize femininity and sexuality, you have to wonder, "Why would she do that?" And when you learn the answer, you have to think, "Do I have that gene too?" Coutless people all over the world were educated about a gene mutation that devastates unsuspecting families generation after generation. If you have a BRCA mutation, you can remove the organs at highest risk, namely breasts and ovaries, before cancer ever begins.

Bilateral Prophylactic Mastectomy (BPM)

To maximally reduce chances of getting breast cancer, some high-risk women choose to have what's known as a *bilateral prophylactic mastectomy* (BPM), also called a preventive double mastectomy, which means the breasts are removed without any known cancer within them, solely for the purpose of preventing cancer from ever happening. In a contemporary series of skin-sparing (removes the nipples) and nipple-sparing (preserves the nipples) mastectomies, the incidence of breast cancer after BPM stays under 3 percent, and with a truly excellent mastectomy technique the risk should be zero, even when keeping the nipples.[26]

Two realities might put you at high enough risk to seriously consider BPM: (1) inherited genetic mutations and (2) elevated risk with marker lesions and/or a strong family history. BPM reduces the death rate due to breast cancer,[27] and I recommend it whenever a high-risk woman wants it after age twenty-one. For BRCA carriers, I suggest BPM prior to age forty (the average age at diagnosis is forty-five years) or ten years younger than the youngest affected relative with breast cancer. Why the ten years advice? An MD Anderson study showed that the current generation of BRCA mutation carriers gets cancer 7.9 years earlier than the prior generation.[28] Also, cancer cells mutate years before we detect them. Ten years should effectively stop cancer before it starts. Some women find out about their BRCA status much later in life; for example, at age 70 you have unwittingly escaped so much risk that your lifetime breast cancer estimate is now less than 12 percent, so rather than surgery, perhaps surveillance fits just right.

Contralateral Breast Cancer (CBC)

If you have cancer in one breast and are considering a mastectomy to treat it, should you remove the other breast as well? Removing the healthy breast in this situation is called a *contralateral prophylactic mastectomy* (CPM). To answer the CPM question, you should understand contralateral breast cancer (CBC) risk, which predicts the development of a second cancer in the opposite breast, the one that didn't have the original cancer. CBC incidence has happily declined 3 percent per year for ER(+) cancers ever since the widespread use of tamoxifen in 1985.[29] Chemotherapy use also reduces CBC incidence by about 20 percent for at least a decade after receiving it.[30] On the flip side, a number of factors increase contralateral breast cancer risk: young age at first breast cancer diagnosis,[31] ER(–) first cancer,[32] lobular first cancer,[33] family history,[34] genetic mutations,[35] young age at menarche,[36] never childbearing,[37] and obesity.[38] Except for BRCA mutation carriers whose lifetime CBC risk averages 40 to 65 percent, the most predictive power regarding CBC risk is held by your current age and the estrogen status of your first cancer. Here's a useful table I created for cancer patients faced with the CPM decision based on an analysis of US cancer databases from 2001 to 2005.[39] The numbers assume appropriate chemotherapy and antiestrogen use. If you look at the CBC risk over the next three decades for both ER(+) and ER(–) tumors, the numbers are not astronomically high.

CONTRALATERAL BREAST CANCER (CBC) PERCENT RISK IN ESTROGEN RECEPTOR-POSITIVE ER(+) AND ESTROGEN RECEPTOR-NEGATIVE ER(-) WOMEN 10, 20, AND 30 YEARS AFTER DIAGNOSIS

AGE AT DIAGNOSIS	ER(+) RISK/ YEAR	CBC IN 10 YRS	CBC IN 20 YRS	CBC IN 30 YRS	ER(-) RISK/ YEAR	CBC IN 10 YRS	CBC IN 20 YRS	CBC IN 30 YRS
25–29	0.45	4.5	9	13.5	1.26	12.6	25.2	37.8
30–34	0.31	3.1	6.2	9.3	0.85	8.5	17	25.5
35–39	0.25	2.5	5	7.5	0.64	6.4	12.8	19.2
40–44	0.24	2.4	4.8	7.2	0.53	5.3	10.6	15.9
45–49	0.24	2.4	4.8	7.2	0.47	4.7	9.4	14.1
50–54	0.26	2.6	5.2	7.8	0.45	4.5	9	13.5
55–59	0.30	3	6	9	0.45	4.5	9	13.5
60–64	0.34	3.4	6.8	10.2	0.47	4.7	9.4	14.1
65–69	0.36	3.6	7.2	10.8	0.51	5.1	10.2	15.3
70–74	0.37	3.7	7.4	11.1	0.55	5.5	11	16.5
75–79	0.33	3.3	6.6	9.9	0.60	6	12	18
80–84	0.26	2.6	5.2	7.8	0.63	6.3	12.6	18.9

Contralateral Prophylactic Mastectomy (CPM)

As you might guess based on the relatively low CBC numbers in most of this table, no study conclusively shows a survival advantage in those opting to remove the breast without cancer with a contralateral prophylactic mastectomy (CPM). Of course, I support anyone's "I'll do anything to survive" attitude, but you survive the same with or without CPM.[40] And that's a huge relief for women who don't want to lose both breasts, but they don't want to *die*, either. I know some of you aren't numbers people; you make decisions from your gut, and I hear it saying, "Take that breast off, girl. The other one tried to kill you." Others might not want to deal with surveillance and the anxiety and possible biopsies that go with keeping the good breast. For them, it's emancipating to choose CPM and live without looking over their shoulders, waiting for cancer to creep up again.

A poll of 81 Australian and New Zealand breast surgeons revealed that after genes and family history, it was simply "fear and anxiety" that drove their patients toward CPM.[41] Maybe peace of mind explains why the US rate of CPM tripled in women under forty-five years old from 9.3 percent to 26.4 percent between 2003 and 2010.[42] Among all ages, 11.2 percent choose CPM.[43] What's interesting is that you are three times more likely to choose CPM with a female surgeon.[44] Perhaps you explore the option more openly or thoroughly with a surgeon you consider a female confidant—or maybe you ask her what she would do in your shoes and she says CPM. An informal poll at the 2015 annual American Society of Breast Surgeons meeting revealed that 5 percent of male surgeons would suggest CPM to their wives, but over 20 percent of female surgeons would choose it for themselves. In Europe, CPM rates have not changed at all, attributed to different public perceptions of breast cancer and plastic surgery.[45]

I can tell you another reason patients might vote for contralateral prophylactic mastectomy—looking lopsided from the mastectomy on the cancer side. CPM can make your new breasts more evenly matched. On the other hand, procedures like a reduction, lift, or implant can also create symmetry and don't require mastectomy, so again, thorough discussions are key. Not worried about any of it? Keep your breast—it's yours!

Difficult Decisions

Only very small studies exist looking into patient satisfaction after bilateral prophylactic mastectomy (BPM), and they all make me sad to write, but you should know the truth. Averaging twenty-nine months after BPM, fifty-five patients answered a questionnaire: 87 percent reported chest wall pain/discomfort; 36 percent said pain affected sleep; 22 percent noticed negative effects on daily activities; and 75 percent had decreased sexual pleasure. But there was one blazing ray of hope: 0 percent agreed with the statement: "I regret the decision I made."[46] On the other hand, most published studies show long-lasting overall *satisfaction* with the choice to have a contralateral prophylactic mastectomy (CPM).[47] One reason BPM patients might feel more dissatisfied with their results than the CPM group does is that none of them had cancer, whereas everyone choosing CPM had endured a breast cancer diagnosis and its treatment, so perhaps the CPM group's appreciation for merely being alive eclipses the nagging, undesirable, and permanent effects of surgical decisions.

Deciding whether you should have a bilateral prophylactic mastectomy or contralateral prophylactic mastectomy is no small choice. Both require fully informed decision making that discusses your actual risk for getting cancer, your perceived risk, your desire and ability to tolerate that risk, the prognosis of your current cancer, cosmetic expectations, and possible surgical complications that are always a risk and become exacerbated by other illnesses or risk factors like obesity or smoking—not to mention the physical, emotional, and financial implications of it all. Prophylactic mastectomy virtually eliminates cancer threats forever: no frequent imaging, no monthly breast exams, no cancer, no chemo, no fear. It's an attractive option to many, but certainly not all, of the women I see. I want to be clear: prophylactic surgery is a very personal, irreversible choice that women must consider thoroughly and carefully. After they learn all about it, some say, "Let's do it!" Others hedge, "Maybe down the road." And still others declare, "Never!" I stand by my patients no matter what their choice, and you should expect the same from your doctor too.

Bye, Bye Ovaries

Now, about bidding your ovaries farewell, we can prophylactically remove them in a procedure called a bilateral *risk-reducing salpingo-oophorectomy* (RRSO). Since the risk of ovarian cancer runs as high as 54 percent in BRCA carriers and increases rapidly after age forty, eliminating this risk by removing your ovaries becomes a lifesaving proposition—and happily, there's a breast benefit too. A prospective study of nearly 2,500 BRCA carriers found that RRSO prior to age fifty drops *breast* cancer rates 37 percent in BRCA-1 and 64 percent in BRCA-2; however, RRSO after age fifty does not significantly reduce breast risk.[48] Even after you remove your ovaries and fallopian tubes, a less than 2 percent chance of primary peritoneal cancer remains, which is cancer in the thin membrane that covers the inside of your abdomen and organs.[49]

National guidelines recommend RRSO by ages thirty-five to forty for BRCA-1 and -2, and when childbearing is complete; BRCA-2 carriers who already had mastectomies can delay RRSO until ages forty to forty-five.[50] You don't have to be miserable in menopause. Taking hormone replacement therapy after RRSO does not increase breast cancer risk in BRCA-1 and -2, nor does short-term use negate the breast cancer *reduction* I just mentioned about RRSO under age fifty.[51] Taking hormones lifelong after RRSO reduces life expectancy by about one year, so consider discontinuing treatment at the time of expected natural menopause, around age fifty years.[52]

Make your choices with both your present and future in mind. Some patients ask about removing only fallopian tubes and leaving their ovaries, knowing that the tubes make most of the cancers, so they keep the ovarian hormones flowing. This is currently not advised. If you're high-risk, approaching thirty-five years, and just aren't ready for biological children of your own but might want them one day, I suggest you consider freezing eggs or embryos and get those ovaries out. With an intact uterus, you can implant embryos and carry your baby whenever you're ready, without the threat of ovarian cancer. Unfortunately, this option may not be covered by insurance, and neither is preimplantation genetic diagnosis (PGD), a controversial procedure that allows a BRCA carrier the option to *not* pass on a faulty gene by using *in vitro* fertilization (IVF) techniques to identify embryos without the mutation for freezing and/or implantation into the uterus.

PICTURE PERFECT

We've covered quite a bit of ground. Now that you understand how complex and interactive all the risk factors from food to family history can be, what's the best strategy to screen the girlfriends to be sure nobody in there is misbehaving? In chapter 8, I will outline the state-of-the-art and standard-of-care for early detection and diagnosis of all the benign and malignant lumps and bumps that breasts can make.

PART 4

MAKING MEDICAL CHOICES AND LIVING WITH RISK

CHAPTER 8

Breast Cancer Screening and Detection

Most women assume that if you endure squashing the girls between two plastic plates in a mammogram machine, at least you receive a definite yes or no, cancer found or not. Unfortunately, complex and confusing issues surround the screening and diagnosis of breast cancer. We have no foolproof way to examine the breast to reliably find early cancers or to hone in on just the threatening ones that need treatment. I wish we did. Who needs to know about a bunch of benign things that don't matter? Who cares about a lazy cancer that won't go anywhere for a hundred years? We can eradicate smallpox, land on the moon, perform robotic surgery from thousands of miles away, and hurl through the air at five hundred miles per hour seated in an upright position . . . yet we can't image a breast and know, for sure, what's inside.

Alas, you must use accurate and balanced information to make informed choices about whether, how, and how often to screen your own breasts. Depending on your risk factors, anxiety level, finances, and personal philosophy about health care, your choice might not be another's. In this chapter, we'll take a close look at your options.

HANDS-ON ACTIVITY

Before we jump into imaging, let's talk about hands-on detection tactics—yours and your doctor's—and how accurate they are at finding cancers and differentiating them from benign lumps. We talked about the importance of a breast self-exam (BSE) in chapter 1, and I stand by that. Now, I know large studies show that women who do BSE have the same mortality from breast cancer as those who do not, and actually, they undergo twice the number of needless biopsies.[1] Similarly, studies show that if you get regular imaging, seeing your doctor for a clinical breast exam (CBE) contributes little to cancer detection.[2] (Wait a minute. Did somebody just call me useless?) Yet with all that said, I've seen *far* too many women with a self-detected lump, or an intuition that things weren't right, or with a prescription to see me for something her doctor found . . . and sure enough, cancer. So, I can't advise against self-exams or clinical ones, and I actually think that if we all did a good BSE consistently, we'd find more tumors at smaller sizes. As it is, the average tumor felt by both doctors and women stays in a narrow range around 22 millimeters,[3] and while mammograms *can* find tumors a quarter of that size, a mammogram's average detected cancer size is 21 millimeters[4]—so tell me, *why are women told that BSE doesn't help* when the average tumor size at detection is the same as imaging?

Since you're with your breasts all day and night, I think you should be familiar enough with them to notice a change, because doing so could save your life. Besides, it's free. In countries where women aren't getting regular imaging, performing diligent BSE and training health professionals in CBE might be the only reasonable way we can improve the dismal fact that between 50 and 90 percent of the breast cancers in places like Kenya, India, Egypt, Tunisia, Saudi Arabia, Syria, and Palestine present at stages III and IV.[5] Case in point: in Sarawak, Malaysia, late-stage cancers declined from 60 percent to 35 percent *in just four years* when doctors trained their health staff in CBE and raised public awareness.[6] So reread chapter 1 to be sure you're doing your exam correctly, and begin monthly BSE by age eighteen, CBE at age twenty-five, and get it every one to three years. Then once you hit forty, CBE should become an annual thing, just like your birthday.

TESTING, 1 . . . 2 . . .

Let's now get into specifics about the three screening processes used to detect benign and cancerous concerns. I find that women from all walks of life have a sophisticated appreciation for health issues. I'm always impressed with how much my patients know and *want to know* about their breast health. So I'm not going to dumb this section down because I know you can handle it, and you want to understand it.

Houston . . . We Have a Problem

Instinctively, you might think it would be great to have regular screenings with *all the imaging* we have for breasts to identify cancers at any size imaginable. Yet while there are three great imaging modalities we use to identify breast cancer and I review them all next—mammography, ultrasound, and MRI—none of them is perfect. Each of them comes with problems you need to understand.

First, there are false positives and negatives with these three imaging tools, plus toxic exposures in two of them. *False positives* occur when the imaging doctor (radiologist) sees something that may or may not be cancer, so she does more imaging and possibly a biopsy to be sure . . . only to conclude that it's nothing, a benign something, or she's still not sure and wants to check again in three to six months. This anxiety-provoking drawback leads to additional exposures, stress, unnecessary procedures, and wasted dollars. *False negatives*, on the other hand, send a letter in the mail that says, "Great news. Your imaging is normal. See you next year," when in reality a cancer exists and escaped detection. Unless a symptom calls your attention, false negatives lead to a delay in diagnosis and possibly worse outcomes. As for toxic exposures, these include gadolinium contrast given with MRI and radiation from mammography, which we'll discuss in a bit.

There's also the problem of *overdiagnosis*. This refers to the detection of cancers that would never have posed a threat to your life because of their indolent, slow-growing biology, but now that we know they exist, we overtreat them with the same arsenal of weapons used against the bad actors, often including surgery, radiation, and antiestrogens, but rarely chemotherapy. How do oncologists know they don't need treatment? Tumor characteristics and genomic tumor testing determine treatment (discussed in chapter 9), but we usually remove the whole cancer to figure this out, so whoops, we already surgically overtreated you. Even if we glean this information off the core biopsy (the needle biopsy that diagnosed the cancer), repeat imaging to assess for growth and change brings constant concern and cost.

How often does overdiagnosis happen? The reality only recently gained serious attention and recognition. Estimates by a UK panel reviewing three randomized trials place overdiagnosis rates at 19 percent for stage 0 (DCIS, ductal carcinoma *in situ*) and early invasive breast cancers, and estimates that doctors overdiagnose three women to save one life.[7] And when it comes to surgical overtreatment, how many breasts are removed entirely due to overdiagnosis? Let's plug in some numbers and find out. A review of 1.2 million US cancer patients diagnosed 1998 to 2011 shows that even though they could have kept their breasts, 29.3 percent of DCIS (and 35.5 percent of early stage) patients chose mastectomy over breast-conserving surgery, and 11.2 percent removed the opposite breast.[8] Let's use round numbers: in the United States, we diagnose 60,000 DCIS per year, and apparently overdiagnose 12,000 of them (20 percent); 3,600 choose mastectomy (30 percent); of these, 400 remove both breasts (11 percent). That's 4,000 "unnecessary" mastectomies per year for DCIS, not considering all of the overdiagnosed invasive disease. Overtreatment also presents a dilemma for the woman who has other illnesses more likely to cause her death than this newly identified breast cancer, which has led to the recommendation to limit screening to women expected to live at least another five years.[9] This problem of overdiagnosis will intensify as we welcome new technologies that find smaller, earlier cancers.

Currently, we accept this imperfect reality of false positives, false negatives, and overdiagnosis with overtreatment in the name of early detection—because that's what we have to offer, and drawbacks aside, early detection beats finding out too late.

HOW DO YOUR BREASTS STACK UP?

When your breasts are assessed using a mammogram, ultrasound, or MRI, imagers use a scale called the Breast Imaging Reporting and Data System (BI-RADS) that rates the level of suspicion for cancer on any given study and standardizes reporting to improve communication about findings (not to be confused with cancer staging, which is 0 to IV, and an entirely different scale). Categories range from 0 (incomplete study, more information needed) to 6 (known biopsy-proven cancer). In between, the numbers are as follows:

1 = normal

2 = benign finding (like a cyst)

3 = indeterminate (needs repeat imaging in 3 to 6 months, less than 2 percent chance of cancer)

4a = suspicious (biopsy recommended, 2 to less than 10 percent chance of cancer)

4b = suspicious (biopsy recommended, 10 to less than 50 percent chance of cancer)

4c = suspicious (biopsy recommended, 50 to less than 95 percent chance of cancer)

5 = malignant (biopsy strongly recommended, 95 percent or greater chance of cancer)[10]

The Magnificent Mammogram

Mammograms gently but firmly compress (that is, squash) the breast between two plastic plates, and a small dose of radiation beams between the plates, producing an image with patches of bright breast tissue interspersed between darker fat. Since cancers appear white, the goal is to find a snowball in a snowstorm. Doctors perform *screening* mammograms when there isn't an issue to investigate; *diagnostic* mammograms magnify an area of concern in an effort to diagnose its cause. Any finding, such as a breast or axillary lump, nipple discharge or inversion, pain, or skin changes like redness, retraction, or thickening, as well as hunting down the finding of another study such as an MRI, will likely benefit from a diagnostic mammogram.

Fast, cheap, and widely available with most radiologists able to read them, mammograms find cancer and absolutely save lives. Mammography is best at finding suspicious calcifications, a harbinger for the earliest stage 0 cancers (DCIS) that never need chemo and never kill. So even though mammograms have shortcomings, they find DCIS better than any other tool we have. Screening 1,000 women generally reveals 3.6 cancers, or *true positives*, and misses 1.2 cancers, or false negatives.[11] In the United States, the average size of all invasive cancers detected by mammography is 21.2 millimeters.[12] One study that examined the relationship between late-stage breast cancer and mammogram screening found that 50 percent of women diagnosed with advanced breast cancer did *not have a mammogram* in the preceding two years; factors associated with the absence of screening included any one of these: age over seventy-five years old, unmarried, no family history of breast cancer, a low-income status, or less education.[13]

Since the dawn of routine mammography in 1976, no one has disputed that mammograms save lives, but they do debate the *degree* to which mammos help. People bemoan their downsides, and with better treatments being introduced at the same time, mammo detection has to share kudos for saving lives with factors like chemo and tamoxifen. Nevertheless, one of the most telling reports on the lifesaving benefits of mammography comes from comparing breast cancer deaths in the twenty years before screening was introduced (1958–77) with those diagnosed in the twenty years after screening (1978–97) in 210,000 women in Sweden. Death rates dropped 28 percent solely due to mammography, and in just the forty-to-forty-nine-year-olds (an age group often told not to bother with imaging), mortality plummeted by 48 percent.[14] Death rates also fell 16 percent in women who did not get imaging at all, which tells you the contribution of better treatments after 1977. By contrast, death rates *increased* continuously in Japan by 1.1 percent annually and in Korea by 2.1 percent per year from 1994 to 2011.[15] It's key to note that these high-income countries have cancer treatment available, but they do not widely embrace mammography screening. So as women in Asia adopted Westernized lifestyles, they died more often from breast cancer, which they did not detect early with screening mammography.

Pooling estimates from all the relevant mammogram trials shows that fewer women aged forty to seventy-four die when receiving them, averaging a highly significant 20 percent mortality reduction, and this benefit holds true when singling out forty-to-fifty-year-olds as well.[16] So why do certain screening recommendations exclude this younger group? American women under fifty annually claim 60,310 new cancer spots (21 percent of total) and 4,700 cancer deaths (12 percent of total). Mammography screening for normal-risk women should begin at age forty, period. On the other side of the age rainbow, randomized prospective trials exclude women over seventy-four years old—why? Consider this: American women aged over seventy-four annually claim 58,885 of the new cancer diagnoses (20 percent of total) and 14,880 cancer deaths (37 percent of total). Furthermore, half of women over eighty are expected to live another ten years. Mammography screening for women over seventy-four years of age should continue until they don't expect to make it another five years, period.

We implemented 2-D *digital* mammography in 1998, which is the main technology widely used throughout the United States. Just as you can manipulate, store, and send smartphone photos, we can do the same to your 2-D digital mammo, which enhances cancer detection among menstruating women, those under fifty, and those with dense breasts—all women whose breasts generally like to hide tumors.[17] In 2011, the FDA approved 3-D tomosynthesis (3-D tomo), performed in exactly the same way as a normal mammogram (squishing and radiation—sorry, ladies). Whereas 2-D smashes a whole loaf of raisin bread end-to-end, takes a picture, and expects us to find the raisins, 3-D tomo takes ten to fifteen thin slices of bread, giving us a much better look at those raisins. How much better? In a 2013 comparative study, 3-D tomo reduced false alarms by 17 percent, and found 34 percent more cancers than 2-D (8.1 cancers per 1,000 screened versus 5.3 cancers for 2-D).[18] Particularly if you have dense breasts or elevated risk, ask your doctor for 3-D tomo instead of 2-D mammograms.

One other mammogram newbie, contrast-enhanced spectral mammography (CESM), takes advantage of the fact that blood vessels form around cancers (remember angiogenesis?). After injecting IV iodine contrast, a normal mammo is taken, but instead of seeing a snowstorm as with 2-D and 3-D, CESM highlights the blood flow pattern around a cancer (making it white) while all the confusing benign breast in the background fades to dark. It's like a blazing star against the night sky. A review of eight studies shows that CESM wins the cancer detection award, sniffing it out 98 percent of the time, but it also sniffs out a bunch of stuff that isn't cancer, doing so 42 percent of the time.[19] The Pink Lotus Breast Center was the first center to offer CESM technology in North America, unveiling it in 2012. Consider CESM as an alternative to MRI (see below) and use it to clarify abnormal findings on your 2-D or 3-D mammogram.[20]

What are the drawbacks to screening mammograms, and are they ever bad enough to make you bail on mammos altogether? The most anxiety-provoking drawback is the false positive, but do not let the fear of a false positive keep you from finding a curable cancer. Your radiologist analyzes mammogram images side-by-side, comparing the left to the right. She looks for areas of concern like what's called a *spiculated mass* (imagine a smashed spider with its legs splayed out); a new subtle change or distortion in one area of tissue seen this year and not prior years; or calcifications, white specks of calcium that cluster tightly together or branch inside milk ducts. Findings like these occur in about 80 per 1,000 screening mammograms, resulting in an 8 percent chance of being called back for additional views. Don't fret if you're called back—I know, easy for me to say—but really, 97 percent of callbacks are for benign things detailed at the end of this chapter. When you're called back, there's a 10 percent chance you will need a biopsy, and only two to three of those people will have cancer.[21] In summary, if you're called back, there's a 3 percent chance it's for cancer. After ten years of annual mammograms, 49 percent of women will endure a false positive result, so you have a lot of "false" company![22]

Want to know how to lower your chances of a false positive? One study looked at nearly ten thousand screening mammograms and found that the following factors led to an increase in false positives: younger age, a history of breast biopsies, a positive family history of breast cancer, estrogen use, an increasing time interval between screenings, no comparison of the current mammogram with previous mammograms, and a radiologist's personal tendency to call mammograms abnormal. So first, if you still menstruate, time your mammogram to the second half of your menstrual cycle (the two weeks before starting your period). During this luteal phase, lower estrogen levels might decrease the density of your breast tissue on the mammogram, making it easier to read. This timing also correlates to less breast sensitivity, which allows better compression, and a more detailed image. Second, make sure you hand-carry all prior mammograms that you have had to your appointment. Ideally, you would be getting your annual mammograms at the same institution each year so that they already have your prior images; but if not, make sure you give the radiologist previous mammograms against which he can compare your current ones. Finally, be on time. Mammograms are most effective when women stick to a twelve-month interval between screenings.

False *negatives* represent another mammography shortcoming. Yes, despite a normal mammo report, you could still have breast cancer. I wish mammos were that accurate and awesome. Dense breast tissue, breast implants, cancers located at the edges of the breast, hormone replacement therapy, and poor imaging quality all contribute to the failure of mammography to detect an existing cancer—which it does around 28 percent of the time.[23] Imagine two thousand women getting screening mammograms. We should expect eight to ten cancers, and two to three will be missed, mostly because they are difficult to distinguish from normal breast tissue. This 28 percent miss rate reaches 37 to 52 percent for women with cancer within extremely dense breasts and falls to 13 percent for women with cancer and predominantly fatty breasts.[24] I'm frequently asked whether implants affect cancer detection. Implants can affect accurate detection in a number of ways, the most significant being the presence of a thickened capsule around the implant, making it difficult to compress the breast thin enough to get a good look at the tissue. Even with the extra images always taken with implants, we miss 30 to 50 percent of cancers; I suggest adding screening ultrasound for women with augmentation mammoplasty.[25] Whenever you find a new lump or concern in your breast, even if you got the A-OK on a recent mammogram, see your doctor.

Sometimes patients decline mammography, fearful that radiation exposure causes breast cancer. You know what I tell them? They're right. A number of studies employ computerized risk models to estimate the numbers of radiation-induced breast cancers and deaths. In a lifetime's worth of mammogram screening, 8.6 out of 10,000 women will get a radiation-induced breast cancer; however, screening finds about *one hundred times more cancers* than it causes.[26] An even more important question is, "How many lives are *saved* by screening for every one life lost *because of screening*?" Numbers vary, but a risk model from England calculated 312 saved lives, and an American one concluded 60.5 saved lives for each single radiation-induced death.[27]

The US Food and Drug Administration (FDA) strictly regulates radiation doses, and when compared to other life exposures, mammography doses are fairly low. The average person in the United States essentially receives the equivalent of one mammogram every seven weeks from naturally occurring radioactive materials and cosmic radiation from outer space, so we all tolerate radiation exposures that don't even have the possible benefit of saving our lives.[28] The reduction in death thanks to mammogram screening greatly outweighs the risk of death due to radiation-induced cancers. If you were to be the unlucky 1 in 1,162 women whose mammo exposure causes a breast cancer, it wouldn't look any different than a "normal" breast cancer, so you actually wouldn't know your mammograms caused it. Just pointing that out.

HOW DOES MAMMOGRAPHY COMPARE TO OTHER IMAGING?[29]

One whole body PET/CT = 62.5 mammograms

One CT angiogram looking at coronary arteries = 30 mammograms

One chest CT = 17.5 mammograms

One chest X-ray = 4 mammograms

Eighty dental X-rays = 1 mammogram

Seven weeks of living = 1 mammogram

Enough said!

If you're hesitant to get a mammogram because it hurts, sometimes in life, the pain is worth the gain. Studies show it's painless for about 45 percent of women, a little painful for 40 percent, and rather painful for the rest, but pain disappears within seconds to minutes for 89 percent of women.[30] Try timing your mammo to the third week of your menstrual cycle to lessen sensitivity. Also, taking acetaminophen (like Tylenol) or NSAIDs (Advil, Motrin, ibuprofen) thirty minutes prior to imaging might help.

Conflicting guidelines exist between different US organizations and international recommendations about what age to begin mammography for those at normal risk, how often to perform it, and when to stop it. To the committees assigned to set these guidelines, it all comes down to a cost/benefit analysis: how much downside (money, false positives, unnecessary biopsies, overtreatment, anxiety) should we tolerate to justify the upside of saving one life? For example, when the US Preventive Services Task Force looked at this issue, they asked, "Is it worth 1,339 mammograms to save one life?" If yes, screening starts at fifty. "Is it worth 1,904 mammograms?" If yes, screening starts at forty.[31] (By the way, they chose age fifty, and said to do it every other year, and to stop at age seventy-four.) In a study of attitudes toward false positive mammograms, the majority of women (who all experienced a false positive callback) felt that 5,000 mammograms would be worth saving one life.[32] Using a computer model to analyze all the conflicting starting ages and screening intervals out there, it turns out that mortality reduction is greatest with annual screening starting at age forty.[33] And as far as false positives go, a woman getting annual mammograms would be recalled once every thirteen years and undergo one benign biopsy every 187 years—she's therefore very unlikely to ever get a biopsy.

All options considered, assuming normal cancer risk, I suggest you begin annual mammography at age forty, and don't stop and don't skip years until you plan to die in the next five years. But what do *you* think? I really want to know, so please tell me at pinklotus.com/beginmammos.

The Ultra Great Ultrasound

Widely available, inexpensive, well-tolerated by patients, no deep compression, no radiation, no claustrophobia, and immediate results—*oh, how I love ultrasound*. I have one in every exam room and operating room and consider it my magical third hand. A flat probe with gel glides across the breast skin, sending sound waves that reflect off tissues to a variable degree depending on what makes up those cells. This yields an instant image of whatever we feel, so within seconds of my putting a probe to skin, we know what needs to be done: aspirate a cyst, biopsy a solid mass, or forget about it. I just described a *diagnostic* ultrasound, which spot-checks an area of concern. With *screening* ultrasound, there's no particular area of concern, and your doctor (or tech) systematically rolls the probe everywhere over both breasts looking for trouble. Screening can be done with a handheld probe, or it can be an automated breast ultrasound (ABUS), whereby a machine directs the probe in uniform fashion across your breasts. Either way, screening ultrasound is a must if you have dense breasts or implants. Read on for the proof.

In 2016, a study took 3,231 dense-breasted women with negative 2-D mammograms and added 3-D tomosynthesis (discussed previously) and handheld ultrasound.[34] They found twenty-four additional cancers that regular mammo missed: 3-D tomo identified thirteen whereas ultrasound detected twenty-three of the twenty-four cancers. The false positive callback rate was a tolerable 3.33 percent. To summarize, for every one thousand regular mammogram-screeners, if you add 3-D tomo, you find 4.0 more cancers, but ultrasound finds 7.1 more. So, if they don't have 3-D tomo where you live, and if you are at elevated cancer risk, have dense breast tissue, or implants, just add screening ultrasound to your regular screening mammogram—don't drive fifty-plus miles to get all fancy with 3-D tomo.

The Magnetic MRI

Breast magnetic resonance imaging (MRI) involves an IV contrast injection and uses a magnet to obtain breast images; it has no ionizing radiation. MRI evaluates the blood flow pattern throughout breast tissues and detects areas where blood rapidly pools and then washes away; this happens at cancer locations due to angiogenesis, which is the formation of new blood vessels at the behest of tumor cells. MRI basically doesn't care about breast density, so it's really good at finding cancer with an over 90 percent ability to do so, outperforming 2-D mammograms, 3-D tomo, and ultrasound (but not CESM, the contrast mammo).[35] Problems? Well, besides costing eight times more than a mammogram and requiring forty-five minutes lying face down in a claustrophobia-inducing clanging tube, when MRI sees something suspicious, you need additional tests and biopsies, which cost more money, time off work, and anxiety—all for a fifty-fifty chance that the MRI was correct.[36] MRI has twice the callbacks and thrice the unneeded biopsies as mammography.[37] It's not a sustainable way to screen millions and millions of women. Nevertheless, MRI has a place, so what is it?

MRI helps plan for cancer surgery by providing more information about the known malignancy, and also by finding additional cancer about 14 percent of the time in the affected breast and 4 percent in the opposite breast.[38] As fortunate as one might feel finding additional cancers, MRI delays surgery and increases mastectomy rates without evidence that it improves outcomes, so routine preoperative use likely causes more harm than benefit.[39] *Diagnostic* MRI is ordered when looking for something specific, such as: (1) additional disease in those with invasive *lobular* cancer (a subtype that hides on other imaging methods, which often underestimates its size); (2) cancer in extremely dense breasts; (3) the response of cancer to chemotherapy prior to surgery; (4) the primary cancer location in patients with cancer in their nodes but normal mammo and ultrasound; (5) masses underneath Paget's disease (cancer of the nipple); and (6) implant rupture.[40] Aside from these reasons, diagnostic MRI remains controversial.

We advise *screening* MRI for those with: (1) a lifetime risk exceeding 20 percent based on computerized models that include family history and personal factors; (2) chest wall radiation prior to age thirty; (3) untested first degree relatives of BRCA, Li-Fraumeni, and Cowden carriers; and (4) gene mutation carriers, starting at the ages noted below or ten years before the youngest breast cancer in the family: BRCA carriers (start age twenty-five), Li-Fraumeni (ages twenty to twenty-nine), Cowden (ages thirty to thirty-five), ATM (age forty), CDH1 (age thirty), CHEK2 (age forty), PALB2 (age thirty), and STK11 (age thirty).[41] Hormonal fluctuations can cause contrast to flow into dense or fibrocystic tissues, so to minimize false positives, time MRI to days seven to ten of your menstrual cycle (day one is the day you bleed) or go off HRT for three weeks prior to scanning. You could drop your annual ultrasound if you get screening MRI, as ultrasound does not add value to mammo plus MRI screening regimens.[42] Contrast enhanced mammograms (CESM, see above) offer a comparable way to screen those who can't get an MRI, including women with the presence of MRI-unsafe metal devices in the body, claustrophobia, morbid obesity, gadolinium concerns, or MRI unavailability.[43] I also want you to be sure your facility uses the safest contrast: macrocyclic gadolinium. This is thought to accumulate in the brain less so than other gadolinium solutions, a health risk that's currently unknown and under FDA investigation.[44]

Thermography

Thermography has resurfaced in the modern technological era. A camera uses infrared technology to identify skin temperature changes that allegedly guide us like a treasure map to an island of increased blood flow and metabolic activity, signifying the presence of an underlying angiogenic tumor. Heat patterns are displayed in a psychedelic swirling image of your breasts with colors indicating the levels of emitted heat. I have chased down countless swirls of hyperthermia, and I have never found them to rival all the imaging tools I already have. The FDA approved thermography for use, but it didn't require thermograms to be effective. No randomized controlled trials of thermography have ever evaluated its impact on breast cancer detection or mortality. Until those exist, thermography will remain unadvised.

This Biopsy Won't Hurt a Bit

What's the next step after BSE, CBE, mammogram, ultrasound, or MRI finds a suspicious area? Your doctor can guess all day long about what something might be, but the only way to know for sure is to get a piece of *that* out of you and under a microscope. Percutaneous (through the skin) needle biopsies use real-time imaging to ensure precision and accuracy as a needle passes into the target and samples the tissue. It's easier for you if ultrasound can be used, but sometimes only a mammo or MRI sees the concerning area, so those things need to guide the needle.

No patient enjoys having her breast clamped in position for a mammo-guided biopsy, or lying in an MRI tube with her breast hanging through the table, but in the end, radiologists and surgeons diagnose a breast lesion with biopsy techniques that barely leave a scar and allow you to go right back to your day's demands.

There are two types of minimally invasive breast biopsies: fine needle aspiration (FNA) and core needle biopsy (CNB). Both biopsies yield tissue samples that get analyzed under a microscope, the results of which need to be compared to the original target to make sure it all makes sense. *Discordance* means that the pathology report states "benign" but the clinical or imaging findings say "suspicious for malignancy." Discordance requires either a repeat biopsy with a different needle type or a surgical excision. *Concordance* means that pathology and imaging match as expected, and either you have cancer or you don't. The more suspicious the target, the more likely a CNB will be done rather than an FNA.

FNA swiftly collapses benign fluid-filled cysts and can also diagnose solid lesions. Your doctor will poke a thin needle attached to a syringe through the skin and into the target, pulling thousands of cells out of the mass that are then sent to pathology for cell analysis called *cytology*. A review of 31,340 FNAs showed that the ability to correctly diagnose cancer when it's present ranges from 65 to 98 percent, depending on the skill of the person doing the FNA and the pathologist reading it.[45] FNA looks at single cells divorced from the context of all of the cells immediately next to it, so they can look weird even when benign. When this happens or when there are too few cells, we usually upgrade to a core needle biopsy (or we just start with a core and skip the FNA option, particularly when the lesion looks like cancer).

Core biopsies obtain tissue samples the size of a grain of rice, so unlike an FNA, specimens contain sheets of cells, which allow for an accurate diagnosis 95 to 99 percent of the time.[46] After numbing the skin, the doctor inserts a needle into the mass and takes a sliver of the target, preferably using ultrasound to guide the needle; when using a mammogram for guidance, the biopsy is called a *stereotactic* core needle biopsy.

When breast MRI detects a lesion that can't be found by ultrasound or mammo, then MRI-guided needle biopsy can be performed.

When women have FNA and core biopsies done, they might worry that the techniques will spread cancer cells, so let's address that. When my son Sebastian shows up with a smear of chocolate on the corner of his mouth, you know and I know and he knows that he ate something chocolate, and yes, probably without permission. Similarly, a biopsy needle withdrawn from a mass can potentially migrate cells once located inside the mass to areas outside the mass. In this way, the adjacent tissues and skin can theoretically harbor seeded tumor cells as a consequence of smearing cells along the needle track. If that tumor turns out to be benign, as it does in over 80 percent of biopsies, tracking benign cells ultimately doesn't matter. However, tracking *malignant* cells is a whole other ball of chocolate.

Ten papers addressed tumor seeding potential, totaling 3,643 women with needle biopsies and track site analysis.[47] The authors concluded that tracked cancer cells infrequently spread to form a new cancer, and this rare event has little direct impact on patient outcome. Although a treatable cancer recurrence along the track uncommonly happens, *seeding* cells actually occurs about one-third of the time.[48] But even when cells seed a track, because they are separated from their blood supply, these displaced cells literally die in their tracks. Even if a few stragglers persist, the vast majority, if not all of these, are excised with the subsequent cancer operation, or get nuked by breast radiation, or starve with antiestrogen pills. I'm wiping that chocolate off your face one way or another. There's no way you're walking around looking like that!

After patients understand the insignificance of cell tracking, they often trade that concern for worry over pushing cancer cells directly into the lymph nodes or bloodstream. Spreading tumor cells out of the breast as a direct result of the biopsy happens uncommonly: an Austrian review on the matter examined 1,890 patients with breast cancer who underwent surgery with sentinel node biopsy. They concluded that preoperative breast biopsy does *not* cause artificial spread of tumor cells to the lymph nodes.[49] In contrast, others have reported that FNA and core biopsy *can* transport cancer cells into nearby lymph nodes or blood vessels, but how this impacts a cell's behavior remains unclear and no studies show a decrease in survival because of it.[50] Also, since animal studies document that invasive breast cancers continually shed millions of malignant cells into the bloodstream, it makes sense that getting poked once by a needle doesn't elevate the survival stakes at all.[51]

Despite assurances, some women simply say, "I don't want a biopsy; I just want it out." I allow women to call shots like these, but having a core biopsy instead of going straight to surgery has so many advantages. Let me count the ways: (1) A benign diagnosis often eliminates the need for surgery altogether. And that lump of yours is over 80 percent likely to be benign. (2) We perform 1.6 million breast biopsies annually in the United States.[52] Imagine the justified outcry over 1.6 million *open* biopsies being done in an operating room every year, the majority of which would be for benign disease and entirely unnecessary. (3) Avoiding surgery with an open biopsy means avoiding anesthesia, a breast scar, surgical pain, infection risks, hematoma risks, possible breast deformity, missed work or other responsibilities, inconveniencing others who have to drive and care for you, and avoiding a number of fees, from the facility to anesthesia to the surgeon to the pathologist. In fact, one 2008 study showed that the 30 percent open biopsy rate in Florida led to $112.7 million in annual charges just in that state alone.[53] If we extrapolate this data to the world, then reducing the number of unwarranted open biopsies would yield annual savings of trillions. (4) If open biopsy shows cancer, we probably have to do a second operation to clear margins and check nodes. You rack up number 3 again. (5) Open biopsies have twenty to one hundred times more hematomas (bleeding at the operative site) than cores.[54] (6) Open biopsies have thirty-eight to sixty-three times more infections than cores.[55] (7) If core biopsy diagnoses a cancer, we have the ability to obtain a complete, personalized treatment strategy prior to rushing into an operation.

Take Elizabeth, for example: a fifty-two-year-old attorney who came to me with an ultrasound showing a suspicious solid mass. To my eye, it appeared to be a complex cyst, not a solid mass. I showed Elizabeth my images and offered an FNA. She protested, "What if it's cancer? You will push cells out into my body! Just take it out with surgery." In my view, I could do a ten-second scar-free aspiration and the whole story would come to a happy cystic ending. To be clear, a radiologist had deemed the mass suspicious, so I felt obligated to get a sample somehow (meaning, it wasn't definitely a benign cyst). The art of medicine isn't "my way or the highway"; it's a two-way street. So, off to the OR we went, and the final pathology report simply stated: "Benign breast tissue with cysts."

SO WHAT IS IT?

Now that you understand how we locate and interrogate lumps and bumps, let's get to the actual diagnoses themselves. Breasts confuse everyone, and misinformation abounds, which escalates uncertainty. Let me clear up a few things.

Painful Pearls of Wisdom

Who keeps telling all my patients, "If a lump hurts, that's a good sign, because cancer never hurts"? False. Breast cancer can absolutely declare itself with pain as the only symptom. I actually wish all breast cancers hurt. We would find more of them at early stages and would not have to rely so heavily on imperfect screening. Be mindful of soreness in one spot that persists throughout menstrual cycles and does not wax and wane.[56] Studies from the United States and the United Kingdom report breast pain as secondary to an underlying malignancy in 2 percent to 7 percent of patients; an Australian guide for practitioners warns that 10 percent of cancers masquerade as pain.[57] If women wrote a novel called *How I Found My Own Breast Cancer*, pain would hold the number-3 spot (6 percent of patients) far behind "palpable mass" (83 percent) and right next to "nipple changes" (7 percent).[58] When pain coincides with another sign, such as a palpable mass or bloody nipple discharge, the risk of breast cancer rises significantly.[59] In less developed countries, we see a much higher correlation with pain and cancer due to the fact that the majority of women present with large tumors and late-stage disease. A Nigerian clinic reported breast pain in 23.1 percent of patients, and 74.3 percent of them had cancer.[60] Always see your physician for persistent breast pain, especially when in a focal, reproducible spot, or associated with a breast lump, bloody nipple discharge, or redness and swelling.

If breast cancer causes breast pain less than 10 percent of the time, then the opposite statistic—benign things cause breast pain 90 percent of the time (when it's the only symptom)—should bring welcome relief to the 69 percent of premenopausal women who experience breast pain at some point in their lives.[61] In fact, *mastodynia* or *mastalgia* (fancy words for "breast pain") accounted for 47 percent of all breast-related doctor visits in a study following 2,400 women for a decade.[62] Two-thirds of breast pain is cyclical, meaning monthly hormonal changes in a woman's menstrual cycle cause breast tissue to swell and hurt for a few days before menstruation and midcycle at ovulation.[63] The other one-third of breast pain is noncyclical and can be constant or intermittent, associated with a host of possible causes: OCPs, HRT, stress, chest wall muscle strain (intercostal neuritis), bone pain (costochondritis), weight gain, ill-fitting bras, and breast inflammation or cysts, to offer a handful of benign etiologies.[64]

Most patients stop holding their breath after clinical exams and imaging show there's nothing of concern in areas of tenderness, and will not desire any specific interventions.[65] But others often ask, "What can I do for this annoying pain?" To be honest, the literature lacks conclusive scientific investigation into the effectiveness of the nonpharmacologic and simple analgesic interventions listed below, but they frequently improve breast pain in clinical practice, and some studies do support their use. This list offers low risk and fairly inexpensive suggestions, so if your breast pain bothers you enough, I suggest you give some of these ideas a try, starting with the first two in combination: evening primrose oil plus vitamin E.

HOW TO BREAK UP WITH BREAST PAIN

CONSIDER THIS	WITH THIS ADVICE	BECAUSE THIS HAPPENS
Evening primrose oil	1,500 milligrams twice a day for 6 months (avoid if pregnant, lactating, or taking anti-seizure medication)	Gamma-linolenic acid restores the fatty acid balance in tissue, decreasing nerve sensitivity[66]
Vitamin E	1,200 IU once a day	Anti-inflammatory; works synergistically with evening primrose oil[67]
Chasteberry, a.k.a. vitex agnus-castus	3 milligrams of dried extract of agni casti fructus twice a day	Binds to opioid, histamine, and estrogen receptors[68]
Soy in food form: tofu, edamame, tempeh	1–2 servings (1/2 cup) a day	Decreases midcycle hormonal surges,[69] lowers estrogen levels[70]
Low-fat diet	Eat fruits, vegetables, fiber, and grains	Lowers estrogen levels[71] and mammographic density[72]
Reduce caffeine intake	Minimize coffee, tea, soft drinks, and chocolate	Methylxanthine restriction can resolve fibrocystic nodularity[73]
Limit sodium/salt intake	1,500 milligrams per day or less (3/4 teaspoon) during the two weeks before menses (luteal phase)	Decreases fluid retention in breast tissue[74]
Chill out	Try muscle relaxation, acupuncture, yoga, or mindfulness meditation	Breast pain may subside by reducing anxiety and tension[75]
Find fitted, supportive bras	Wear daily and with exercise	Decreases nerve compression, improves support, and tempers breast mobility with exercise[76]
Exercise	Walk, run, bike, swim, hike, play sports	Endorphins hit opioid receptors in the brain, reducing perceptions of chronic pain[77]
Topical NSAIDs such as Voltaren, Aspercreme and Capzacin-HP	Apply to painful areas as needed	Anti-inflammatory[78]

For the uncommon situation involving severe, debilitating pain, ask for a referral to a breast specialist who can review the use of prescription medications and surgical approaches to mastodynia.

The Deal on Discharge

Let's talk about discharge for a minute, because this comes up a lot with my patients. In the office, I can squeeze drops of fluid from over 50 percent of nipples; it's *that* common.[79] You can ignore discharge (other than bloody, red, brown, or clear like water) as long as it only happens when you squeeze around your nipples. Discharge can be thick and sticky, or thin and watery. Colors include amber, yellow, green, blue, gray, white, and black. These colors, when associated with discharge *only* elicited by pressure and squeezing originate from benign conditions such as cysts, hormonal imbalances, fibrocystic change, and ductal ectasia (dilated, twisty ducts with inflammation).[80] Discharge from these conditions generally occurs in both breasts and comes from multiple duct openings on the surface of your nipples. If you don't like the fact that discharge comes out of your nipples when you squeeze them, just stop squeezing them. Breast ducts naturally contain tiny amounts of fluid, even if you've never been pregnant, so you aren't going to squeeze yourself dry; it just comes back. Sometimes the fluid loses most of the water component and plugs the ends of the nipple ducts, looking like a tiny white dot on the nipple surface. When you squeeze, it pops out (you know who you are). I've seen many panicked women over these spots of gunk, so maybe I just saved you a trip to the doctor.

Now, when discharge comes out *spontaneously*, that's a different story. Something inside the milk duct pushes the fluid out, and while that something could be cancer, it's more likely to be a papilloma (one of those marker lesions from chapter 6), infection, abscess, mastitis, a response to breast injury or trauma, the result of medications or herbs or marijuana, hormonal imbalance, endocrine disorders, or a number of other benign conditions.[81] An analysis of the discharge, appropriate imaging studies, and possibly a breast biopsy should lead you to a definitive diagnosis.

IS YOUR BREAST LEAKING?

See your doctor when discharge appears

- all by itself, staining the inside of your bra cup or nightgown, or you see it drip out of your nipple
- clear like water
- bloody, pink, red, or brown in color; when these colors result from cancer, there is usually a lump present as well[82]
- any color associated with breast pain or a lump
- with a visual change to the nipple, such as retraction or inversion, or thick, scaly, cracked, or itchy nipple skin
- in a man—any duct, any color, from squeezing nipples or not
- milky white with copious amounts coming from both nipples, but there's no baby you're planning to feed (this can be a sign of a noncancerous brain tumor in your pituitary gland called a *prolactinoma*, diagnosed with a blood hormone level and a brain scan, treated with medications or surgery)

If you've ever felt an obvious breast lump, your mind likely unraveled to the worst-case scenario. Yet 95 percent of palpable breast masses in women under forty are not cancer,[83] and in women of any age who get a biopsy for a palpable mass, over 80 percent are benign.[84] So when's a girl to panic? Okay, never panic. Anxiety adds nothing useful to the situation. But when do you head to the doctor? Start by knowing your usual breast terrain (see BSE, chapter 1). Then, if a mass persists throughout your cycle, feels gritty and firm, doesn't hurt at all, can't be defined at the edges because it blends into the surrounding tissue, or it has no matching lump in the same place in the opposite breast, check in with your physician. Even then, it's more likely to be benign than malignant, and some benign lumps even go away on their own (but let your doctor tell you that).

The Lowdown on Benign Breast Lumps

When you're talking to your doctor, she may use the terms *lump*, *mass*, *lesion*, *tumor*, *neoplasm*, and *growth* interchangeably—none of them is a synonym for cancer. In fact, these terms apply to both benign and malignant masses. Here's a comprehensive guide to noncancerous lumps, should your doctor mention one in an appointment or the terms show up in your radiology or pathology report.

CYSTS: Cysts are the most commonly diagnosed palpable breast masses, found frequently in women between thirty-five and fifty years old.[85] These benign, fluid-filled sacs likely develop from blocked milk ducts. They usually feel round and a bit squishy, like a tiny water balloon, but can also be quite firm. A galactocele is a milk-filled cyst found in women who are breastfeeding. Cysts can be singular or too numerous to count, spaced apart or clustered together, microscopic to larger than 10 centimeters (4 inches). They generally come and go with your menstrual period, getting larger and tender when you start menstruating, then regressing over a few days. They are readily identified and diagnosed by ultrasound. One large study identified cysts in 65.1 percent of premenopausal compared to 39.4 percent of postmenopausal women, and half had cysts in both breasts.[86] Women on HRT demonstrated cysts at the premenopausal rate of 66 percent, which makes sense, since cysts are very hormonally sensitive.

The natural history of cysts is to develop and regress, with about half completely disappearing within a year and 70 percent within five years.[87] Even though most cysts disappear, draining them via aspiration takes mere seconds with a tiny needle. Reasons to aspirate a cyst include: (1) patient desire, usually because a cyst is particularly large or painful, or even bulges the skin; or (2) the cyst appears "complex" on imaging, meaning, it might actually be solid, or there is something solid-appearing within the cystic fluid. Of 475 complex cysts found in the above study, two (0.42 percent) harbored a cancer, a percentage reflected by similar studies.[88] The presence of benign cysts does not elevate your cancer risk.

FIBROCYSTIC CHANGE: Affecting at least half of all women, fibrocystic change (FCC) is the most common breast condition seen, and it often feels like a lump. However, because FCC frequently fluctuates in size, when a prominent area of palpable tissue suddenly arises, it must be distinguished from cancer using clinical exam and imaging. FCC can appear vague and indistinct, or organized and masslike. FCC often swells and becomes tender during ovulation (mid cycle) and before periods, and with influences such as hormonal supplements, stress, caffeine, or salt intake. Tenderness can be in one breast or both, intermittent or constant, in one spot or everywhere. FCC often increases as you approach middle age and then disappears with the withdrawal of estrogen influences after menopause (one benefit).

FIBROADENOMA: Due to poorly understood hormonal stimuli on the lobular (milk producing) part of the breast gland, lobules sometimes morph into a benign solid mass, called a *fibroadenoma* (FA). Stick your tongue into your cheek and feel your tongue by rubbing your cheek. FAs feel like that: a spherical marble, or a rubbery firm eraser. FAs most commonly occur in the upper outer quadrant of the breast, flipping away from fingers when pressed. They persist during the reproductive years, can increase in size during pregnancy or with birth control pills, and often regress after menopause. FAs typically do not cause pain, but may be uncomfortable for a few days before periods. It's a young ladies' thing, found in 7 to 13 percent of women between fifteen and thirty-five years.[89] When found, they are solitary 75 to 90 percent of the time, with multiple masses in one or both breasts 10 to 25 percent of the time.[90] When they occur in adolescents, they are termed *juvenile* FAs and account for half of the breast lesions in young girls.[91] They are more common in those who use birth control pills before age twenty. When they persist past menopause, FAs can calcify, creating a chunky popcorn-like appearance on a mammogram.

The diagnosis of an FA in adolescents can be safely presumed with classic features on clinical exam and ultrasound images. You should get an exam and ultrasound every six months for two years to make sure nothing changes. In women over twenty years, the only sure way to confirm a benign diagnosis is with a needle biopsy or excision. However, you can manage a well-defined solid mass with benign imaging features with a follow-up regimen of repeat breast examination and ultrasound in three months (if no biopsy were done) or in six months (with a biopsy).[92] About half of FAs disappear over a fifteen-year period, 25 percent remain the same, and 25 percent grow.[93] The reported odds of finding cancer within an FA range from 1 in 10,000 to 50,000.[94] Highly in your favor.

Reasons that you might want an FA removed include focal pain, anxiety, cosmetic reasons, sudden growth, or precancerous cells found on a biopsy.[95] Excision can be accomplished through a small, well-hidden scar.[96]

PHYLLODES: Phyllodes tumors come in three types: benign (50 percent), borderline (25 percent), and malignant (25 percent). They present as a palpable, firm, mobile, painless mass 80 percent of the time, with 20 percent found by imaging and not palpable.[97] They occur at any age, but most often in women in their early forties, and in men with gynecomastia (man breasts).[98] Benign phyllodes look and feel a lot like FAs; even pathologists cannot always differentiate between these cousins on core biopsy, mistakenly calling them FAs 25 to 30 percent of the time.[99] The thing about phyllodes, though, is that they tend to get really big, really fast. So if your biopsy report says "I don't know, maybe phyllodes, maybe not" or if a so-called FA grows rapidly on follow-up exams, it should be removed. Phyllodes want to recur and usually do so within the first two years after removal, so you should be followed every six months for two years with exams and imaging to make sure they don't come back.[100] Benign phyllodes are not associated with increased future cancer risk. Borderline and malignant phyllodes require wide excision with a generous rim of normal breast around them (and sometimes mastectomy), but *very* rarely spread outside the breast or require chemo.[101]

ADENOMA: Adenomas look, feel, and behave a lot like fibroadenomas, but have less connective tissue (the "fibro" part). Lactational adenomas occur exclusively in pregnant or nursing moms and often disappear once breastfeeding stops and that supercharged hormonal state resolves.[102] Tubular adenomas tend to occur in younger women and often have tightly packed calcifications inside of them. Although adenomas may require excision because of their size, they do not have malignant potential and, once biopsied, can safely be ignored.[103]

NIPPLE ADENOMA: As the name implies, this lump forms under or in the nipple, and also goes by "florid papillomatosis of the nipple ducts" and "erosive adenomatosis." Nipple adenomas arise most commonly in women thirty to forty years old but can show up in men. Even though they are benign, they tend to invade the local tissues, and cells can even grow into the nipple skin surface, causing skin changes and nipple erosion. Nipple adenomas can bleed and become painful, making doctors confuse them for a nipple cancer (Paget's). Most nipple adenomas are excised due to the symptoms you feel and the very remote possibility of coexisting cancers within or around them.[104]

INTRADUCTAL PAPILLOMA: Papillomas are benign, solid, wart-like masses that grow from the cells that line milk ducts. They generally arise in women thirty-five to fifty years old and can sometimes be felt as a pea-sized lump under the nipple or areola. Most papillomas, however, are not palpable; they get identified during an investigation of bloody nipple discharge, are found on breast imaging studies, or are incidentally discovered when something else was biopsied.[105] Atypical, palpable, and multiple papillomas are marker lesions, discussed in chapter 6; they should always get removed because they upgrade to cancer up to 67 percent of the time.[106] By the way, skin and genital warts caused by the human papilloma virus have no connection whatsoever to breast papillomas. They just sound the same because of a similar cell structure.

FAT NECROSIS: That's doctor talk for "dead fat" that forms a round, firm ball in the breast. Fat necrosis is always benign but can masquerade as cancer on imaging, so sometimes only a needle biopsy can confirm that it really is just fat.[107] Fat necrosis can develop after blunt trauma to the breast, such as a car accident, fall, or something as innocent as moving boxes that bump into your breast as you carry them. Usually you notice bruising on the skin at the time trauma occurs. Other causes include injection of substances such as fat,[108] paraffin,[109] or silicone[110] (incidentally, injecting free silicone into your breasts to enlarge them often forms rock hard balls, probably not the look you intended); operations such as lumpectomy or breast reduction[111] or breast reconstruction after mastectomy;[112] and radiation therapy to the breast.[113] If fat liquefies, it becomes oil and is easy to aspirate with a thin needle, but if it stays solid, just leave it, unless it bugs you.

MASTITIS: Because the nipple surface contains the openings of eight to twelve milk ducts, bacteria can crawl down them and set up shop deep inside the breast ducts. When nursing, milk can pool inside blocked ducts, and the bacteria become even happier with the free food. Mastitis begins as inflammation and can quickly evolve into a bacterial infection accompanied by a palpable red, warm, tender breast lump with body aches, fever, and chills. In advanced situations, that lump represents a breast abscess, which is a pocket of pus. While mastitis occurs most commonly in breastfeeding women, it happens to non-breastfeeding women as well. In the latter group, women often smoke or have diabetes, obesity, chronic illnesses, or weak immune systems. Cancer, especially inflammatory breast cancer (which looks like a breast infection), must always be ruled out in a nonlactating woman with mastitis that lasts more than a few days with appropriate treatment.

Treatment for all mastitis involves warm compresses, both acetaminophen and ibuprofen, breast massage, and antibiotics. Vibration therapy over the mass can stimulate the circulation and loosen blockages—you can actually use a back vibrator or vibrating toothbrush for this. A breast surgeon can unclog any plugged ducts found at the nipple surface and aspirate galactoceles (milk-filled cysts) or inflamed cysts in the office. Nursing moms should continue to pump and breastfeed, as this helps release duct blockages; consider seeing a lactation specialist to review optimal latch and nursing techniques. Many antibiotics are safe for the baby while nursing.

ABSCESS: A breast abscess occurs when mastitis progresses, and bacteria form a contained pocket of pus that is usually palpable and accompanied by red, warm skin and focal pain. Abscesses in breastfeeding moms occur 3 to 11 percent of the time.[114] Risk factors include age over thirty, first pregnancy, and smoking. Abscesses occur more frequently in nonlactating women than lactating, especially those with the following risk factors: African American, obese, or smokers.[115] Treatment always involves antibiotics and some form of drainage: either repeated aspirations every two to three days until it's gone or via open incision done either at your surgeon's office or asleep in the operating room.[116]

GRANULOMATOUS MASTITIS: This is a rare, benign inflammatory breast condition that presents as a palpable hard mass in the breast with or without other symptoms such as nipple discharge, nipple retraction, pain, inflamed skin, ulcerated skin, abscess formation, and enlarged lymph nodes. Although benign, it is indistinguishable from cancer or abscess until a biopsy confirms the diagnosis.[117] Granulomatous mastitis can be caused by numerous conditions—tuberculosis, sarcoidosis (see following pages), diabetes, or as a reaction to injected foreign bodies like free silicone (I warned you about that stuff).[118] Without having a cause identified, the condition is termed idiopathic granulomatous mastitis (IGM) and can resolve spontaneously after an average of nine to twelve months.[119] Don't bother to try excision, steroids, or medications, since granulomatous mastitis is known for poor wound healing and rebound inflammation in these situations.[120] Granulomatous mastitis poses no increased cancer risks.

DIABETIC MASTOPATHY: Diabetic mastopathy—a.k.a. lymphocytic mastitis or lymphocytic mastopathy—accounts for less than 1 percent of all benign breast disease and occurs infrequently in 0.6 to 13 percent of premenopausal women with long-standing type 1 diabetes.[121] Diabetic mastopathy typically appears as a firm, mobile, palpable, painless breast mass or masses in one or both breasts.[122] Core biopsy confirms the diagnosis, and no treatment is needed, and no increased risk of subsequent breast cancer exists.

LIPOMA: Breast lipomas present in the same way they do everywhere in the body—as semi-squishy, non-tender lumps of mature fat cells organized together with a thin capsule around them. If in doubt, a needle biopsy might confirm the diagnosis, but realize that the pathologist usually just reports "mature adipose cells" (fancy words for fat), and not a lipoma. Excision can be performed if lipomas grow rapidly, cause pain, or otherwise concern you. There is no increased risk of subsequent breast cancer.

HAMARTOMA: These are benign lesions composed of the normal tissues found in the breast, but the cells grow in a disorganized manner. A pathologist might also call them a fibroadenolipoma, lipofibroadenoma, or adenolipoma.[123] These appear as soft, discrete, and painless masses with a capsule around them, and they can be quite large. Since the cells inside don't have distinctive features (they look like normal cells found in a breast: ducts, lobules, fat, connective tissue), a diagnosis cannot be made short of complete excision. Although malignancy rarely occurs mixed within hamartomas, we always excise them.[124]

PSEUDOANGIOMATOUS STROMAL HYPERPLASIA: Pseudoangiomatous stromal hyperplasia is a ridiculous thing to pronounce and takes too long to say, so we call it PASH. Microscopically, PASH has little slits in the tissues that look like blood vessels but aren't, hence the description pseudoangiomatous—meaning, fake appearance of vessels. Because of this fake-out, core needle biopsies with PASH are sometimes mistaken for a cancer made from the lining of blood vessels, called *angiosarcoma* (if that happens, get a second opinion on those slides).[125] PASH occurs most frequently in perimenopausal women around fifty years old and also in men. Although most commonly found incidentally with other biopsies, PASH also presents as a palpable, non-tender thickening 30 to 44 percent of the time.[126] Imaging with mammogram and ultrasound often shows a solid, well-defined mass that looks like a fibroadenoma or sometimes carcinoma.[127] A diagnosis of PASH by core biopsy precludes the need for surgical excision, as long as imaging is not suspicious.[128] Women with PASH seem less likely to develop breast cancer.[129]

SARCOIDOSIS: Sarcoidosis, a chronic noncancerous inflammatory disease most commonly affecting the lungs, only rarely originates in the breast. When it does, sarcoidosis presents as a firm, hard mass that mimics a carcinoma. The imaging also shows suspicious spiculated masses. Core biopsy confirms the diagnosis, and once obtained, excision is not necessary.[130] Sarcoidosis occurs most commonly in women in their thirties and forties.[131] There is no increased risk of subsequent breast cancer.

BREASTS CAN REALLY GET BUSY

As bothersome as this exhaustive list of lumps can be, when one of them shows up in your breast, there is *one more* diagnosis that would make you embrace any and all of the above. . . . In the next chapter, we face cancer head-on, and as we do, let's already decide to emerge from the journey victorious, instilled with newfound purpose and joy!

CHAPTER 9

Cancer Happens: A Newly Diagnosed Starter Kit

It doesn't matter if your doctor is upbeat or serious, whether she touches your shoulder or tells you on the phone, or if you're an innately confident or fearful person—hearing the words *It's breast cancer* universally shakes every woman to her very core. If this should happen to you, or is currently happening, for that matter, I want to help you do a few things to make your journey from cancer to cure as fruitful as it can be.

First, take a deep breath, and on the exhale, think, "I will survive." This will become your mantra. Believe it, all day and every day. Know that it's not just a feel-good epithet—it's the truth. Most women with breast cancer *do* survive, so why not you? I'm not minimizing the strength and endurance it takes to get from here to cure—but you must believe that you will get there. You're about to assemble a family (true, one you've never wanted) including a surgeon, plastic surgeon (as needed), medical oncologist, radiation oncologist, and hopefully a Chinese medicine doctor, nutritionist, physical therapist, support group, and psychologist (as needed) to make sure you recover wholly and intact. You'll also want to collect important notes as you move from decision making to decisive action: imaging reports (mammogram, ultrasound, breast MRI, PET/CT, bone scan, brain MRI), images on a CD, pathology reports, consultation notes from each doctor seen, operative reports, special study reports (like genetic testing, MammaPrint, Oncotype Dx, BCI—don't worry; we're getting to all of these foreign words shortly), radiation summary, chemo summary, and lab results—and then pretty soon you can put that binder somewhere out of sight to collect a bunch of dust while you get busy embracing your new life.

Let's talk about what you can expect between now and the day you see your journey in the rearview mirror. This chapter provides a crash course explaining what breast cancer is and all the different ways we treat and, yes, cure it. I intend to infuse confidence and hope in you through education; together, let's make sure you get the care you deserve. So read on, and live long!

THE FIRST FEW DAYS

Breast cancer is like the weather. Sunshine-and-rainbows stage 0 DCIS never needs chemo and behaves differently than a rainy-day stage IIA recovering from her mastectomy but who can't even imagine the blizzard swooshing around stage IV who just enrolled in a promising trial. Yet when you first receive a diagnosis, your instinct is to gobble up as much information as you can about breast cancer as a category so that you feel in control. But sunshine shouldn't get too much advice from clouds, and vice versa. Some ways to do this are better than others.

It's only natural that when you're trying to wrap your head around upsetting news, you want to gather as many details from as many sources as you can. To be honest, I caution against random Internet searches before you know more staging details about your cancer and outline a plan of attack with your doctors. Reading horror stories on message boards from strangers that may or may not relate to your specific cancer could start this off on a terrifying foot. I'd be selective about sharing your situation with people. By all means, remain true to your personality and do what empowers you, but as a general rule, I find this advice, when followed, brings more clarity to the decision making at hand. Hearing well-intentioned tales about Aunt Diana's friend's daughter whose journey was fraught with setbacks won't help. (One of my favorite greeting cards says: "When life hands you lemons, I promise I won't tell you a story about my cousin's friend who died from lemons.") You'll want to minimize as much outside noise as you can so that you can get your calmest head in the game, so to speak—ready to act strategically and with correct information, hope, and encouragement from the most informed and experienced voices.

When sharing your diagnosis with family members, I'd be careful about how you approach children and aging parents. You know your family best in terms of how they handle uncertainty, rely on your presence, or possess the maturity to cope with tough news. Usually, if you don't need the advice of these family members to help you make decisions, I find it's wise to wait until you clarify your treatment strategy. This way, you won't drag loved ones into what may feel like an interminable wait for pathology details and body scans as your life seems to hang in the balance. My patients often say that the waiting, the *not knowing*, is the worst of all, so if you can spare others the worst of it (and potentially spare yourself from their fears reflecting back at you), that's preferable. Better to present your news fully packaged with the prettiest bow that matches the situation. This is especially the case with young children, and I might even wait until after surgery, if that makes sense for you. I also recommend using the word *cancer* with kids, because hiding your illness with vague terms and secrecy gives it power and makes others fear it. Kids figure it out eventually, so it should come from you; receiving the truth from you in this moment increases the transparency and trust they will feel in future moments. "Mommy had a little sickness in her breast called cancer," you might say to your six-year-old, "but it was only in one tiny spot, and it's already gone. Remember that shot you got in your arm so that you never catch chicken pox? I'm going to take some medicine now so this won't come back. The doctors told us to expect a long, healthy life, so don't worry; I will be here to tell you to clean your room and eat your vegetables!"

WHAT IS BREAST CANCER, REALLY?

Much of why the word *cancer* holds so much power is because, until you understand what's happening in your body, it's shrouded in an opaque drape of mystery. But when you realize the biological progression from normal cells to cancerous ones, you can look at this for what it is—an anatomic hiccup that needs to be removed from your body. Stripped of its anonymity, cancer looks less daunting. Let's strip it down then, shall we?

If you recall from chapter 1, our breasts have milk-producing lobules and thin tubes called *ducts* that coalesce as they carry milk down toward the nipple (see picture on page 4). This path ends with eight to twelve ducts traversing the nipple itself to open on the surface. Duct size varies from 1 millimeter at the lobules (lobules average 3 millimeters) up to 5 to 8 millimeters near the nipple. About 75 percent of all breast cancers originate inside those spaghetti-sized ducts, 10 percent begin in lobules, and 15 percent involve less common subtypes that usually also initiate in the ducts but have unique features about them that make us give them descriptive names like *mucinous* or *tubular*, but it's all *breast cancer*.[1]

Imagine cutting across one of those normal ducts in the breast and looking through it like a telescope (or for lobular cancers, slicing across a lobule and peering into it like a little bowl). When normal, you see a single layer of cells lining the inside, appearing uniform and orderly, one to the next, like the left circle in the picture below.

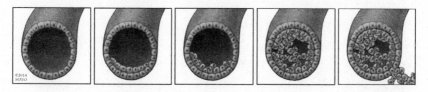

Left to right: Normal breast duct; usual ductal hyperplasia (UDH); atypical ductal hyperplasia (ADH); ductal carcinoma *in situ* (DCIS); invasive ductal carcinoma (IDC)

When something stimulates those cells to proliferate (mutations, estrogen, IGF-1, and so forth), and they form a second layer that's also orderly, we name that *usual ductal hyperplasia* (UDH)—the second circle in our picture. Like skin making a new freckle, UDH is not melanoma, and nobody cuts it out; it's just part of aging. However, when those UDH cells become disorganized, growing without control or order, creating multiple layers and changing their shape, they're called *atypical*. Atypical ductal hyperplasia (ADH)—the third circle—needs to be removed when identified. ADH is a marker lesion, discussed in chapter 6. Eventually, if enough atypical cells encroach upon the duct's empty space so it expands past 2 millimeters, or if two adjacent ducts contain ADH, then the pathologist labels it breast cancer.[2]

More specifically, ADH evolves into the earliest form of breast cancer, *ductal carcinoma in situ* (DCIS), which is diagnosed in 1 in 33 women—the fourth circle. When left untreated, 36 percent of DCIS eventually breaks through the duct wall, invading the surrounding breast tissue.[3] Catch that? So, 64 percent of DCIS could stay put for the rest of your life and never cause harm. The problem is, we've tried and tried to figure out which third invades and which two-thirds don't (patient age, tumor grade, size, and so on), and all DCIS seems to have the same proclivity to invade.[4] So, yes, we overtreat two-thirds of all women with DCIS.[5] If cancer cells break through the duct wall by 1 millimeter or less, we term this DCIS with microinvasion.

Once a volume of cells greater than 1 millimeter breaks the duct wall, it's called *invasive ductal carcinoma* (IDC)—the fifth circle. The same story applies to cancer progression in a lobule that becomes *invasive lobular carcinoma* (ILC). That ominous word *invasive* simply refers to cells once inside an intact duct now being immediately on the other side of that duct wall, right there in your breast where it started. Although we're using the word *invasive*, we have no idea at this point whether or not the cancer invaded anywhere else, like your lymph nodes or liver. A pathologist only looks at the little slice of tissue from the tumor that someone biopsied—she has no idea if this cancer spread outside the breast. Invasive cancers (IDC/ILC) can *potentially* enter the lymphatics or bloodstream and travel to other organs (metastasize), but at the moment of diagnosis, only 5 percent of all cancers have metastasized past lymph nodes into organs like lung or bone. Are you with me so far?

A quick word about ILC as compared to ductal. ILC tends to invade the breast in single-file fashion, like kids lining up for recess in a straight line. This pattern doesn't readily declare its presence with a mass on imaging or exam until it finally starts taking up enough space to get recognized. That's why ILC tends to be a lot larger than IDC at the time of diagnosis.[6] Despite this fact, stage-for-stage, ILC has an equal or even better survival rate than IDC, owing to mellower biology.[7] IDC and ILC are treated in the exact same way.

One other sneaky subtype deserves special mention: inflammatory breast cancer. This tumor often presents without a mass at all, and the first sign is a suddenly swollen, red, painful breast with thickened pitted skin that looks like an orange peel. This can be mistaken for a breast infection, so if antibiotics don't clear it up entirely in a few days, urgently consult a breast surgeon because inflammatory breast cancer needs treatment ASAP.

THE CORE REPORT

Now that you have a basic understanding of how normal cells progress to abnormal, fill up your ducts or lobules, and then break the wall (i.e., invade it), let's explore the nitty gritty details. The core biopsy pathology report ("path") reveals a lot about the inherent biology of your cancer, and this information helps guide our treatment strategy. Your path report defines the type of cancer, the grade, and whether it's in the lymphatic or blood vessels of the breast tissue; it also provides a biomarker profile composed of four biological markers, all of which we'll discuss next. The tumor then gets categorized into a *molecular subtype* that your doctors use to formulate a plan.

RIGHT BREAST 11 O'CLOCK 4 CM FN (CORE BIOPSY)

- Invasive ductal carcinoma
  - Modified Bloom-Richardson histological grade 2 (out of 3); Total score: 6/9
    - Nuclear grade: 2 (out of 3)
    - Tubule formation: 3 (out of 3)
    - Mitotic index: 1 (out of 3)
  - No lymphovascular invasion identified

Let's start at the top. Doctors document an area of interest as if your breast is a clock seen from their vantage point. So, in our report above, "Right Breast 11 o'clock 4 CM FN" (centimeters from the nipple) puts this mass in the upper outer quadrant of the right breast. The "worst" news is always written first in a path report, so here, it's an "invasive ductal carcinoma." Next, we learn the grade. Grade compares features of the cancer cell to a normal cell, giving us insight into how hostile the cells might be. Grade can be called 1, 2, 3; low, intermediate, high; or well, moderately, poorly differentiated (it's all the same). Grade 1 looks similar to the original breast cell, grade 2 is more altered, and grade 3 appears wild. If you see the Nottingham or Modified Bloom-Richardson score on your path report, this details how the pathologist arrived at your final grade. Bottom line: the higher the grade, the angrier the cancer, but grade is just one of many features we examine.

Some pathology reports specifically note whether or not cancer cells are seen parading into breast vessels or nerves, termed *lymphovascular invasion* or *perineural invasion*, respectively. Even when present, this does not mean the cells spread outside the breast, but it's another sign of aggressiveness.

About a week after receiving your initial biopsy report, you'll also get information called the *tumor profile* (or *biomarker profile*) that provides critical insight into your cancer's biology. Let's go line by line through an example tumor profile so you can learn to unravel the mysteries hidden in there.

BREAST BIOMARKER PROFILE FOR
INVASIVE CARCINOMA

PROGNOSTIC MARKER	RESULTS (% POSITIVE)	STAINING INTENSITY	TEST RESULT
Estrogen receptor	98%	3+	Positive
Progesterone receptor	79%	2+	Positive
HER2 IHC test		2+	Equivocal
HER2 (FISH)			Negative
Ki-67 antigen	26%		High

Most importantly, is the cancer fueled by estrogen and progesterone? Ideally, we see a high percentage (ranges 0 to 100 percent) of estrogen receptors (ER) and progesterone receptors (PR) with a strong staining intensity (ranked 1 to 3+, 3+ being strongest). In this example, estrogen fuels 98 percent of the cancer cells and progesterone stimulates 79 percent of them. Some labs report an Allred score instead, which ranks ER and PR on a 0 to 8 scale; higher is better. When circulating hormones hit these receptors, they signal the cancer cells to multiply and divide, so when your ER percentage is high, this means the cancer is highly fueled by estrogen. Remember, even postmenopausal ladies have plenty of estrogen thanks to the aromatase enzyme hanging out in fat cells, converting steroids into estrogen. While this might not sound so great to have a bunch of estrogen flying around an estrogen-driven ER(+) tumor, we love these receptors, present in about 80 percent of cancers. First of all, they associate with less aggressive, more curable cancers.[8] Second, if estrogen feeds them, we can starve them with endocrine therapy using an *anti*estrogen pill. Finally, if you *don't* have ER, you probably need chemotherapy as part of your cure, but (silver lining) chemo is very effective against most estrogen-negative ER(−) tumors. We don't have any therapy strictly aimed at PR, but the higher the PR, the less aggressive the cancer.

With invasive cancers, your tumor profile includes a gene in charge of cell growth and repair called the *human epidermal growth factor receptor*, or *HER2/neu* (a.k.a erbB-2), or—most commonly—*HER2*. HER2 gets amped up in 15 percent of cancers. It's tested in two ways, so you will first see the IHC (immunohistochemistry) test; IHC shows the *absence* of HER2 with a 0 or 1+ score, the *presence* of HER2 with a 3+ score, and confusion with 2+. So in this case, it's tested again using FISH (fluorescence *in situ* hybridization), which usually yields a definite answer. HER2 positive [HER2(+)] cancers are more aggressive than HER2 negative [HER2(−)] ones, so they almost always need chemo. The great news here: if you've been diagnosed with a HER2(+) invasive cancer, targeted treatments like Herceptin and Perjeta so effectively and precisely destroy this subtype that, once treated, HER2(+) actually has the *best outcome of all subtypes*.

One of the most aggressive subtypes of breast cancer bears the name *triple negative breast cancer* (TNBC). "Triple negative" refes to the *absence* of these three receptors we just discussed from the surface of the tumor cell: estrogen, progesterone, and HER2 receptors. It's true that TNBC generally carries the worst prognosis of all subtypes, but as mentioned above, chemotherapy works well against ER(-) tumors, including TNBC. In fact, when TNBC patients receive chemotherapy *before* removing the cancer, we find that chemo literally destroys every last cancer cell in the breast and lymph nodes nearly 30 percent of the time.[9] When this happens, it's called a *pathologic complete response*, or pCR. Those with a pCR show dramatically improved survival rates, mirroring those with ER(+) subtypes.[10] With TNBCs, the majority of your recurrence risk falls into the first three years—and after five years cancer free, you're pretty much golden.[11] Definitely pop open the champagne on that day.

The final part of the tumor profile analyzes the Ki-67 antigen. Ki-67 answers the question, "How many cells are actively dividing here?"— that is, one cell turning into two cells, rather than lying dormant. The percentage of proliferating cells ranges from 1 to 100 percent. Ideally it's less than 11 percent, and we consider more than 20 percent high (labs vary, so check your report). The lower the number, the lazier your cancer. We love couch potatoes! But certain treatments (silver lining) work better against fast dividers, so don't get scared if your Ki-67 is sky high.

If you're looking at a path report from your entire cancer being removed after lumpectomy or mastectomy, then your report includes additional information: final tumor size, number of tumors found, other lesions such as DCIS, the margin status (whether cancer landed at the edge or is clear from the edge of removed tissues), how many nodes were removed, and if any nodes contain cancer.

MOLECULAR SUBTYPES: PROFILE OF A VILLAIN

Although it's all called breast cancer, at least twenty-one unique subtypes exist under the microscope. How cells *behave* matters much more than how they look. A serial killer can appear handsome and friendly—show me his intentions and capabilities, not his photograph. That's what molecular profiling does: using the four biological markers we just discussed, doctors categorize tumors into one of five distinct molecular profiles, each with its own genetic propensity to present, respond, and recur in variable ways. Molecular subtyping combines the presence or absence of ER and PR into one category called *hormone receptors* (HR+/HR–) with overexpression of HER2 protein (HER2+/HER2–) and Ki-67 to determine the subtypes as follows:

Luminal A (HR+/HER2–): 74 percent of cancers, lots of ER(+), low grade, lower Ki-67, better prognosis; treated with endocrine therapy, chemo less commonly advised; associated with early menarche, late menopause, HRT, late childbirth.

Luminal B HER2+ (HR+/HER2+), also called *triple positive*, and **Luminal B HER2-(HR+/HER2-):** 10 percent of cancers, fewer ER(+) cells, grades 2 to 3, higher Ki-67; treated with endocrine therapy, usually chemo, add anti-HER2 drugs for triple positives; associated with weight gain after age eighteen.

HER2 enriched (HR-/HER2+): 4 percent of cancers, high grade, aggressive; treated with chemo and anti-HER2 drugs.

Triple Negative (HR-/HER2-): 12 percent of cancers, includes basal-like tumors, high grade, high division, poorer survival with no targeted therapies available; treated with chemo; less common with prior lactation, more common in African Americans.[12]

With some of the more favorable subtypes like Luminal B (HR+/ HER2–) cancers with 0 to 3 involved nodes, molecular profiling leaves us with a blurry image of our villain; we need a clearer mug shot to know whether chemotherapy should be used against this cancer. We gain insight into what genes drive a particular cancer using *genomic profiling* from one of several commercially available tests: Oncotype DX, MammaPrint, EndoPredict, PAM50/Prosigna, or Breast Cancer Index. These assays interrogate cancer cells for the presence or absence of a number of biologic markers—some are good to have, some bad—and depending on what your personal tumor expresses or doesn't, it's all thrown into an algorithm that spits out the percentage chance that this villain will come back within the next ten years in a more ominous place like lung, liver, brain, or bone. If recurrence risk is high, chemo can make it lower; but when risk is low, *chemo can't make a low number lower*—so keep that hair, girlfriend.[13] More on chemo in a bit.

YOUR CANCER'S STAGE

Begun in 1959, the TNM staging system provides an international cancer language for doctors to communicate clearly about tumor anatomy and extent of disease: T = tumor size; N = nodes; M = metastases. Since the value of staging lies in predicting survival and guiding treatment, in 2018, biologic factors (grade, ER/PR, HER2) and genomic profiles (Oncotype, MammaPrint) were incorporated into the staging system. Adding this biologic and genomic data makes staging much more meaningful in terms of prognosis than anatomy alone (the TNM part). However, most of the world cannot afford the technology to stage beyond the anatomy features in TNM, so it will take some time before the new staging criteria are applicable globally.

No one knows how long she will live—cancer or not—but sometimes predictions bring comfort. One prefers not to know her prognosis; another needs a general sense of what to expect. Remember, you are not a statistic. Survival percentages reflect the outcome of large numbers of women with the same stage as yours; your oncology team can help you arrive at a more personalized outlook, if you desire. In doctor talk, "five-year survival" (5YS) tells the percentage of patients alive five years later—this does not mean you die year six! We publish 5YS, 10YS, 15YS rates because treatments improve all the time; a 15YS reflects treatments that are at least fifteen years old, which is less relevant to you than the 5YS data. What follows reflects anatomic staging (TNM) with 5YS, and then we review examples of how the newer staging system incorporating genomic info can turn TNM staging on its head. No matter what your cancer stage, every stage has hope.

STAGE 0: DCIS (ductal carcinoma *in situ*). Cancer cells trapped inside breast ducts with no ability to spread. LCIS (lobular carcinoma *in situ*) is not cancer, despite the name. 25 percent of breast cancers. 100 percent 5YS.

STAGE IA/IB: Cancer cells invade the walls of a duct or lobule, but the total size is under 2 centimeters; cells have not spread to lymph nodes. 48 percent of invasive cancers. 99 to 100 percent 5YS.

STAGE IIA/IIB: Cancers over 2 centimeters that have not spread to nodes or invaded chest muscles; cancers under 5 centimeters in size that have spread to one to three axillary (armpit) lymph nodes. 34 percent of invasive cancers. 93 percent 5YS.

STAGE IIIA/IIIB/IIIC: Cancers of any size that spread to *four* or more armpit lymph nodes, the nodes around the clavicle (collarbone), and/or the nodes under the sternum (internal mammary nodes); cancers over 5 centimeters that spread to any nodes; and tumors that have grown into the chest muscles. 13 percent of invasive cancers. 72 percent 5YS.

STAGE IV: Cancer has metastasized beyond the breast and nearby nodes to other organs or distant nodes. The most commonly involved areas are lung, liver, brain, and bone. I often hear people say that a relative had breast cancer, but died of lung cancer. She probably died of breast cancer that *went to* the lung. When breast cancer metastasizes to the lung, it still looks and acts like breast cancer, not lung cancer. 5 percent of invasive cancers. 22 percent 5YS.[14]

When you throw biology into the staging mix by incorporating molecular profiles (MammaPrint, Oncotype), predicted survival rates supersede what the TNM anatomy foretells. For example, it's worse to have a tiny, aggressive triple negative (TNBC) than it is to have a 5-centimeter luminal A cancer—because the biology of TNBC makes it worse, and biology matters more than size. So, for example, in the new staging system, a 1-centimeter TNBC becomes stage IIA even when it's less than 2 centimeters and node negative (TNM stage IA). On the flipside, a 4-centimeter grade 2 triple positive [ER(+), PR (+), HER2(+)] invasive cancer with a low-risk genomic profile that spread to *nine axillary nodes* is now stage IB (TNM stage IIIA). Whoa—that lady just went from a 72 percent 5YS to 99 to 100 percent because we weight tumor biology more heavily than anatomy.

The unequal distribution of cancer stages around the world at the time of diagnosis parallels global economic disparities, as you can see from the table on the next page, which shows TNM staging at the time of diagnosis in a sampling of women from around the world. The lower the income, the higher the cancer stage.

I often hear this logical inquiry: "How do you know for sure that the tumor hasn't gone anywhere else in my body?" Well, we take a good look with body scans, and we check your blood for tumor markers that elevate in the presence of stage IV metastases. Patients with positive nodes or aggressive profiles should consider whole-body staging, whereby your doctor will order imaging of your entire body hoping *not* to find distant metastases. Potential scans include positron emission tomography (PET); computed tomography (CT) of the chest, abdomen, and pelvis; brain

MRI (for TNBC and HER2+); and bone scans. You don't truly know your cancer stage until these scans are done, but in favorable profile, node-negative cancers, the radiation exposure from scans probably isn't worth the risk since they will almost certainly be negative.

AROUND THE WORLD: STAGE OF BREAST CANCER AT TIME OF DIAGNOSIS (PERCENT)[15]

COUNTRY	STAGE I	STAGE II	STAGE III	STAGE IV
Brazil (2008–2009)	20	47	28	5
Canada (2000–2007)	41	38	13	8
China (1999–2008)	19	55	23	3
Denmark (2000–2007)	29	47	16	8
Egypt (South Cancer Inst., 2001–2008)	11	39	25	25
Iraq (Kurdistan, 2006–2008)	5	53	32	10
Libya (2008–2009)	9	26	54	12
Malaysia (E. coast and Kuala Lumpur, 2005–2007)	5	39	45	11
Nigeria (Lagos, 2009–2010)	6	15	63	16
Thailand (2009)	12	38	41	9
United Kingdom (2000–2007)	40	45	9	5
United States (2004–2010)	48	34	13	5

Percentages rounded to the nearest number and may not add up to 100; DCIS and unknown stage are excluded.

HOW LONG HAVE YOU HAD CANCER?

Once patients understand the continuum of disease that defines all cancer cell formation and progression, nearly everyone asks, "When did this thing start?" Actually, your cancer cells invaded the wall anywhere from three to twenty years ago—and because I know you're wondering, neither you nor your doctor would have been able to feel or find them back then. Even prior to that, cells might have mutated into atypia as far back as when you were in your mother's womb (remember DES exposures that caused vaginal cancer?).[16] It all has to do with how many cells are actively dividing at any given time, and at what rate. Cells replicate differently based on their biology, but on average for those who are younger than fifty years, they double once every 80 days; for those fifty to seventy years, 157 days; and for women over seventy, 188 days. So it takes around three to six months for one cell to become two, and not all the cancer cells are actively dividing.[17] Mind you, a sugar cube–sized cancer houses one billion cells.[18] So, for example, in a sixty-one-year-old with a 1-centimeter mass and 20 percent of her cancer cells actively dividing, that first cell mutated 10.3 years ago. Clearly, the HRT she took for the last three years didn't create this cancer, but it might have fueled it to show up sooner. That also goes for the morning-after pill someone took two months ago, and the steak you ate last week.

The truth is, some women live and die with, but not from, cancers they never knew they had, and other cancers might even disappear on their own. How do I know this? From autopsies on women *without* known breast cancer who died from something else, like an accident. A combined autopsy series on 852 women showed that 39 percent ages forty to forty-nine years had DCIS—and this is wild—only 10 percent aged fifty to seventy had DCIS.[19] Where did all the DCIS go? Similarly, researchers in Norway and Sweden have postulated that some of the cancers detected through mammography may spontaneously regress.[20] They randomized over 600,000 women into two groups: regular mammos for six years starting now or starting four years later. You would expect that the delayed group would have fewer cancers found in those first four years, since they weren't getting imaged, which is what happened (they had 49 percent less cancer than the mammo group). But once they start mammos, they should catch up in number to the other group, right? They didn't. The group that began later had 14 percent *fewer* breast cancers found, suggesting that a certain number of cancers go away.

Don't misunderstand. Once you're diagnosed with cancer, we aren't smart enough (yet) to know which ones will regress with no treatment at all, so "better safe than sorry" becomes the best course of action.

DID YOU CAUSE YOUR CANCER?

We probably can't identify exactly how or why this cancer showed up in your breast. The answer harkens back to our seed and soil discussions, knowing that cancer results from a perfect storm forming between carcinogenic influences, genetic factors, and the tumor microenvironment. Rather than obsess over "Why me?" and introduce feelings of futility or guilt, I prefer for us to focus on strategy. Admittedly, some cancers outwit the best army you send after them, but the momentum of other subtypes can be halted or reversed—like all that DCIS in the autopsies I just mentioned. Our bodies are not defenseless against this disease.

Do you remember the study from chapter 4 in which *diet and exercise* transformed the blood of obese women into a cancer-fighting machine in just two weeks, destroying breast cancer cells in a petri dish? How about when diet and lifestyle *reversed* biopsy-proven prostate cancer in men? And two chapters ago, retinoic acid turned atypia and *in situ* cancers back to normal? We all have room for improvement, and now that you know your breast cells are capable of generating a cancer, let's hit the reset button and start making sure our bodies become inhospitable to cancer's return. You have the power to change your body's future.

But first, let's get rid of this thing.

WHAT ARE YOUR TREATMENT OPTIONS?

In the United States, we're pretty good at treating and curing this disease. Want proof? Just ask the 3.5 million women running around with a personal history of breast cancer in the US today![21] Breast cancer death rates crept up 0.4 percent per year until 1975; after 1989, mortality pulled a one-eighty among all races and ages, dropping 36 percent.[22] Kudos go to early detection and better treatment.[23] We have five effective tools in our toolbox, not that you need to use all of them: chemotherapy, surgery, radiation, hormonal therapy, and targeted therapies. Let's dive into all of these options and explore what makes sense for which tumors.

CHEMOTHERAPY

First up, we address the concern I hear the most: "Do I have to do chemo?" Well, you don't *have* to do anything you don't choose to do, but to safely avoid a chemo recommendation, we generally need to have all four of the following factors be true of your cancer: ER(+), HER2(-), less than four involved nodes, and a low-risk genomic assay score (MammaPrint, Oncotype). In any given situation, having a low-risk genomic score could trump any of the other factors and land you a get-out-of-chemo card. The opposite usually clinches a recommendation to pursue chemo, except this time, you need only one of them: ER(–), HER2+, four or more nodes involved, and a high-risk genomic assay score.

No one ever wants chemo, but they also don't want to die; while chemo doesn't come with a cancer-free guarantee, many choose it when the benefit outweighs the risk. To arrive at this conclusion, your medical oncologist will analyze all the variables he knows about your cancer, entering your data into computer models like Adjuvant! Online, and weighing results of genomic testing (MammaPrint, Oncotype) to predict the benefit you'll receive from endocrine therapy with or without chemotherapy. We rely on genomics now more than ever, but unfortunately, most of the world cannot access this expensive tool that often reverses what our intuition tells us to do. For example, the MINDACT trial showed that 23 percent of women had a low risk MammaPrint and didn't need chemo, whereas using the computer models entering data like high tumor grade and positive nodes would have led to advising chemo.[24] The study took these 1,550 women with conflicting "advice" regarding the need for chemotherapy and randomized them into chemo versus no chemo, then followed them for ten years—and no significant difference in survival emerged. In other words, chemotherapy can't make a low recurrence risk even lower, so don't do it. In general, most people lean toward chemotherapy for a 5 percent or better survival benefit;[25] others pull a Dr. Seuss and categorically declare, "Not here, not there, not anywhere."

Chemotherapy is usually given into your veins every one to three weeks for up to six months and takes about four hours to administer. A 2017 meta-analysis included twenty-five trials in which 34,122 patients with early-stage breast cancer were treated with a "dose-dense" regimen, meaning chemo was given every two weeks.[26] Dose-dense yielded less recurrence (by 4.3 percent) and higher survival rates (by 2.8 percent) at ten years compared to the standard every-three-week regimen. Given that the cycles were tolerated the same, I would favor dose-dense—why not get all the benefit you can out of this unwelcome experience?

Chemo doesn't aim at a target or receptor; it just flies around your bloodstream trying to destroy cells that move quickly. Since it doesn't know the difference between fast-moving cancer cells and high-turnover normal cells, collateral damage abounds to all the normal cells that move fast. Hair follicles? Bald. Fingernails? Brittle. GI tract? Barf. But now for the great part—TNBC? *BAM*. HER2(+)? *Annihilated*. This also explains why certain tumors get to skip chemo; for example, ER(+) low division rate? *Boring, slow-moving, chemo overlooks it*. So, you see, the more aggressive the tumor, the more effective the chemo, which brings welcome news to the googler who just read she has "the worst type" possible. Chemotherapy suddenly seems worth the temporary side effects of hair loss (alopecia), fatigue, nausea, vomiting, and infection risk (from immunosuppression); even potentially permanent complications such as nerve damage to hands and feet (neuropathy), chemo brain (foggy thinking), osteoporosis, heart damage, infertility, early menopause, and acute leukemia sound better than possibly dying.[27]

Speaking of chemo brain, which is when your mind feels slow and forgetful from the chemo treatments, ask your doctor about the safety of combining methylphenidate, aspirin, and erythropoietin with your chemotherapy treatment,[28] and if antioxidants (vitamins A, C, E, gluta-thione, selenium, coenzyme Q-10, melatonin, and N-acetylcysteine) are okay in between cycles.[29] Mounting evidence suggests that these interventions can help prevent the fuzzy head that comes after chemo treatments.

We have fixes for many of chemo's unwelcome side effects, and complementary and integrative therapies often provide a world of supportive care during this challenging time. You can even wear an ice cap on your head that shunts chemo away from the scalp to prevent hair loss. Another trick is to keep your fingers and toes in ice water to divert the chemotherapy-saturated blood away from your digits to help avoid neuropathy. Most women work through chemo, with a few days off as needed after each treatment cycle. Patients often tell me that they know someone who died from doing chemotherapy, and not from the cancer itself. Statistically, 1.3 per 1,000 receiving chemotherapy die because of the treatment received, so I'm not sure how so many people know some-one to whom this happened, but chemo *won't kill* basically 999 of every 1,000 who choose it.[30]

Just because I know you're wondering, if you do radiation, no, you can't skip chemo. Why not? Surgery and radiation keep cancer from coming back locally *where it started* in the breast, skin, chest muscles, or nodes. In contrast, chemo, hormonal, and targeted therapies (which we'll discuss soon) reduce the risk of recurrence *where it's going* (like to the liver). Chemo improves survival rates (and also decreases local recurrence in the breast, but that's not why you do it). So if you need chemo to make its way into all your distant cells (systemic therapy), radiation doesn't obviate that need, nor does surgery (local therapy).

What should you do first—chemo or surgery? You want to do what-ever makes you live longer. Turns out, it doesn't matter which you do first, so there's no wrong choice.[31] Even though survival remains the same, if you definitely need chemo (say, for TNBC), there are benefits to chemo before surgery (called *neoadjuvant* chemotherapy):

1. A large cancer that needs mastectomy might shrink enough to make lumpectomy cosmetically feasible.
2. It's all happening too fast, and you don't know if you want a mastectomy or not. Chemo buys you four to six months to get your genetic mutation panel back (BRCA and so on) and to meet plastic surgeons to consider your reconstruction options without haste.
3. It's reassuring to measure the tumor's response to treatment to be sure the drugs are working (downsizing makes it all seem worth it; growth makes us change our strategy).
4. Perhaps you can join a clinical trial that requires the tumor be present to monitor response.
5. You find out if the cancer totally disappeared with the chemo— called a *pathologic complete response* (pCR), which you find out after surgery when the pathologist cannot find any cancer cells left in the removed tissue. A woman with a pCR has higher survival rates, but you would not have this information if you took the tumor out and then did chemo (you would have the same higher survival rate, but you wouldn't know it).[32]

If you decide to have surgery first—and we'll discuss that next—do not allow more than ninety days between your last operation and the start of chemo. Analyzing 24,843 patients from the California Cancer Registry diagnosed with stages I to III breast cancer, researchers found equivalent survival rates when women started chemo within ninety days of surgery. After ninety-one–plus days, you pass the window of equal opportunity: 34 percent decrease in survival across the board, and 53 percent worse for TNBC as compared to starting within ninety days.[33]

LET'S TALK SURGERY

You remember that I'm a surgeon, right? I've been waiting nine chapters for this part! It's time to chat about what it takes to remove your tumor with the intention to cure it, in a way that instills you with confidence about your future and leaves you feeling like *you* inside your own skin.

Should You Do a Lumpectomy or Mastectomy?

Everyone with breast cancer needs an operation if they want to remove cancer from their bodies for sure, since everything else we aim at cancer may or may not (generally *not*) make every last cell disappear. We have two ways to get that intruder out of your breast: (1) *lumpectomy* (also called partial mastectomy, or breast-conserving surgery), which removes the cancer with a rim of healthy breast surrounding it; and (2) *mastectomy*, which takes all the breast tissue with none or some of the overlying skin.

Ready to hear something shocking? When treating invasive breast cancer, removing your entire breast does not add one more day to your life as compared to keeping your breast. You read that right. Six landmark studies radically altered the landscape of breast cancer surgery in the 1980s by unveiling this truth: removing the breast with mastectomy or keeping the breast with lumpectomy (with *or without* radiation) yields identical breast cancer survival rates.[34] Wowza. There's one exception here: adding radiation after lumpectomy in higher-risk cancers did add a 5.3 percent survival benefit fifteen years later.[35] What about local recurrence rates—i.e., cancer coming back again in the breast or axilla? *Nearly identical* whether you choose to have a lumpectomy with radiation or mastectomy. Shocking, right? To reiterate, both survival and local recurrence rates are essentially identical whether you keep your breast and radiate or remove your entire breast with mastectomy. Although lumpectomy *without* radiation has similar survival rates, the local recurrence rate will triple compared to adding radiation or choosing mastectomy. Therefore, lumpectomy *without* radiation is usually too risky—exceptions discussed below.

We have all this proof because researchers followed thousands of women for decades after randomizing them into one of three treatment groups: lumpectomy alone, lumpectomy with radiation, or mastectomy; they tracked who lived, who died, who had it come back, and who didn't—and over twenty years later, we still see equal survival, and essentially equal local recurrence between mastectomy and lumpectomy with radiation.[36] Mastectomy had slightly lower long-term local recurrence rates, but this didn't impact survival—and remember, modern adjuvant therapies (a catchall term for postoperative chemo, radiation, anti-estrogens, and targeted therapy) all decrease local recurrence more than before. These studies began in the 1980s, so women received treatments nearly forty years ago. For example, 10 percent of HER2(+) cancers used to recur within three years in the breast after lumpectomy with radiation, but the recent addition of anti-HER2 drugs—*not mastectomy*—now makes it 1 percent.[37]

Whether choosing lumpectomy with radiation or mastectomy, if you accept adjuvant treatments, expect that cancer to stay far away from your breast or chest wall for many years to come—and most likely, forever. For all stages combined, the five-year local recurrence rate is 1.8 percent,[38] and 0.8 percent for stage I cancers.[39] Remember, these are not metatstatic predictions but refer to cancer recurring in the breast or chest skin or nodes near where it all started. Farther down the road of life, as the effects of medications and radiation wear off a bit, and certain cancer cells have a chance to regroup, cancer recurs within ten years 4 to 6 percent of the time,[40] and lifetime rates cap at 10 to 20 percent.[41] So once removed, cancer stays gone from your breast or chest wall 80 to 90 percent of the time—that's pretty good, especially when you remember that local recurrence doesn't mean you will die, although you do have to deal with the tumor all over again. The following increase local recurrence rates, but in most studies, they do so equally for lumpectomy with radiation and mastectomy, so surgical choices remain equivalent: positive nodes, positive margins, age less than forty, lymphovascular invasion, TNBC, untreated HER2(+), more than one tumor in the same quadrant (multifocal) or different quadrants (multicentric), and extensive DCIS.[42] We'll walk through the mastectomy-or-not decision in a minute.

Everything we just discussed pertained to invasive cancer. For DCIS, survival approaches 100 percent no matter what surgery you have, but dealing with it all over again isn't fun. So, fifteen years out, adding radiation after lumpectomy cuts local recurrence from 19 percent to 9 percent (it's probably a smart decision to radiate),[43] whereas local recurrence after mastectomy approaches zero (but that might be rather extreme, all things considered—which we do consider below).[44] By the way, half of those DCIS recurrences are now invasive, so that's disappointing since invasive cancer can become a bigger deal to treat. Local recurrence rates double for positive margins, but bigger is not better; the margin just needs to be "clear" (it's on your path report). Regarding margins, think of a hard-boiled egg. The yolk is cancer, the white part represents a margin of normal cells excised around the cancer. How much white is enough? It turns out, just as long as there's no yolk exposed anywhere, we're good, assuming radiation follows surgery; it's called "no ink on tumor."[45] If you are not radiating, your surgeon will plan to get a bigger margin (more of the egg white around that yolk).

You might be thinking, "Rewind. How do you get breast cancer after mastectomy if there isn't a breast?" I know, it feels unfair. You can still recur where the breast used to be, or in distant metastatic locations. Even in meticulous surgical hands, the skin cannot be scraped clear of every last breast cell. If surgeons did that, you would lose your skin's blood and lymphatic supply, and skin would not survive. Scattered microscopic breast cells remain here and there under the skin and in the axilla, and tumor cells can persist inside the skin vessels (more likely with involved nodes). As stated above, DCIS recurrence after mastectomy is almost zero, but for invasive cancers, residual cancer cells in skin, muscle, or axillary nodes recur 10 to 20 percent over your lifetime, depending on the cancer profile and stage.[46] Regarding metastatic recurrences, when women die from breast cancer, it's because cells leave the breast and land in an organ that they cannot live without: lung, liver, brain, or bone. It stands to reason that if cancer cells are flying around your bloodstream at the time of surgery, whether we scythe around a little tumor or get aggressive with mastectomy, neither operation removes those rogue cells.

Around 28 percent of breast cancers will eventually return with a distant recurrence, but this number is improving.[47]

Knowing that survival and recurrence rates are equal, your surgical choice becomes exactly that—a *choice*, with equal outcomes. Yet many women take off their breasts even if there's no survival advantage. In the United States, 65 percent choose lumpectomy, 35 percent mastectomy.[48] Here are six reasons why you might choose mastectomy:

1. Small breast relative to cancer size, or multiple cancers. While technically possible, lumpectomy will be significantly deforming (and then you have to radiate what's left, *eeek*), so mastectomy looks prettier.

2. Positive margins after attempt(s) to clear them.

3. Not interested in radiation after lumpectomy: already had radiation for a previous cancer, believe it's too toxic, medically unwell (e.g., bad heart disease), don't live where it's offered, have ATM mutation or collagen vascular disease (skin handles radiation poorly).

4. BRCA, other gene mutation, or strong family history of breast cancer.

5. Inflammatory breast cancer always requires mastectomy.

6. Personal preference: "It's my breast, and I just don't want it!" Zoom in. This is the number-one reason I perform mastectomy. This sister likely fears recurrence or clings to a perceived survival benefit that defies statistics (she isn't a numbers person, or she already feels like "1 in 1,000," so stats go out the window).[49] I get it. Your breast has betrayed you, and it has lost its appeal. Perhaps the idea of surveillance, of exams, mammograms, ultrasounds, MRI, and biopsies every time there's a blip on the radar looms as an exhausting eventuality, filling you with anxiety. Or maybe this whole nightmare makes no sense—you're young, no family history, super healthy—and it's as if there's something wrong with your breast DNA; whether we can prove that or not, you know your life will become more peaceful without breasts.

Where Will Your Incisions Be?

Your surgeon will make sure incision locations take into consideration a cancer location (if present), existing scars, cosmetic goals, and breast size reduction (if desired). Ideally, incisions are hidden from view at the border of the areola where skin naturally changes color, or underneath the breast in the inframammary fold, where an underwire sits. When meeting your surgeon, be sure to discuss these details if they're important to you. For example, even when removing the nipple, a slash across the entire chest should only be used when necessary; I often remove just the nipple itself when it has disease close by, and take the breast away through the inframammary incision, leaving the pigmented areola in place—it just looks like you have flat nipples. We can even borrow half of the other nipple and graft it there, so it's all real. Attention to incision location, coupled with the diverse reconstruction techniques available today, will hopefully leave you feeling sexy and strong inside your own skin.

What About the Lymph Nodes?

If cancer exists in the breast, it might escape to axillary lymph nodes via lymphatic vessels. The first node(s) that receive this drainage are called *sentinel nodes*. You have about twenty to forty nodes in each axilla, but you only want to know about the sentinel nodes. Your surgeon will perform a sentinel lymph node biopsy (SLNB) at the time of your breast surgery by injecting blue dye, radioactive tracer, or both, into the breast prior to lumpectomy or mastectomy. The dye/tracer then travels into the armpit, turning an average of two nodes bright blue/radioactive; these are the sentinel nodes that get removed via a small incision in the axilla and tested by a pathologist. Everyone has sentinel nodes. Turning blue/hot doesn't mean they have cancer; these are just the nodes that would have cancer *if cancer spread*, so we test them, and you don't get them back.

"Negative" nodes means cancer didn't spread. "Positive" nodes contain cancer cells. (I know, how confusing: it's a negative thing to have positive nodes.) What happens when they're positive? Well, with three or more sentinel nodes involved, or when your nodes were biopsied and positive before surgery, your surgeon will do a complete axillary lymph node dissection (ALND) removing at least ten nodes. ALND results in complications in up to 84 percent of patients (most are mild and resolve): pain, numbness, fluid buildup (seroma), limited arm movement, infection, or permanent arm swelling (lymphedema).[50] The most feared complication of axillary surgery, lymphedema, occurs in 13 percent ALND and 2 percent SLNB;[51] SLNB reduces all complications to less than 10 percent.[52] When only one or two SLN have cancer, you'll usually be advised to just radiate the whole breast, which usually hits some of the lower-level nodes in the axilla. This radiation leads to the same survival and nodal recurrence as ALND, so of course you'd rather avoid ALND.[53]

Approximately 20 percent of DCIS upgrades to invasion after excision. SLNB at the time of lumpectomy for DCIS is controversial; your surgeon might advise it if you're under fifty-five, planning mastectomy, or if you have disease spanning at least 4 centimeters on mammogram, palpable DCIS, or high-grade DCIS.[54] Most surgeons do *not* perform SLNB in conjunction with prophylactic (preventive) mastectomies, but we find cancer in 2 to 8 percent of removed breasts that weren't expected to have cancer.[55] In this scenario, we can't perform SLNB because there isn't a breast into which dye/tracer can be injected. Now you have to decide: do you want to go back for an ALND to be sure this cancer didn't spread (yikes, elephant arm), or radiate, or just hope for the best? Prophylactic breast dye injection (PBDI) resolves this dilemma by injecting dye at the time of mastectomy, and tagging next to the true sentinel node with a suture or clip, but not removing it. In the rare instance we find cancer, we can go back and just take the correct node or two, but we didn't subject 98 percent of women to an unnecessary node excision. PBDI gives more control and peace of mind to women. I developed this technique in 2013 with the hope that PBDI would give more control and peace of mind to women. Since that time, I have returned to the operating room only once to retrieve the SLBN due to a surprise cancer—and there it was, sitting next to my suture like a little blue pearl.

Can You Spare Your Nipples During a Mastectomy?

Nipple-sparing mastectomies (NSM) allow you to keep all of your breast skin exactly the way you see it in the mirror now—nipples, freckles, scars, and all. The nipples are not taken off you and reattached; through a pencil-thin incision, your surgeon takes all the breast away from underneath the blanket of skin, and then (usually in the same operation) a plastic surgeon puts an implant or tissue under that skin. *It's you*, just with a fake-out of a breast under the skin. NSM have increased by over 200 percent since 2005, with a reported 0.4 percent chance of cancer recurrence in the nipple itself.[56] Unless you have Paget's disease (nipple cancer), inflammatory breast cancer, or cancer cells smack under the nipple ducts, you can safely keep your nipple without compromising survival or recurrence rates. Cosmetic results are usually superior with NSM; you look in the mirror and see a fuller, rounder version of yourself, harkening back to pregnancy days, if you had them, but implants sit higher than your breast likely did. And large-breasted ladies used to being ptotic (droopy) might look and happily think, "Wow, perky!" Drawbacks to NSM: (1) preserved nipples have no sensation or function; (2) it's challenging to lift droopy nipples into a central, symmetrical location; and (3) some skin has terrible blood flow and nipples don't survive postoperatively. I know some tricks.

To this last point, skin or nipple loss, called *necrosis*, occurs from compromised blood supply to the skin. Smokers, diabetics, those with prior radiation, multiple breast scars, severe drooping, obesity, breasts that are larger than a D cup, stretch marks, or vascular disease can have a wimpy skin blood supply. I've actually come up with a fix for this, so if this applies to you, talk to your surgeon about what I'm about to say next. He may already have his own technique to mitigate this issue, but he's welcome to use mine too. Just snap a pic of this page and hand it over!

When you have high-risk skin, and then take the breast with all its blood flow away, that skin becomes a skin-thin parachute hanging over air. How's it even alive? Existing vessels dilate and new ones form to send a rush of blood to the site of injury and trauma to help heal and repair it.[57] In 2008, I heard about surgeons in Italy who had published a few years earlier about using laparoscopic tools through a tiny incision to lift the nipple off the breast weeks prior to mastectomy in an effort to stimulate blood flow to the skin.[58] Later, when the mastectomy happened, the skin said, "I have tons of blood flow; we just did this last week." The idea of ramping up blood flow in tissues prior to moving them has been used by plastic surgeons for centuries.[59]

Using these concepts, I created an open *nipple delay* technique that works like a charm. In the operating room, one to three weeks prior to the actual mastectomies, I make the planned mastectomy incision (a slit in that parachute) and lift half of the skin off the breast surface. I also excise the ducts behind and within the nipple, which get analyzed by pathology, thereby confirming that the nipple is safe to keep from a cancer point of view. Then I put the skin right back down and sew the incision closed. Over the next week or two, that lifted skin automatically recruits all the extra blood flow we will need when we do the mastectomy—so now, women with challenging breasts that would have been denied NSM can preserve their nipples 99 percent of the time.[60] For large or very ptotic breasts, I do the nipple delay through a central incision that curves around the top of the areola and remove a half-moon crescent of skin above this border so that the nipples get lifted higher when the edges are sewn back together. For *very* large-breasted patients who want to keep nipples, we can first do a reduction/lift, taking them down to a C-cup, while removing the cancer and nodes as well. We wait ten weeks (or longer if chemo is needed), do a nipple delay, and then perform NSM—nipples are viable and in great position.[61]

I also keep hyperbaric oxygen therapy in my back pocket, just in case the skin limps along after surgery. This therapy increases the amount of oxygen your blood can carry to struggling skin flaps, further decreasing the likelihood of nipple and skin necrosis.[62] Be sure to put hyperbarics in your back pocket too.

Breast Reconstruction Techniques to Consider

After breast-conservation surgery and radiation, you might desire reconstruction to correct indentations or asymmetry. Your breast surgeon may be skilled in oncoplastic techniques or enlist a plastic surgeon to help, but oncoplastic surgery mobilizes surrounding breast tissue at the time of lumpectomy to reshape the breast. Plastic surgeons use fat grafting (fat harvested from your abdomen, buttocks, or thighs via liposuction gets injected into areas of the breast needing more volume), reduction/lift, tissue rearrangement, scar revision, and other secrets to improve the cosmetic outcome after breast conservation. If your nipples get removed, a projecting nipple with no sensation can be made from the breast skin itself (like origami) or by using skin from elsewhere on the body. Tattoos can recreate a tinted areola as the pigmented circle around a reconstructed nipple, or you can opt for a surprisingly realistic 3-D–appearing tattooed nipple.

Gone are the days of an unrealistic grapefruit stuck onto your chest, meant to replace a shapely sloping breast that once held that place. Reconstruction options vary depending on your desired aesthetic outcome, body size, general health, prior breast operations, and radiation exposures. Two broad categories of reconstruction exist: implants and flaps, or a combo of both. You'll discuss all the options relevant to you personally with your surgical team, but I will give you a broad-strokes overview of what's possible.

Preferably, surgeons reconstruct immediately during the same operation as mastectomy rather than delay this process weeks to years later. Implants are the most common reconstruction method in the United States.[63] During what's called *one-step* or *direct-to-implant operations*, your plastic surgeon places the permanent implant at the time of mastectomy. Sometimes it's too risky to push an implant snugly against a skin flap that just had most of its blood supply stripped away fifteen minutes ago by a mastectomy. One-step works well for smaller breasted women who don't care to be bigger. Otherwise, we find a majority of patients back in the operating room to tweak things: too big, too small, too far apart, nipples didn't align symmetrically, they need fat grafting around the edges . . . one-step actually becomes two.

More often, implant reconstruction involves placing what's called a *tissue expander*, which is basically a deflated implant, under the skin or behind your chest muscle. Expanders maximize blood flow to the breast skin and nipple because they remain deflated after placement and don't squish the tiny blood vessels in the skin. They get slowly inflated with saline or air over a period of one to three months until you reach the desired volume. Expanders allow your surgeon to optimize the final implant size, location, appearance, and nipple position because there's a second operation. The expanders get swapped out for the permanent implant, which is usually silicone, since saline ripples and sloshes too much without a breast over it.

Another option, called *autologous flaps*, use your own skin, fat, and sometimes muscle from the abdomen (TRAM or DIEP flap), back (latissimus), thigh (gracilis), or buttock (gluteal) to create a more natural breast reconstruction than implants can achieve, since body tissues and fat slope more like a breast. Flaps, however, create scars and potential weakness at the donor site and require longer operations than implants, with lengthier hospital stays and recovery periods. With the rise in bilateral mastectomy, sometimes there isn't enough tissue to recreate two breasts. You will find a lot of variation in reconstruction across regions in the United States and internationally, depending on where you live. There's no better or worse choice—just the right one for you.

Despite the fact that US state and federal laws mandate insurance coverage for reconstruction, 65 to 75 percent of women who have a mastectomy do not undergo it.[64] In a multiethnic survey of over 2,200 mastectomy patients from Los Angeles and Detroit, factors associated with not undergoing reconstruction included lower educational level, increased age, competing illnesses, African American race, and chemotherapy. The most common patient-reported reasons were the desire to avoid additional surgery (48.5 percent) and the belief that reconstruction wasn't important (33.8 percent).[65] To be sure, I have a growing number of "flat and fabulous" patients who were fully informed about their options, opted out of reconstruction, and love their choice.

WHEN SHOULD YOU OPERATE?

Although a cancer diagnosis feels like an emergency, it's more of an emotional emergency than a biological one, so you have some time to put your ducks in a row. However, don't let those ducks wander all over the place. A 2016 analysis of US cancer databases shows that you want to move toward surgery or chemo within four weeks of diagnosis.[66] In 94,544 cancer patients over sixty-six (average age: seventy-five), five-year survival rates were 4.6 percent lower in those waiting over three months versus less than one month; this was only seen for stages I and II, not III. So ironically, when your cancer is diagnosed early, you're the one who doesn't have as much time to waste. In 115,790 women ages eighteen-plus (average age: sixty) the 5YS rate dropped 3.1 percent by waiting over three months versus less than one month, and again only for early stages.

Lumpectomy with any axillary surgery, nipple delays, tissue expander swaps, as well as mastectomy without reconstruction are outpatient operations and take one to two hours. You head home an hour after surgery armed with ibuprofen and maybe a small handful of narcotics. The next day you can shower and drive, if you feel like you can operate a vehicle safely and aren't taking narcotics. You can even work, although more extensive operations or axillary dissection might keep you home a week.

Mastectomy with implant reconstruction can also be outpatient, but is more often done with a one-to-two-day hospital stay or recovery in an aftercare facility. Flap reconstructions are done in the hospital with variable lengths of stay. Expect to be sore, gradually improving, feeling fine two weeks after, and feeling great four to six weeks later, at which time you can return to work—except for housework. None of that for five years. (Joking!)

What About Pre- and Post-Op Meds and Supplements?

Many of my patients take daily supplements, so they like hearing what might support their body during the surgical process. I'm sharing my favorite perioperative support supplements here, but be sure to run this list by your surgeon for approval. You really don't need to consider doing any of this for a simple lumpectomy, but for longer cancer operations and especially mastectomies, I find that women enjoy contributing to their healing process in a proactive way, and employing some or all of these suggestions allows you to do exactly that. Also, as soon as you schedule surgery, show your surgeon a current list of medications and supplements, as some promote bleeding and need to be stopped seven days pre-op, such as aspirin, ginkgo, and vitamin E.

Consider taking the following supplements beginning two weeks before surgery. Continue them until one week after lumpectomy or four weeks after mastectomy.

These supplements enhance wound healing (I realize this is a ridiculous number of pills, so try blending them into my Antioxidant Smoothie each morning):

- Vitamin A: 25,000 IU daily
- Vitamin C: 1,000 milligrams daily
- Zinc: 30 milligrams daily
- Glucosamine: 1,500 milligrams daily
- High-potency multivitamin: 1 daily
- Aloe vera gel: ¼ cup inner fillet daily[67] (Acemannan in the gel revs up the immune system with inflammation-reducing cytokines; side benefit: anthraquinones suppress breast cancer activity by decreasing ER-alpha.)[68]

To help detoxify after anesthesia, hydrate with a glass of water every two hours while awake. You'll also want to avoid meat, dairy, refined sugar, and alcohol for forty-eight hours, since fat-soluble anesthetics are excreted in the bile, and these foods slow bile down. I also suggest bumping up the fiber (think broccoli, beets) and sulfur-rich foods (garlic, onion). Take ¼ teaspoon turmeric daily, and sip on three to six cups of green or dandelion teas for forty-eight hours.[69] For operations that will last longer than three hours, I recommend supplementing with a lipotropic detox combo one week before and two weeks after surgery: choline (1,000 milligrams) and methionine (1,000 milligrams) daily,[70] which move the fat and bile along, plus milk thistle (silymarin, 140 milligrams) three times daily.[71]

And as you heal, I'd recommend a few things to reduce swelling, bruising, and nausea. To reduce swelling and bruising, put five dissolving granules of arnica under your tongue just before heading off to the OR, and take five more when you awaken. Begin bromelain (1,000 milligrams) daily after surgery for inflammation.[72] And as a quick fix for nausea, take ginger root powder (1,000 milligrams)[73] and noni fruit extract (600 milligrams)[74] one hour before surgery, and ginger root once more after you're fully awake. You can't eat or drink anything for eight hours prior to surgery, but I allow these supplements with a tiny sip of water.

Finally, you'll want to do all you can to keep the site of your surgery as clean as possible. Showering with chlorhexidine-based skin antiseptics like Hibiclens once a day for three days prior to surgery decreases infection rates.[75] Put it on dry skin, neck to belly button, hang out for three minutes, and rinse. Be sure to tell your surgeon if you develop a fever, infection (skin, tooth, urine), or illness in the days prior to surgery, since an infection elsewhere in your body increases surgical breast infections, and your surgeon might prefer to postpone until you're feeling better. Lastly, a number of silicone-based creams and adhesives directly applied to healing incisions prevent upraised scars, or keloids. Start using these one week post-op, and continue twice a day for twelve weeks.

Bogus Surgical Myths That Won't Help You One Bit

There are a number of surgical claims related to breast cancer that really mess with the preoperative zen I try to create. Here are the two I debunk most.

I often hear patients express concern that exposing cancer cells to air makes them spread. Tumors actually flourish in a *low* oxygen environment. This fact has driven an entire movement focused on the delivery of oxygen to cancer cells in an effort to destroy them.[76] Yet in a questionnaire survey of 626 cancer patients, 38 percent of patients stated they believe air exposure at surgery causes tumor spread.[77] If held strongly, this belief would have devastating outcomes as women decline lifesaving surgery.[78] Cancer cells metastasize out of the breast via lymphatics and blood vessels, and exposing cells to air doesn't suddenly escort them into lymphatics or blood; if anything, a blast of O_2 would kill cancer cells on the spot.

Another request patients sometimes make is that I operate according to their menstrual cycle, claiming this improves survival. This concept originated in 1988 when experiments noted a timing correlation in mice with breast cancer.[79] In the 1990s, this tale I call "Of Mice and Women" enthused dozens of researchers as they set out to investigate the surgery/menses hypothesis. It's pretty funny, actually. Studies from Camp Follicular Phase stated that operations during cycle days zero to fourteen led to lower local recurrence rates and higher survival rates.[80] "Not so fast!" said Camp Luteal Phase, confirming that operating during days fifteen to thirty-two actually led to longer lives.[81] "Hold the phone!" cried Camp Any Phase, concluding that no association exists.[82] Further complicating matters, these studies assumed every woman ovulates like clockwork on day fifteen. (Really? And after a cancer diagnosis?) Shifting the natural cycle length in these same studies by a few days up or back suddenly jumps many patients from Camp Luteal to Follicular, or vice versa.[83]

To prove the surgical timing theory, three prospective studies defined the menstrual phase by blood hormone levels, not by asking frazzled cancer patients to recall their last menstrual period.[84] Guess what? They all side with Camp Any Phase. When phases were biochemically defined, no difference in recurrence or survival emerged between Camps Luteal and Follicular.

WHEN IT'S TIME FOR RADIATION

What is radiation exactly, and how does it work? Radiation uses high-energy X-rays (photons) precisely targeting the breast itself, the chest wall after mastectomy, and/or surrounding lymph nodes in an effort to "sterilize" any straggler cancer cells that want to make a repeat appearance at some point in your future.

There's no question that radiation helps vanquish remaining sinister cells. In the 1990s, large trials showed that lumpectomy without radiation led to local recurrence in 35 percent of cases twelve years later, but adding radiation dropped it to 10 percent.[85] As noted above, modern radiation techniques place ten-year recurrence at 4 to 6 percent. Recurrences happen because residual microscopic disease exists in the breast despite a lumpectomy with clear margins. Upon evaluating three hundred mastectomy specimens with cancers smaller than 4 centimeters, spots of cancer were noted more than 2 centimeters away from the main cancer in 43 percent—meaning, had they chosen lumpectomy, those cells would never have been removed, and everyone would have thought the margins were fine.[86] Added bonus: breast cancer–specific survival (as opposed to dying of a heart attack or something else) at fifteen years goes up 5 percent in women who receive radiation after lumpectomy (many women choose *chemo* for 5 percent).[87]

Even after mastectomy, you sometimes need radiation for invasive tumors larger than 5 centimeters, skin or muscle involvement, four or more positive nodes, positive margins, positive nodes after chemo, and extensive lymphovascular invasion.[88] Case-by-case consideration is given to one to three positive nodes or close margins after mastectomy, since modern-era chemo and endocrine therapies leave little opportunity for radiation to improve numbers.[89] By the way, if you require radiation after mastectomy with implant reconstruction, be sure to follow this regimen in order to minimize the skin and muscle tightening that leads to capsular contracture (squeezing of the implant): starting day one of radiation, take Singulair 10 mg, one tablet a day for three months; starting one week after radiation, take Trental 400 mg one tablet three times a day for six months; starting one week after radiation, take vitamin E 1,200 IU, one tablet a day for six months.[90]

Radiation energy sources can be external, from a large machine outside your body sending beams into your breast, or internal, from a small device temporarily placed inside the breast where the cancer used to be, sending a circumferential ring of radiation from the inside out. Your radiation oncologist will suggest one of four radiation options for both invasive and DCIS cancers—two external, two internal: (1) whole breast irradiation (WBI); (2) accelerated whole breast irradiation (AWBI); (3) accelerated partial breast irradiation (APBI); or (4) intraoperative radiation therapy (IORT). IORT happens during surgery, but the other three are delivered after surgery; if chemo is planned, APBI comes before, and WBI/AWBI come after chemo.

WBI has been the standard for eons, and it remains the *only radiation option* for breast cancers invading skin or chest wall, positive lymph nodes, postmastectomy, or inflammatory subtype. Additionally, nodes near your sternum and above and below your collarbone get radiated along with the axilla if you had four or more positive nodes, and possibly with one to three nodes as well. Starting three to six weeks after surgery, WBI happens every day, Monday through Friday, for five to seven weeks. It takes about twenty minutes for setup and delivery of a painless, invisible beam to your breast as you lie on a table, but these daily interruptions are exhausting and inconvenient.

Do we really need thirty-three sessions? Not always. An accelerated version (AWBI) cuts thirty-three treatments to fifteen or sixteen over three to four weeks, otherwise delivered the same way as WBI, with the same safety and cancer-killing efficacy.[91] To be eligible for AWBI, cancers must be smaller than 5 centimeters, in only one quadrant of the breast, with clear margins, negative nodes, and a breast width less than 25 centimeters. Two delivery techniques—3-D–conformal radiation therapy (3DCRT) and intensity-modulated radiation therapy (IMRT)—minimize collateral damage to innocent surrounding organs, such as lung and heart (especially for left-sided cancers, since your heart is on the left). The last few doses of WBI/AWBI hit only the cancer site to give it an extra punch, called a boost. *Proton therapy*, with even more precision and less collateral damage, is still emerging in breast cancer treatment, with only a handful of centers offering it and an absence of trials comparing results to tried-and-true photons.

Is three weeks still too long for you? Ask your doctor about these forms of APBI: (1) catheter-based techniques (SAVI, MammoSite, and Contura devices) require percutaneous insertion of the device into the empty space where the cancer used to be. This can be done under local anesthetic in the office (just like a core biopsy). Part of the catheter sticks out of your skin through which we thread radioactive iridium seeds; you're plugged in for ten minutes twice a day (separated by six hours) for two to five days, done. (2) Multicatheter interstitial brachytherapy involves placing fifteen to twenty catheters around the lumpectomy site (in and out of the skin like a safety pin). Then we do the radioactive seed thing as above. I am not a big fan of the second method when we have the first, because I just worked really hard to make your breast look beautiful, so why make thirty to forty entrance/exit scars like a railroad track on your skin? It works, though. (3) You can also use the same 3DCRT and IMRT external beam machines, but aim *only* at the lumpectomy site twice a day for five days.

Seven randomized clinical trials all show nearly identical local recurrence rates for all three forms of accelerated partial breast irradiation as compared to WBI/AWBI, but APBI inclusion criteria must be met: at least age forty (some radiation docs want you to be fifty), tumor smaller than 3 centimeters, node negative, ductal subtype (not lobular), margins negative, and no lymphovascular invasion.[92] APBI works because 85 percent of cancer recurrences occur within 2 centimeters of where they started, so in properly chosen patients, you just need to blast that area, not the entire breast.[93] APBI limits implant contracture (tight squeezing) in women with augmentation. Psst . . . keep this tidbit handy: APBI can treat local recurrence in the breast even after WBI; so, if you really don't want a mastectomy despite a recurrence, repeat radiation is possible—you can have WBI once, and APBI once.[94]

IORT delivers a single dose in the operating room at the time of lumpectomy (not applicable to mastectomy) by wrapping a device in the space where the cancer used to be, and then radiating the site for twenty to twenty-five minutes (you snooze through the whole show). Since we don't have confirmation of the final pathology at the time of radiation, you may not have actually qualified for IORT; nevertheless, you can move on to WBI and consider the IORT your boost. Two trials comparing whole breast irradiation (WBI) to IORT show local recurrences at five years that are quite low, but still higher than WBI,[95] so it's not ready for prime time, but you can join trials.[96]

You are not radioactive during or after any chosen radiation, so hug your kids or grandkids with abandon. Radiation can feel isolating and depressing in the moments of receiving it, but I encourage you to feel grateful for this important therapy; the International Atomic Energy Agency (IAEA) estimates that the world lacks at least five thousand radiotherapy machines in developing countries. As a result, up to 70 percent of cancer patients who would benefit from radiation do not receive it.[97]

Most short-term side effects resolve after a month of external radiation: fatigue (the biggest complaint); "sunburned" skin appearing red, darkened, blistered, warm, itchy, dry, tender, or peeling (apply Aquaphor, argan oil, or vitamin E); heavy or swollen breast. Potential long-term side effects include: shrunken, firmer breast; nerve damage (knife-like stabbing "zingers" last seconds, maybe twice a week, forever); lymphedema (swelling) of the breast, chest, or arm; fractured ribs.[98] Radiation-induced cancers of the lung, esophagus, thyroid, and connective tissues or vessels are rare (e.g., lymphangiosarcoma risk is less than 0.5 percent),[99] but they are 23 percent higher than general female population risk and peak ten to fifteen years following treatment.[100] You can't produce milk from radiated breasts. APBI complications include telangiectasias (little spidery red vessels on the skin at the treatment site), infection, trapped fluid, and forming a firm ball of palpable or tender fat necrosis.[101] Once radiated, especially with WBI/AWBI, your skin and muscle never forget that insult, losing elasticity and vascularity, which can complicate reconstruction if future mastectomy is needed for a recurrence.

Can certain women safely avoid radiation altogether? Yes. In fact, National Comprehensive Cancer Network (NCCN) treatment guidelines advise women over seventy years to entirely skip radiation for estrogen-positive tumors less than 2 centimeters, and negative nodes on endocrine therapy.[102] In this group, WBI only reduces five-year recurrence from 4.1 percent to 1.3 percent with the same survival rates, so many women decide to skip six weeks of heat and avoid all those side effects.[103] For women older than twenty-six with DCIS, your breast recurrence at eight years will be 6.7 percent without radiation, and 0.9 percent with it, but your DCIS must be smaller than 2.5 centimeters, grade 1 or 2, with at least a 3 millimeter clear margin.[104] If we allow DCIS of any grade up to 5 centimeters and any margin, fifteen years later, radiation will have dropped recurrence from 31 percent to 18 percent.[105] Genomic assays (Oncotype DX, PreludeDx) predict local recurrence of DCIS on an individualized basis and can add value when debating the benefit of radiation.[106] The critical ingredient to successfully avoiding radiation in reasonable candidates is to achieve 5 to 10 millimeters of clear margins.

ENDOCRINE/HORMONAL THERAPY

Despite the fact that hormonal therapy can cause menopause déjà vu or this-girl-is-on-fire feelings, most women feel rather relieved that they can take a little dose of something working against cancer everyday. There can be some serious peace of mind that comes in the shape of a pill.

Approximately 80 percent of all breast cancers demonstrate estrogen receptors ER(+) and progesterone receptors PR(+), and when naturally circulating hormones trigger these receptors, cancer cells multiply and divide.[107] Endocrine (hormonal) therapies either block estrogen at the receptor itself, or eliminate estrogen production in the body. If your cancer demonstrates ER(+) or PR(+), your medical oncologist or surgeon will definitely be talking to you about endocrine therapy. Here are the most common, so you can familiarize yourself with their names and actions.

Endocrine therapy usually comes in the form of pills, although there's liquid too. They're taken daily for five to ten years and include tamoxifen and aromatase inhibitors (AI). Tamoxifen works by fitting into the estrogen receptor to inactivate it, like gum pressed into a lock, so cancer cells peter out without their fuel; however, in the uterus and bones, it's proestrogen. This is to say, it's a *selective* estrogen receptor modulator (SERM). Another SERM, toremifene (Fareston), is only approved for metastatic breast cancer. The AIs—anastrozole (Arimidex), exemestane (Aromasin), and letrozole (Femara)—halt the conversion of androgens into estrogen by shutting down the converting enzyme, aromatase, in your adrenals, ovaries, brain, liver, skin, and fat. Fulvestrant (Faslodex) tags estrogen receptors for destruction and is the only ER-downregulator (ERD) prescribed for the treatment of postmenopausal breast cancer. Faslodex adds 20 percent more disease-free time (months without any sign of cancer in your body) than Arimidex (16.6 months versus 13.8) in those with locally advanced or metastatic ER(+) HER2(-) cancers.[108] It's given monthly by intramuscular injection. Hormonal therapy usually begins after completing surgery, radiation, and chemo. The main goal is to prevent recurrence, but sometimes we give these medications neoadjuvantly (prior to surgery) to shrink a cancer, and occasionally they keep cancer in check for those with other illnesses that prevent us from treating the breast with curative intent.

For invasive cancers, irrespective of chemo use, age, node, or PR status, tamoxifen reduces in-breast recurrence by 47 percent, new cancers in the opposite breast by 50 percent, and improves survival by 29 percent.[109] (Interestingly, these numbers look nearly identical to those reported in all the soy studies we reviewed in chapter 3, further validating the tamoxifen-like behavior of that little bean.) AIs are more effective than tamoxifen in postmenopausal women and should be preferentially chosen for this group.[110] If you have functioning ovaries, taking an AI won't stop your ovaries from churning out estradiol, so you either take tamoxifen, or shut your ovaries down and then take an AI. Why do that? In premenopausal women at high risk for recurrence, ovarian suppression plus an AI keeps them breast cancer–free by another 1 to 15 percent over tamoxifen.[111] We can put ovaries to sleep *reversibly* with monthly subcutaneous injections of goserelin (Zoladex), leuprolide (Lupron), or triptorelin (Trelstar), or *permanently* with chemo (sometimes) or oophorectomy (surgical removal). Extending endocrine therapy an additional five years reduces recurrence at the ten-year mark from 25.1 percent to 21.4 percent, and death from 15 percent to 12.2 percent.[112] A number of combinations exist using tamoxifen followed by an AI (once postmenopausal), or vice versa, or tamoxifen for ten years.[113] The genomic assay Breast Cancer Index (BCI) analyzes your cancer cells, personalizing the benefit from an additional five years of endocrine therapy; the side effects might not be worth the benefit depending on your cancer's unique genetic makeup. Since endocrine therapy improves survival by reducing metastases, you need to consider taking it even after double mastectomy for invasive cancer (which could have escaped the breast), but not for DCIS. After lumpectomy with radiation for DCIS, tamoxifen drops breast recurrence by 42 percent, and contralateral cancers by 50 percent, but it doesn't add benefit after double mastectomy for DCIS.[114] AIs have not been formally studied in DCIS.

Endocrine therapy side effects look annoyingly like menopause with hot flashes (30 percent of women), insomnia (20 percent), weight gain (20 percent), decreased sex drive (16 percent), and fatigue (20 percent).[115] Women can also experience night sweats, vaginal dryness, vaginal discharge, leg cramps, mood swings, dry skin, and thinning hair. Tamoxifen complications occur in fewer than 1 percent of users and include cataracts, blood clots in large veins (deep vein thrombosis, DVT) or lungs (pulmonary embolism, PE), stroke, and uterine cancer. Notably, tamoxifen-induced uterine cancer prior to age fifty is so rare that the American College of Obstetricians and Gynecologists does not even recommend monitoring for it. Joint pain and osteoporosis are frequent AI issues. Zoladex, Lupron, and Trelstar can cause bone pain, weight gain, hot flashes, nausea, and pain where injected. Faslodex-takers might notice joint pain, hot flashes, fatigue, and nausea. I feel bad leaving you hanging here at the end of this paragraph after listing all of those miserable symptoms, but never fear—I have some remedies to share in chapter 10.

TARGETED DRUG THERAPIES

Targeted drug therapies behave like medicinal arrows slung at specific receptors or proteins critical to cancer's survival. They can be used before or after surgery, or newly called into action against local recurrence or distant metastases. Most side effects are tolerated well.

Let's start with HER2 therapies, which lock onto HER2 receptors with such precision that they have taken what was once a highly fatal subtype and turned it into a highly *favorable* subtype. You get a flu shot to make antibodies that recognize and destroy an antigen, right? Similarly, trastuzumab (Herceptin) is a man-made antibody against the HER2 protein, which fuels about 15 percent of cancers. Given through an IV, initially with chemotherapy, Herceptin continues once every three weeks for a year after chemo stops. In metastatic cancer, it continues indefinitely. A 3 percent cardiac toxicity exists when combined with doxorubicin or epirubicin (chemo drugs), so your heart gets monitored with an echocardiogram or MUGA scan every three to six months.[116] An FDA-approved medication biologically similar to Herceptin can be used instead and is called trastuzumab-dkst (Ogivri).[117]

Pertuzumab (Perjeta) attacks HER2 at a different spot than Herceptin; it's given through an IV before surgery with Herceptin due to synergistic effects and sometimes after surgery or in advanced-stage cancer. A third HER2 antibody IV drug, ado-trastuzumab emtansine (Kadcyla, a.k.a TDM-1), treats advanced-stage cancer. Other anti-HER2 arrows include the daily pill kinase inhibitors, lapatinib (Tykerb), and neratinib (Nerlynx). Tykerb treats advanced cancers after Herceptin fails, and Nerlynx helps early stages after Herceptin's year is up.

Next: cyclin-dependent kinase (CDK) inhibitors. These are arrows flung into two proteins, CDK4 and CDK6, to slow or stop cell division. Palbociclib (Ibrance) or ribociclib (Kisqali) works alongside aromatase inhibitors to halt ER(+) HER2(-) advanced cancer cells from growing in both premenopausal and postmenopausal women, and they have been shown to *double* the amount of time it takes for disease to progress.[118] If you are taking this combination of palbociclib and an AI, I have a word of caution: some natural estrogen-like compounds in food can interfere with these medications. Avoid all soy (genistein) and all conventionally raised cow products and corn (zearalenone), which inactivate this powerful drug combo in tissue cultures.[119] These pills are taken daily for three weeks, with one week off before resuming again.

Your doctor may also recommend mTOR inhibitors such as everolimus (Afinitor), which send arrows into the mTOR protein, involved in cell division and angiogenesis. When advanced ER(+) HER2(-) cancer cells grow despite letrozole or anastrozole use, postmenopausal women can switch to the daily pills Aromasin and Afinitor to block the mTOR protein.

Finally, PARP inhibitors fling arrows into poly (ADP-ribose) polymerase (PARP), an enzyme involved in DNA repair. The pill, olaparib (Lynparza), slows down progression of stage IV cancer in BRCA-1 and -2 carriers with metastatic TNBC or ER(+) HER2(-) disease, possibly by preventing cancer cells damaged by chemo from repairing themselves.

Bull's-eye! Target reached and destroyed, or at least effectively disabled.

IS IMMUNOTHERAPY THE ANSWER?

Cancers are resourceful enemies, creating resistance to our poisons by manipulating the very immune system designed to seek and destroy them. A functional immune system sets off the car alarm when intruders like bacteria, viruses, parasites, and cancer try to hijack what belongs to you, in order to fuel themselves and leave you stranded. The goal of immunotherapy is to boost your body's innate immune system such that it actively identifies and neutralizes micrometastases while leaving healthy cells unharmed. Herceptin is a *passive* immunotherapy agent, useful only when repeatedly injected into you. In contrast, *active* immunotherapy and breast cancer vaccines initiate a sustained immune activation so your body continually fights cancer long after traditional treatments have been completed. Ongoing immunotherapy and vaccine trials investigate ways to prevent breast cancer from starting, returning, and/or metastasizing.[120] To see if a trial exists for you, visit breastcancertrials.org.

Immunotherapy holds tremendous promise on the breast cancer front as both a life-extending treatment in metastatic patients and as a cancer-prevention vaccine, as evidenced already in these immunotherapy successes: a preventive vaccine for cervical cancer and the first-ever therapy proven to extend the lives of patients with metastatic melanoma.

COMPLEMENTARY AND ALTERNATIVE MEDICINE (CAM)

Complementary and alternative medicine (CAM) integrates an array of therapies and botanicals with the typical Western offerings. CAM helps you better prevent, treat, and recover from illness, sometimes with evidence-based certainty and other times with a can't-hurt-might-help attitude. CAM should not be confused with "alternative therapy," which rejects standard treatments altogether in favor of something unproven. Especially with a nonterminal invasive cancer diagnosis, dismissing therapies that have been repeatedly proven to lead to a cure is usually dangerous and unwise. Still, it's always your cancer and your breast and your life and your choice—and others should support you as best they can.

I routinely integrate complementary and alternative medicine (CAM) into my surgical practice. I remember a patient on tamoxifen who complained miserably about hot flashes every time I saw her. For four years she ignored my suggestions to try acupuncture. One day, she unexpectedly stopped by the office just to tell me, "Doctor Kristi, I finally went to Dr. Mao two months ago—one time—and I haven't had a hot flash since!" A randomized trial compared twelve weeks of venlafaxine (Effexor) to acupuncture for the treatment of hot flashes in women on an antiestrogen.[121] Both groups equally reported fewer hot flashes and less depression, but get this: the venlafaxine group had side effects like nausea and dizziness, and two weeks posttreatment, hello, hot flashes all over again. Meanwhile the acupuncture group not only stayed flash-free without side effects, they had side *benefits* including increased sex drive, more energy, clearer thought, and a sense of well-being.

A survey of over four thousand cancer survivors showed the following CAM methods being sought: prayer/spiritual practice (61.4 percent), relaxation (44.3 percent), faith/spiritual healing (42.4 percent), nutritional supplements/vitamins (40.1 percent), meditation (15 percent), religious counseling (11.3 percent), massage (11.2 percent), and support groups (9.7 percent).[122] The least prevalent interventions included hypnosis (0.4 percent), biofeedback therapy (1.0 percent), and acupuncture/acupressure (1.2 percent). Those seeking complementary practices were more often female, younger, white, higher income, and more educated. In an MD Anderson Cancer Center survey, 83.3 percent had used at least one CAM approach,[123] 82 percent reported doing so in Canada,[124] and in fourteen European countries, CAM use ranged from 15 to 73 percent.[125] There is tremendous opportunity for cancer centers to fill a CAM void by offering services, providing reliable information, and initiating research.

In addition to the CAM practices listed above, traditional Chinese medicine (TCM), Ayurvedic medicine, mind-body exercise (*qigong, tai chi*), aromatherapy, essential oils, medicinal mushrooms (reishi, turkey tail, shiitake, maitake), milk thistle, mistletoe (iscador), laughter, stress reduction techniques, yoga, art/dance/music therapies, herbal medicine, teas, chiropractic care, kinesiology, osteopathy, Reiki, visualization/guided imagery, psychoactive tetrahydrocannabinol (THC), and nonpsychoactive cannabidiol (CBD) have all been tried with variable success to increase the body's ability to fight cancer and/or improve physical and emotional well-being.

ONE JOURNEY ENDS; ANOTHER BEGINS

Assuming you just delved into the complexities of a cancer diagnosis and pondered all the treatment decisions that follow, you deserve an honorary medical degree right now. But reading it is one thing—*enduring* it is quite another. I wish I could say that once all your active cancer treatments end, you'll heal up as good as if nothing ever happened—the way I could promise you after pulling a piece of broken glass out of your foot. Alas, the majority of warriors must now transition to assuaging lingering side effects and avoiding a recurrence. We have a lot of living left to do, so join me in chapter 10, and let's continue the journey.

CHAPTER 10

Now What? Life After Diagnosis and Treatment

For most women who've undergone breast cancer treatment, the worst of the storm passes and life assumes a new normal. The incessant doctors appointments disappear, and while you're grateful for that, it's a little weird. As you sit on the sidelines catching your breath, you may wonder how to move on with your life. Days ago, the rules seemed pretty clear: accept that a knife will be cutting into your flesh, endure cancer-killing juices through your veins, and tolerate X-rays beaming onto your chest. Perhaps you felt weak and vulnerable or ill, but at least you had a plan and knew what to do and where to go next. But now the inactivity, the silence, *the absence of active illness*, can feel eerie, even frightening. This gives your mind time to wander: Will rogue cancer cells seize this moment to flourish?

This often-bumpy transition must take place in every journey. Nothing feels the way it did before your cancer detour, and it never will. I call it the inevitable BC/AC: Before Cancer/After Cancer. How do you overcome the trauma and assign purpose to the pain? You're not dead, so how do you plan to live? My deepest hope is that women emerge from their treatment phase victorious, recognizing their worth, redefining their beauty, celebrating their resilience, and having the courage to persevere . . . because the journey continues, and it's filled with choices. You cannot control the ultimate outcome of anything, really, but you can choose how you respond to your cancer experience. What attitude will you adopt—grateful, joyful, hopeful, and being a warrior, or angry, fearful, sad, and being a victim? What decisions will you make about medications, surveillance, psychosocial wholeness, relationships, nutrition, fitness, and spirituality? In this final chapter, we will explore posttreatment life: monitoring for recurrence, managing complications, and deepening relationships—with God, with others, and with yourself.

ONGOING SURVEILLANCE

After cancer, it's incredibly important to stay in tune with your body and to communicate anything out of the ordinary to your physician. Health-related inconveniences or oddities that you may have ignored or waited to investigate before cancer now warrant prompt exploration.

Conditions to report to your physician run the gamut from seemingly innocent to clearly dangerous. Not every new ache or pain is cancer knocking, of course—if you nick yourself shaving, you'll get a cut; if you start doing Pilates, your chest muscles will feel sore—but anything that persists deserves mentioning to your doctor. Be sure to ask her, "Could this be from breast cancer?" She might forget that you had cancer a decade ago and miss a true sign of recurrence. Continue, too, to perform monthly breast self-exams to search for anything that wasn't there before—a lump, skin change, nipple discharge—as explained in chapter 1. New symptoms that should raise an eyebrow include:

- bone pain
- fractures
- constipation
- decreased alertness
- extreme fatigue
- difficulty breathing with activities that never caused shortness of breath before (like walking up a flight of stairs)

- a cough without a cold
- dizziness
- blurry vision
- weakness on one side
- headaches
- confusion
- memory loss
- difficulty speaking or moving
- seizures
- nausea
- increased abdominal girth (pants too tight at waist)
- yellow, itchy skin
- swollen hands/feet
- loss of appetite
- unintentional weight loss

The American Society of Clinical Oncology (ASCO) updates evidence-based guidelines on breast cancer follow-up and management in asymptomatic patients after curative therapy.[1] For tumors smaller than 5 centimeters and fewer than four positive nodes, recommendations include physical examination every three to six months for the first three years, every six to twelve months for years four and five, and annually thereafter. Commonly, your medical, radiation, and surgical oncologists will have their own surveillance schedules that make for even more frequent exams, but evidence does not support doing this. For those with stage III or IV cancers, your treatment team will personalize the surveillance plan, and you might find yourself always in some form of treatment, especially if stage IV. Per ASCO, surveillance by any practitioner experienced in examining breast cancer patients, including radiated breasts, leads to identical outcomes as when specialists do the follow-up, and patients are satisfied. You should perform breast self-exams (see easybreastexam.com for video instruction), and be sure to report new lumps, bone pain, chest pain, difficulty catching your breath, abdominal pain, or persistent headaches to your physician.

For women who still have their breasts, mammography is due one year after your last mammo, or six months after completion of radiation therapy, whichever comes first. Continue mammos on the cancer side every six months until stable, and then resume your annual mammography. Don't worry about checking blood panels and tumor markers (CEA, CA 15–3, and CA 27.29), bone scans, chest X-rays, liver and pelvic ultrasounds, PET/CT scans, and MRI as routine follow-up if you're otherwise asymptomatic with no specific findings after your doctor examines you. It seems counterintuitive, but early detection of metastatic disease offers no survival advantage when compared to waiting for symptoms, finding metastases, and then pursuing treatments.[2] Therefore, a routine search for metastatic disease is not recommended without symptoms, such as back pain prompting a bone scan.

Even so, I suggest customizing a surveillance plan with your physicians. For example, if mammograms missed your lobular cancer but MRI detected it, your doctor might choose to add annual MRI to surveillance. In dense-breasted women or gene mutation carriers, he might also add ultrasound. On a more sophisticated level, a prospective study found 24 percent of women with early stage cancers had circulating tumor cells (CTCs) in their blood prior to any chemotherapy.[3] Follow-up showed that CTCs predicted early recurrence and decreased survival, so talk to your doctor about possibly screening for CTCs in nonmetastatic breast cancer to potentially allow for early intervention and a longer life. When cancer cells rupture and die, they release circulating cell-free DNA (cfDNA), genome fragments that float freely through the bloodstream. One study showed that cfDNA predicted metastatic recurrence better than the tumor marker CA 15–3.[4] Finding CTCs and cfDNA via blood sampling is called a *liquid biopsy*; uses for these blood tests are evolving. True, the current methods for identifying metastatic disease (like PET/CT or CA 15–3) do not improve survival over simply responding to symptoms, but liquid biopsies might flip that reality. Ask your medical oncologist if you should get liquid biopsies.

As you ease back into everyday life, don't neglect your overall health either. You're still prone to heart disease, diabetes, high cholesterol, and other illnesses just the same as you'd be without cancer. Your oncology team likely won't focus on general wellness, so it's up to you to keep this ball rolling in the right direction.

STAY ORGANIZED

After cancer treatment, patients can get lost in the transition from being actively treated to passively followed by their doctor. Once cancer becomes part of your past, you still need to keep records of what's been done, what will be done in the future, and who will be doing it.

You can download a free tool at pinklotus.com/thrivership called the "Thrivership Care Plan" that provides a comprehensive list of all the documents you must collect, and the questions you must ask your oncologists and primary care physician in order to create a survivorship plan unique to you. This way, the most important factors to your ongoing wellness won't fall through the cracks, which can happen. For instance, when 11,219 Canadian breast cancer patients were identified through the Ontario Cancer Registry and followed five years posttreatment, researchers found that most women saw oncologists and a primary doctor each year. Is this good news? Well, not if the right hand isn't working alongside the left. One-third of these women had *too few* mammograms, and one-half had *too many* tests for metastatic disease.[5] Without organization, communication collapses and your health suffers.

LET'S BE HONEST: CANCER'S PARTING GIFTS ARE NO FUN

You endure various treatments in the effort to vanquish cancer and keep it at bay, and while sporting battle scars beats losing the war altogether, it's still disappointing and frustrating to deal with many of those daily reminders. In a Livestrong Foundation survey of cancer survivors, a staggering number experienced one or more posttreatment concerns in the following areas: 96 percent emotional, 91 percent physical, and 75 percent practical.[6] On the emotional front alone, anxiety, depression, and distress can affect relationships, body image, and self-esteem. So let's face these common complications from past or ongoing treatments head-on and discover all the areas with room for improvement.

Lymphedema

The breast and the arm on the same side share the same axillary lymph nodes, so tinkering with the nodes during surgery by taking some away and/or radiating those that remain can potentially impede the lymphatic outflow from the arm, breast, neck, or torso, resulting in lymphedema (lymphatic fluid retention) in these areas. Depending on the severity, your symptoms may range from imperceptible to pain and heaviness in the affected area (usually the arm) to impairment of daily function and fine motor skills. Factors that increase lymphedema by two- to fourfold include the number of lymph nodes removed, axillary radiation, a lack of mobility during the healing process, obesity, postoperative infections, and fluid collections or cording (axillary web syndrome).[7]

Especially in those at high risk to develop lymphedema, a simple device called L-Dex can be used at your routine doctor visits to identify the early buildup of lymphatic fluid in your arm before you would ever notice it. The device passes a harmless electrical signal through both arms and uses bioimpedence spectroscopy to compare how quickly the signal travels (fluid buildup will make it travel faster). When a difference is detected, prompt intervention with a compression sleeve and physical therapy results in very low rates of progression to permanent lymphedema.[8] Big Arm averted.

Due to inconsistent definitions of lymphedema, incidence ranges from 0 percent to 94 percent in the literature, but a pooled estimate from thirty prospective studies averaged 21.4 percent, typically developing within two years after surgery.[9] Lymphedema also increases the risk for arm infections and, rarely, lymphangiosarcoma (a cancerous mass in the blood vessels in the arm).[10] Lymphedema prevention and management includes manual lymphatic drainage via massage, compression bandages and sleeves, active exercises, skin care, and education.[11] If you are at high risk for lymphedema based on the criteria above, or if you notice arm changes, ask for a referral to a physical therapist with specialty training in lymphedema, and ideally, begin sessions a few weeks after surgery or radiation. For debilitating cases, using microsurgery to transfer nodes from elsewhere to the axilla, a process called *vascularized lymph node transfer*, can be curative.[12]

By the way, after any axillary surgery, you don't need to be overly vigilant when it comes to taking precautions unless advised otherwise by your practitioner. In the Physical Activity and Lymphedema (PAL) trial, *no increased risk* occurred with same-side blood draws, blood pressure readings, sleeping on that side, acupuncture, burns, bug bites, hangnails, cuts, airplane travel, lifting weights, sunburn, or vigorous exercise in hot weather when compression sleeves were worn during exercise.[13] And in another study that followed 632 patients a median of twenty-four months, without sleeve precautions it was found that blood draws, injections, blood pressure readings, and air travel had no effect on lymphedema.[14] Phew! Relax on all the precautions, except no saunas—sauna use was the only activity linked to lymphedema.

Osteoporosis

During cancer treatment from chemotherapy and AIs, your bones can become so weak that even a simple sneeze can cause a fracture. But there are precautions you can take. If you're lacking natural estrogens thanks to chemo- and endocrine-induced menopause, talk to your doctor about getting annual DXA scans to test your bone mineral density so you can monitor this. To protect your bones, supplement with 1,200 IU of calcium and 2,000 IU of vitamin D daily. Perform weight-bearing exercises like power walking, climbing stairs, *tai chi*, and lifting weights at minimum twice a week for twenty minutes. When needed, bis-phosphonate medications like Fosamax (alendronate sodium), Actonel (risedronate), and Boniva (ibandronate) reduce malignant metastases to bone recurrence and improve survival in postmenopausal patients with nonmetastatic breast cancer.[15] Super low body weight, smoking, and alcoholism exacerbate the risks.

Bone and Joint Pain

Chemotherapy (especially a drug class called *taxanes*), hormonal therapies, and targeted therapies can all cause bone or joint pain.[16] Even bisphosphonates might cause bone pain. Unrelenting pain needs a workup to rule out cancer recurrence, but most of the time it's collateral damage. However, tons of people without cancer have these same complaints— think poor posture, autoimmune disorders, arthritis—and since you're still a person, there's always a chance that your pain is totally unrelated to cancer and its treatments. Amp up your vitamin D and calcium, alternate heat and cold packs, take NSAIDs like ibuprofen, apply capsaicin cream, and/or visit complementary medicine practitioners for acupuncture, massage, physical therapy, chiropractic therapy, *tai chi*, and Reiki. As with any new symptom, always talk to your doctor.

Neuropathy

Chemotherapy sometimes injures your peripheral nerves, which can lead to numbness, tingling, and weakness in your hands and feet. Neuropathy improves with time, but 30 percent of patients report long-term effects.[17] Ask your physician for a referral to a rehabilitation doctor and physical therapist for evaluation and treatment, as well as pain specialists for medications, and look to integrative practitioners for acupuncture and massage. Occupational therapists will educate you on a number of daily living changes and precautions to follow at home and work to ease the pain.

Fatigue

Treatment-related fatigue doesn't go away after a good night's rest. It invades your brain and bones and makes it challenging to keep an interest in conversations and activities. Fatigue can be a slippery slope, compounded by depression and isolation. Among patients actively undergoing chemo or radiation, fatigue affects 99 percent, with more than 60 percent rating it moderate/severe.[18] And years later? The largest study on this subject found that 33 percent of women still have fatigue one to five years posttreatment; depression and pain emerged as the strongest predictors of lasting fatigue.[19] To mitigate this, you really do have to push yourself to move and walk, get serious about nutrition, join a support group, try complementary medicine, and talk about this with your doctor, who will check for medical issues like anemia and thyroid dysfunction. Take baby steps to improve your stamina, a little at a time, and be kind and patient with yourself. Prioritize activities when you do have a burst of energy, like trying something new (yoga?) or visiting family.

Menopausal Symptoms

This won't come as much of a surprise: depleting your body of every last estrogen molecule turns up the heat with menopause, no matter your age. Symptoms include depression, anxiety, insomnia, chemo brain, vaginal dryness, decreased libido, weight gain, osteoporosis, fatigue, bone and joint pain, hot flashes, flushing, sweating, dry itchy skin, and hair thinning. Take heart; chapter 5 is full of effective non-estrogen interventions to try.

Weight Gain

As if a threat to your life isn't enough, cancer and its effects on your psyche can make you gain weight too. Reduced activity, water retention, certain medications, increased eating, and a welcome-to-menopause drop in metabolism can inch up the needle on your scale. You have to limit high-calorie junk food, refined sugar, salt, saturated fat, alcohol, and get moving. Consult a dietician. Flip back to the obesity discussion in chapter 5 to remember how death rates double when you are heavy. No matter how all that adipose appeared, the same rule always makes it disappear: eat less, move more.

Sex, Sexual Dysfunction, Fertility, and Pregnancy Concerns

A lot of patients feel concerned about how cancer has affected their sex and reproductive lives, but they rarely mention it. It's not taboo. Talk about it.

When it comes to getting your mojo back after cancer, a number of issues arise from both emotional and physical catalysts. These include arousal difficulties, painful intercourse, an inability to orgasm, and decreased libido (less interest in sex).[20] In the posttreatment setting, dysfunction can be due to a dry or atrophied vagina (courtesy of chemical menopause and AIs more than tamoxifen); depression; self-consciousness over cosmetic outcomes; feeling undesirable or unsexy; being betrayed by your body; or keeping an emotional distance from your partner. But there are solutions to many of these issues.

Painful intercourse from vaginal dryness or tightness is a scenario that comes up a lot. One option is to buy a dilator set that gradually stretches a tight vagina. Use water- or silicone-based moisturizers and lubricants every day and apply liberally during intercourse. There are also vaginal lasers such as the MonaLisa Touch and ThermiVa that stimulate collagen formation and improve moisture in just a few sessions, so ask your gynecologist about that option. A study looked at topical vaginal estrogen use in sixty-nine women with a history of breast cancer and did not find an increase in recurrence,[21] but that does not mean you should use this, especially when taking an AI.[22] Your medical oncologist needs to approve any hormone use, and it should be a last resort for any ER(+) cancer patient. Try a non-estrogen oral herbal like Menopause Miracle, as users noted 53 percent improvement in vaginal moisture after twelve weeks.[23]

If your sexual block is more emotional, seek out expert advice. Seeing a psychologist, sex therapist, or counselor with or without your partner can offer insight and solutions; with homework assignments and reporting back requirements, the awkward task of relearning your intimate life can be initiated by someone other than you, so you feel less pressure. It might also help to anticipate and plan sex so the prep work can be done: low lights and lingerie if you're self-conscious, extra pillows to cushion painful spots, scene-setting with candles, aromatherapy, music, or movies. It's normal for sex and desire to change after cancer, so gently reintroducing physical touch and making love is worth the effort. Check the American Association of Sexuality Educators, Counselors, and Therapists (AASECT.org) to locate sexual health specialists in your area.

If you're worried about fertility, it's important to know that the closer you are to menopause, the more likely chemo will permanently shut down your ovaries. Since 5 percent of breast cancer occurs prior to age forty, most women interested in childbearing might already be at an age where reproductive assistance (like IVF) would be necessary, and then cancer comes along and really forces the issue. Prior to treatment, always discuss your future childbearing wishes and consider freezing your eggs or embryos as a precaution. Know, too, that if you take drugs like leuprolide (Lupron) that shut down your ovaries during chemo, there's a chance that chemo will pass over them without causing harm, and then months later your ovaries will "wake up." Tamoxifen outcompetes your own estrogen, but your ovaries are still happily pumping out hormones, so once you stop tamoxifen, you will be as fertile as you naturally would have been.

And if getting pregnant is in your future, know that retrospective studies confirm the safety of pregnancy after breast cancer, including in women with estrogen-positive disease.[24] Pregnancy after breast cancer does not increase cancer recurrence;[25] neither does breastfeeding increase the risk of recurrence or pose any health risk to the newborn.[26] I encourage women previously treated for breast cancer and free of recurrence to follow their dreams with respect to childbearing and breastfeeding. Discuss the timing of conception with your doctor.

Insomnia

If you find yourself up at 2:00 a.m. after cancer treatment, you are not alone, sister. Around 70 percent of metastatic breast cancer patients find that they can't fall or stay asleep at some point in the journey.[27] Try your best to catch seven to eight hours of sleep a night or else your cortisol and melatonin hormones will get out of whack; we need melatonin to sing its anticancer lullaby to all your cells. Tips? Wake up and fall asleep at the same times, seven days a week. Keep your room dark. Turn off screens (TV, computer, phone) an hour before bed. Exercise during the day. Try mindful meditative activities to rest your mind. Enlisting naturopathic supplementation with magnesium, coQ-10, ginseng, or cordyceps mushroom might help. Consider prescription medications when all else fails.

Breast, Chest, Axillary, Shoulder, Scar Pain

During the first three months after surgery or radiation, you'll probably experience unsolicited twinges of sharp, stabbing pain and/or a burning discomfort, tingling, pressure, or numbness that commonly occurs as your nerves "wake up" from the trauma and swelling subsides. Some patients also have a more long-term pain that involves damaged or stretched nerves that cannot recover normally, or at all, complete with phantom sensations from a missing breast or nipple. In one breast study, 23 percent of patients reported long-term pain, and predictors included: age less than fifty, more invasive surgery, early postoperative pain, and less analgesic use.[28] All women having a node dissection (ALND) or radiation to the axilla should undergo physical therapy to limit frozen shoulder and axillary web syndrome (AWS), which is when a taut cord pulls like a guitar string from the armpit to the inner elbow.[29,] AWS occurs in 48 percent of women after ALND and usually disappears by twelve weeks.[30] Focal pain at the operative site from scar tissue or radiation-induced fibrosis and muscle soreness can improve with physical therapy, myofascial release massage techniques, lidocaine patches, or acupuncture. Aerobic and resistance exercise, water therapy, and complementary techniques can all improve pain.[31] Combining pentoxifylline, vitamin E, and clodronate might ease radiation-induced neuropathies.[32] You can try capsaicin cream for stabbing pain,[33] while smoldering pains respond better to medications like gabapentin, venlafaxine, and amitriptyline.[34] Painful scars or keloids are treated with direct steroid injections, silicone sheets/gels, cryotherapy (liquid nitrogen), lasers, or capsaicin cream.[35]

When all else fails, surgical revision with the removal of tender areas or altering the reconstruction often provides relief.

Cardiotoxicity

Anticancer therapies, particularly anthracyclines (epirubicin), HER2-directed monoclonal antibodies, tamoxifen/AI, and left-sided radiation all can contribute to reversible or irreversible heart muscle dysfunction, heart failure, and/or even cardiovascular death, with significant cardiac issues occurring in less than 5 percent.[36] Your team will employ strategies to monitor, prevent, or mitigate the effects of cardiovascular damage.

Chemo Brain

Studies on that I'm-just-not-as-sharp-as-I-used-to-be feeling show that brain fog affects 16 to 50 percent of breast cancer patients,[37] but mental acuity seems to improve with time. In one prospective study, 8.1 percent of breast cancer patients met criteria for cognitive impairment one year out.[38] Cognitive decline takes many forms, including impairments in visual and verbal memory, reaction time, attention, concentration, and processing speed. Sometimes you might not even notice you're a bit spacy until you're under pressure, tired, or multitasking. (Or until you realize your kids are taking advantage of you: "Mom, you said yesterday that I could take the car today." *Did you?*)

Although brain MRI, PET, and EEGs confirm unmistakable structural and functional changes after chemotherapy,[39] chemo brain is not exclusively from high doses and longer duration of chemo, despite the name.[40] There are many cooks in the cognition kitchen. Menopause alone can dull your thinking, so just imagine adding an emotional cancer whirlwind, hits of general anesthesia, dashes of chemo, and a decade of endocrine therapy into the menopause mix.[41] Interestingly, cognitive decline shares risk factors for the development of cancer in the first place, such as our old friends oxidative stress and cytokines, with their DNA-damaging activity and inflammation.[42] Acupuncture and exercise can increase blood flow to the brain. Another option is cognitive rehabilitation, which includes working with a therapist on memory and attention training, compensatory strategies (e.g., make lists, don't multitask), stress reduction, relaxation techniques, and problem-solving techniques.[43]

Non-Breast Malignancies

Non-breast malignancies occur for a number of reasons, but particularly as a complication of the initial breast cancer treatment. For example, postmenopausal women with a uterus taking tamoxifen might be screened for endometrial cancer (your incidence goes from 1 in 1000 to 2.6 in 1000); you should report any vaginal bleeding.[44] As discussed in chapter 6, inherited genetic mutations like Li-Fraumeni and Lynch syndrome carry high risks for other organs to get cancer, so your doctors will follow the appropriate surveillance as dictated by NCCN guidelines. And if you haven't already had a consultation for genetic testing or a discussion about screening, be sure to request one. A Dutch study followed over 58,000 breast cancer patients a median of 5.4 years and found that one in twenty developed one of these non-breast malignancies within ten years of diagnosis: esophagus, stomach, colon, rectum, lung, uterus, ovary, kidney, bladder, soft tissue sarcomas, melanoma, non-Hodgkin's lymphoma, and acute myeloid leukemia (AML).[45] AML is a known result of chemotherapy that occurs in patients receiving alkylating agents (cyclophosphamide) and topoisomerase-targeting drugs (anthracyclines). Patients receiving these agents can expect AML at a rate of 0.5 percent without and 2.5 percent with radiation.[46] Symptoms such as infection, fatigue, bruising, or bleeding should trigger a workup. For irradiated patients, second cancers including lung, esophagus, thyroid, and sarcoma peak ten to fifteen years following treatment.[47] Although genetics and adjuvant treatment account for most of these malignancies, the same lifestyle factors that influence the development of breast cancer are often implicated in these cancers as well. Here's good news: healthy lifestyle behaviors like controlling weight and eliminating smoking and alcohol can lower secondary cancer risks.

Emotional Ramifications

Depression, anxiety, and general malaise are extremely common after treatment and stem from a number of causes. Any reason that you might feel blue, however, is not only valid and understandable, but worth exploring further with a professional so that your healing process can be as thorough and complete as possible.

The numbers don't lie. Approximately 20 to 30 percent of breast cancer survivors demonstrate measurable signs of anxiety and/or depression in the year following diagnosis, and up to 15 percent have depressive symptoms five years later.[48] Don't-ask-don't-tell policies in the workforce and elsewhere often fail women who need to address emotional and existential challenges during their cancer experience, to the extent that their jobs and relationships are adversely affected. I remember finishing a postcancer exam of Marlene, and as I was about to leave, I noticed how dejected she seemed. "Is something wrong?" I asked. "You look so depressed." She burst into tears and shared that she and her husband had just separated. "Oh, I know the best marital counselor in town," I told her, and four years later, they've rebooted their marriage. Don't wait for your doctor to notice psychological needs, though; ask around for referrals for counseling, support groups, and stress management if you feel you need a lift.

One common reason for depression is that women feel unsatisfied with their surgical outcome. Unsightly scars or misshapen, mismatched breasts can impact more than your appearance. Feeling unhappy in your own skin exacerbates depression, withdrawal, sexual dysfunction, and relationship struggles—and you can't hide these issues under an oversized sweatshirt. Though a large multiethnic survivor survey showed 66 to 80 percent overall satisfaction with cosmetics, whether choosing to keep or remove the breast,[49] tumor location and size, remaining breast volume, radiation, complications, and expectations all create aesthetic challenges—and what matters is what *you* think when you look in the mirror. If you're unhappy, talk to your surgical team. A number of effective tools lie in their bag of tricks.

Another major contributor is recurrence fear. "If it happened once," you think, "it can happen again." Up to 70 percent of cancer survivors report fear of cancer recurrence even years after diagnosis.[50] Triggers can include hearing about a celebrity or Facebook contact with a recurrence, a news report about cancer breakthroughs, or just showing up for doctor visits. All my follow-up patients who get their mammograms and immediately see me for an exam know I first review it with the radiologist so I can open their exam room door, and shout (if true), "Your mammo is perfect!" Exhale.

Finally, returning to normal often means returning to work—but it isn't always as easy or welcome as it sounds. The Americans with Disabilities Act protects you from discrimination in getting hired or fired and in obtaining affordable health insurance. Admittedly, most oncologists don't know much about this, but legal aid and financial assistance exist should you need it. Employers play a pivotal role in your successful return to work.[51] Don't be afraid to discuss workplace accommodations with the boss, and reach out to coworkers so you can maximize your performance. One of my patient's coworkers all donated a paid time off (PTO) day to her, which made a huge difference in her financial situation.

CANCER, REVISITED

Earlier in the book, we talked about two types of cancer in the breasts that could occur after your initial diagnosis. Contralateral breast cancer (CBC) occurs as a completely new cancer in the breast opposite to your first cancer. Once you've had cancer, your CBC risk averages a 7 percent lifetime chance, but can be much higher in younger women or those with unfavorable biology. You're generally more likely to get a CBC than any other new cancer in your body. If this happens to you, remember that you have beaten it once, and as much as you don't want to, you can do this again.

Locoregional recurrence, on the other hand, means that cancer has shown up again on the original cancer side in the breast tissue, skin, muscle, or lymph nodes in the armpit or above your collarbone. You or your doctor might notice a new lump, thickening, or skin rash, or imaging could show an interval change. This can even happen if you've had a mastectomy—recurrences usually show up as nodules in or under the skin, or in nodes, reconstruction or not.[52] Seventy-five percent of locoregional recurrences happen within the first five years after your original treatment (hence, the significance of the often-celebrated five-year-cancer-free anniversary.)

Whether you half-expected this day might come, or if you thought yourself bulletproof, it's a devastating moment when the news arrives. Did you pick the wrong team? Did you do/think/eat the wrong things? Were the treatments not good enough? Well, maybe, and if any of that's the case, *hooray* because now we have identified something important to change or add that just might kick this thing to the curb for good. It's when you did everything right that we have only the tumor's biology to blame, and apparently this biology likes to come back, no matter what you throw at it. We call cancer near the area where it first happened an ipsilateral breast tumor recurrence (IBTR); when cancer recurs more than 2 to 3 centimeters from the initial cancer location, or if it shows up in the adjacent nodes, it's a locoregional failure (LRF). Within ten years of treatment for negative nodes, IBTR and LRF occur in 6.4 percent and 1.9 percent respectively; with originally positive lymph nodes, IBTR and LRF increase to 8.7 percent and 6.0 percent.[53] Overall, these numbers are pretty low, but when cancer is back in *your* breast, chances become 100 percent—and the blow can make it hard to breathe. LRF carries a poorer survival rate than does IBTR (34.9 percent versus 76.7 percent alive after five years), and when either recurrence occurs less than two years after the initial cancer, survival worsens.[54]

Your game plan has to be curative intent. Be sure your doctor has four key moves in mind: (1) breast MRI; (2) body scans (PET/CT, bone, and brain) to rule out stage IV disease; (3) blood tumor markers; and (4) tumor profile (ER, PR, HER2, Ki-67) on the tissue that was biopsied to diagnose your recurrent cancer. If chemo isn't advised up front, let's get that cancer out. Although the standard of care for either type of recurrence remains mastectomy, for those with a small IBTR and adequate tissue remaining, talk to your doctor about repeating a lumpectomy, followed by partial or whole breast radiation (you can have the opposite radiation from the first time).[55] Otherwise, if your breast is small, or you think, "It's time for mastectomy," then mastectomy it is. If you already had a mastectomy, speak to your doctor about excising the cancerous tissue and closing the skin together, or recruiting tissue from elsewhere on your body, plus radiation if you didn't already have it. Mastectomy or not, any axillary or supraclavicular node recurrence requires node excision, and possibly targeted radiation if it wasn't previously done, and systemic therapy (chemotherapy and/or endocrine therapy).

YOUR WORST FEAR

Inherited and acquired genetic mutations, health behaviors, socioeconomic circumstances, medical care, and environmental exposures all contribute and collide differently within each body to heighten or lessen your personal risk of breast cancer recurrence. No one factor in isolation determines your destiny, nor do we understand the complexity of the interactions.

Despite our best efforts, about 28 percent of women inititally diagnosed with early-stage breast cancer (that is, not stage IV) eventually develop metastatic disease to an organ such as lung, liver, brain, or bone; but remember, increasingly effective therapies and earlier detection continue to improve this number.[56] Approximately 155,000 women in the United States are alive today with metastatic breast cancer (MBC); 75 percent of these women were initially stages I to III, and over 11 percent of them will survive more than ten years.[57] Patients sometimes mistake a metastatic recurrence for a different cancer, like thinking their new problem is liver cancer. Think of MBC this way: if an American travels to Paris, she doesn't become French; she still looks American and speaks English even though she's standing at the base of the Eiffel Tower. In the same way, breast cancer that metastasizes to the liver still looks and acts like breast cancer, not liver cancer.

The truth is, some cancers are more difficult to cure than others, and treatments don't work in every patient or sometimes work for a while and then stop working. The risk of relapse persists decades after the initial diagnosis, so do we have insight into whose cancer is more likely to recur? Well, yes, studies show that tumor details, genomic profiles, and treatments all play a part in recurrence. For example, in an analysis of over 110,000 women treated from 1985 to 2000, chemotherapy decreased mortality 38 percent (age less than fifty years) and 20 percent (age fifty to sixty-nine years), followed by a further reduction of 31 percent from tamoxifen; the final mortality reductions were 57 percent and 45 percent, respectively (and would have been lower with more current therapies).[58] In other words, treatment improves survival, and this protection lasts through fifteen years of observation.

Treatment aside, what else predicts recurrence? Larger tumors, more positive nodes, higher grades, and ER/PR—all have higher recurrence.[59] Interestingly, being ER(+) protects you up to four years after diagnosis but is detrimental after 7.7 years; in other words, ER(–) patients do worse early on—6.5 percent recurrence each year times three years versus 2 percent for ER(+)—but once ER(–) survive past the critical three-year window, recurrence becomes similar to ER(+), with a crisscross happening between years seven and eight when ER(–) tumors show half the recurrence risk of ER(+). This exact same pattern with diminishing risk of the "bad" thing followed by a crisscross around seven to eight years with the "good" thing is evident for large versus small tumors, positive versus negative lymph nodes,[60] high versus low grade,[61] good versus bad subtypes (luminal A/B/HER2/TNBC),[62] and high versus low genomic profiles (Oncotype DX[63] and MammaPrint).[64] To put it another way, aggressive features exert their powers in the first five years, are often subdued by treatment (and if not, then recurrences happen), but after that, it's the more favorable cancer that seems to gain momentum.

Perhaps you've known someone whose cancer happened twenty years ago, and then one day, you hear news that it's back in her liver. How does this happen? The key lies within the original years of a tumor's life. You see, irrespective of growth rates, cancers start from one single cell and grow at constant rates for long periods of time (years to decades) unrecognized by any scan or hand, and they start to metastasize even before getting detected. Plus—and here's the key—the metastases, if not cleared by your immune system, *grow at approximately the same rate as the primary tumor.*[65] Aha. It's the tortoise and the hare. So when "hare" metastases divide quickly, or have targets like a HER2 receptor on their backs, our agents annihilate them pretty handily; but if therapy fails, the hare rears its ugly recurrence head rather abruptly, usually within a few years of diagnosis. Why? Just like their parent cell, those metastatic cells often resist treatment and divide quickly. On the other hand, the plodding, lazy "tortoise" cancer is unrecognized by chemo, which only seeks to destroy rapidly dividing cells; however, endocrine therapies slow its progress. Still, some of these tortoises soldier on, determined to find a resting place in a non-breast land, with recurrence rates at 0 to 5 years: 9.9 percent; 5 to 10 years: 5.4 percent; 10 to 15 years: 2.9 percent; 15 to 20 years: 2.8 percent; and 20 to 25 years: 1.3 percent.[66]

Metastatic breast cancer can show up as solitary or countless metastatic lesions, which can arise in one or multiple organs, most notably in bone, lung, liver, and brain (in descending order of frequency). Overall, MBC survival rates are increasing by 1 to 2 percent each year,[67] largely due to better chemotherapeutic and hormone agents.[68] The most common metastatic site is bone for all subtypes except triple negatives, which favor brain, lung, and distant nodes.[69] HER2(+) also goes to the brain. While most MBC responds transiently to conventional treatments, the majority will show disease progression within one to two years of initiating treatment.[70] However, some cancers go into complete remission after chemotherapy and remain in this state even beyond twenty years. I have inherited MBC patients who have outlived their doctors. A distinctive subset of MBC patients have oligometastatic disease, meaning that one or a few metastatic lesions are limited to a single organ; this potentially *curable* stage IV situation occurs in 1 to 10 percent of MBC patients.[71] Let's say you have an oligometastatic lesion in one spot in your spine. Stereotactic body radiotherapy (SBRT) focuses a radiation beam in five brief treatments to the spot, has almost no collateral damage, relieves pain, and cures the cancer (in that area) in 100 percent of those treated.[72]

Here's what to expect when newly diagnosed with MBC. First, staging scans will be repeated to discover the full extent of disease. Then, whenever possible, we want to get a biopsy of the metastatic cancer to see if its biology matches the original cancer from your breast from years ago. Think about it: if 70 percent of your tumor were ER(+), maybe it's the 30 percent ER(–) cells that have resurfaced. As scientists delve deeper into tumor DNA, the breadth of genetic diversity they are finding *within a single tumor* is shocking.[73] To that end, some centers use the liquid biopsies we talked about earlier to analyze tumor cfDNA that spun off from the cancer. They look for genetic mutations and other drivers of a tumor's growth. In the era of personalized medicine, liquid biopsies allow us to choose which therapies might work best for your particular recurrence, and since it's just a blood draw, we can monitor the response to treatment and catch alterations in the cfDNA, indicating a need for a strategic change.[74] We want to aim targeted drugs, systemic chemo, immunotherapy, and endocrine therapies directly at what you have now, not what you had previously. Surgery and radiation might be used to control local symptoms like pain, or perhaps to eliminate a solitary tumor site, but with MBC we have to expect micrometastatic cells are not far behind the tumor(s) that showed up, and we therefore need to get after them with systemic treatments. I suggest turning back to chapter 9 to refresh your memory about the different chemical weapons we might use in this new war. Your doctor will usually continue with a regimen until disease progresses or markers rise, and then switch to something new. We have a number of tricks in our armamentarium, so don't give up hope easily. Ask your treatment team if there is an open clinical trial you can join, and check for yourself at breastcancertrials.org. The National Comprehensive Cancer Network (NCCN.org) has a free "Guidelines for

Patients: Breast Cancer—Metastatic (Stage IV)" booklet that reviews all the medication strategies available.

In addition to attacking cancer cells, you'll want to preserve your healthy ones, and all the while tend to the physical damage and emotional aspects of coping with MBC. It's difficult to maintain a positive outlook in the face of discouraging circumstances, but you should know that psychosocial interventions can reduce depression, which in turn prolongs survival, so consider seeking out religious or support groups and therapy. In a randomized trial of supportive therapy, 125 MBC patients who improved their depression scores over one year versus those who did not lived a median of 53.6 months versus 25.1 months.[75]

There are many aspects to supportive care. Since bone is the most common metastatic site, not surprisingly bone pain is the most common MBC symptom, and you're at risk for fractures, spinal cord compression, and high calcium in the blood. Bisphosphonates are prescription drugs that stop the breakdown of bone, reduce pain, and prevent fractures. They include zoledronic acid (Zometa, IV over fifteen minutes every three to four weeks) and pamidronate (Aredia, IV over two hours every three to four weeks). You might need supplementation with vitamin D and calcium; denosumab (Xgeva or Prolia, a subcutaneous shot every four weeks) also stops bone absorption.[76] These drugs can break down your jawbone (mandibular osteonecrosis), which reminds us that efforts to prolong life can adversely affect the quality of life. Talk to your doctor about balancing cancer therapies with symptom control, and discuss your willingness to endure collateral damage. Be sure to give your body the support it needs during this time: complementary medicine, nutrition, and psychology plus/minus medications as needed for anemia, anxiety, constipation, depression, infection risk, insomnia, loss of appetite, nausea/vomiting, neuropathy, and pain control.

You know how we said that some oligometastatic disease can be cured, and some women live twenty-plus years? This occurs in 1 to 3 percent of all MBC.[77] Many reports from prospective clinical trials examine the effects of all the therapies we strategically aim at MBC. Despite initial response, most patients will worsen within twelve to twenty-four months; the median (half more, half less) survival after resistance is eighteen to twenty-four months, and less than 5 percent of patients live five years once resistance to therapy develops (not after initial MBC diagnosis).[78] Given what we know, it's imperative that you pursue a reasonable approach with input from your physician team, always being mindful about what you want from what is most likely your last two to four years. Don't get me wrong—I am an eternal optimist by nature, and it isn't easy to limit what God can do; I certainly would want proof that you're not in the 1 to 3 percent before believing otherwise, but in the same breath, it must be said that pretending that most women with metastatic breast cancer live decades steals dreams from those who would live differently had they known that they had closer to three years, not thirty. Choose treatments that align with your desires regarding more- versus less-intensive therapy. In the end, you are not a statistic or a median or a subtype: *you are you*, and you call the shots.

FINDING SUPPORT AND COMFORT WHERE YOU NEED IT

The power unleashed from intimacy with a partner or from friendships and social support and from connectedness to the Creator of the universe brings with it the power to heal. What is it that heals hearts and relationships and pain and loss, and yes, even breasts and bodies? In the vulnerable period that follows cancer treatment, whether cancer has now spread, recurred, or thankfully seems part of your past, what matters most of all . . . is love.

Faith

There's a difference between spirituality and religion, though their purposes can overlap among patients. Spirituality generally refers to connection to a higher power or a feeling of transcendence, whereas religion uses an organized belief system to achieve that sense of transcendence and includes attending services as part of a community in that process. Studies show that spirituality and religion might influence recovery from illness by illuminating life's meaning and purpose, thereby enhancing the will to live.[79] Sixty-nine percent of cancer patients pray for their health, versus 45 percent of the general population.[80] An investigation of the spiritual/existential needs of breast cancer patients showed they desire help with overcoming fears (51 percent); with finding hope (42 percent), meaning in life (40 percent), spiritual resources (39 percent), and peace of mind (43 percent); and with navigating dying and death (25 percent).[81]

Viewed in a spiritual context, the cancer journey strengthens a woman's resolve to emerge from the experience refined, perhaps with more empathy or a renewed sense of passion in life. The interconnectedness between mind, body, and spirit exists. Studies show that *meaning* in life expressed by spiritual cancer patients improves overall *quality* of life. Spirituality correlates to psychological well-being and mitigates the impact of stress on physical health;[82] in fact, when measuring cancer-fighting cells in the bloodstream ("good" white cells and lymphocytes) against self-reports of spirituality, higher functional immunity correlates to greater spirituality.[83] Being religious also elicits feelings of optimism,[84] comforts existential fears,[85] elevates self-esteem, creates an internal locus of control, and reduces anxiety.[86] Breast cancer survivors emphasize the positive benefits of prayer and a relationship with God.[87] On the other hand, spiritual distress and feeling abandoned by God or the religious community causes depression and decreased adherence to medical advice among cancer patients.[88]

It is true that *healthy* church-service attendees have 25 percent reduced mortality compared to nonreligious peers (likely due to adopting a healthier lifestyle: less alcohol and drug abuse, more community/ social connectivity, a stronger sense of meaning in life), but no studies show improved survival or slower cancer progression in religious women with breast cancer.[89] Whatever the number of years remaining for you on Earth, your quality of life improves when you have faith and hope, rather than despair and fear. Ask for a referral to a pastor, minister, rabbi, or other spiritual counselor to explore making this trade: trade away confidence in *your* ability or resources, and accept faith in the goodness and greatness of God. In church recently, my pastor said something that made me think of all my patients and now of you, dear reader. "The number one cause of anxiety is the future," he said. "The future doesn't belong to you. It belongs to God . . . and it might be better than you think!" God leads incrementally, one step at a time. The Bible claims in Psalm 119:105 that "Thy word is a lamp unto my feet, and a light unto my path," not a floodlight onto my highway for the next ten years. All you can do is take the next step that God leads you to take, and you can be sure that firm ground awaits your foot when it lands.

Partners in Sickness and in Health

Partners of women with breast cancer are just as sideswiped by the diagnosis as their wives. One of the largest studies to look at marital relationships observed that a partner's support did not alleviate the breast cancer patient's physical or mental pains ten months after diagnosis. Of course, each relationship is unique, but they conclude that limits exist to the effectiveness of close relationships in times of severe stress.[90] This highlights the importance of a social support network outside the nuclear home for both spouses.

Partners do not have to guess how to be supportive to their wives, because resources exist. It's difficult to navigate a flood of feelings all at once and sometimes at breakneck speed. For example, one moment a discussion about mastectomy pros and cons could take place, and then hours later, a spouse feels conflicted about initiating romance: *If I do, is it insensitive? If I don't, will she perceive it as rejection?* As with any relationship, communication is key, and that includes high empathy, low withdrawal, and just listening.[91] Maybe read those three skills again just to make sure you lock them into your "communication repertoire." Carve out time in an environment conducive to talking: that place might be a park, a restaurant, or the couch. If talking sounds too hard, maybe write down your feelings and desires and share it with your loved one. Working with an expert might help you navigate this more smoothly.

During the cancer journey, partners shoulder a lot. One study inventoried the tasks husbands provided on a daily basis as follows: assistance with dressing (37 percent), eating (31 percent), bathing (21 percent), shopping (66 percent), trips outside (42 percent), taking medicine (46 percent), managing finances (49 percent), and organizing appointments (41 percent).[92] In this study, husbands reported that the highest burdens they endured involved social awkwardness, followed by sex and intimacy, work, household issues, and extended family relations.

I've seen this in my own practice and studies support it time and again: breast cancer never returns a couple to the precancer state. They grow closer or fall further apart.[93] They do not, however, divorce any more frequently than other couples.[94] Marriage counseling offers an excellent way to learn effective coping strategies and to explore helpful communication techniques (even having simple phrases to fall back on can eliminate a number of misunderstandings). Here's a proven fact that will surprise no one: school-age children function better with more interaction from the non-ill parent and when their families cope with their problems.[95] After the storm passes, many survivors and spouses report positive life changes and post-traumatic growth as a result of the journey.[96] Marriages are more likely to emerge intact (1) when couples expressed their satisfaction with the relationship precancer, (2) with less surgery (lumpectomy), and (3) when the spouse reacted supportively.[97]

Positive Relationships

Relationships between you and your family, friends, and community play an integral, critical role—dare I say, *a lifesaving or life-destroying role*—in the story of your life. In fact, breast cancer survivors with "lower social support" prior to their cancer journey experience higher levels of pain, depression, and inflammatory blood markers (IL-6) six months posttreatment, compared to those with more social support.[98] Among breast cancer survivors aged sixty-five and over, having lower social support independently predicted *accelerated decline* in emotional, physical, and cognitive function over seven years follow-up.[99] Over 2,200 early-stage women in the Life After Cancer Epidemiology Study were followed 10.8 years. Those with low, not high, levels of social support from friends and family and lack of religious/social participation were 58 percent more likely to have died during the study period than those with high levels of support. This is important: social networks mattered more for cancer patients who were caregivers versus non-caregivers. In other words, social support helps to offset the physical and emotional burden of your familial responsibilities.[100]

Your relationships influence your behavior, stress level, and beliefs, so choose your company wisely—your health and cancer outcome depend on it. You deserve uplifting, encouraging, honest, and loving friends who desire to see you healthy and joyful. If you're overweight, and your friend knows that you're determined to lose a few for the sake of fighting cancer, she shouldn't derail you by saying, "Aw, you look great. Give yourself a break and have some more fudge on that sundae."[101]

Guess who provides newly diagnosed patients with the most emotional and informational support they crave, improving their quality of life and lifting depression? Breast cancer survivors. Respondents to the Livestrong Foundation survey reported that cancer positively affected their lives in the following ways: 71 percent help other cancer survivors; 85 percent would like to do more to help other survivors; 86 percent advocate for screening for cancer; and 94 percent wish to share their personal story. Survivors participating in a Twitter forum expressed 43 to 85 percent increased knowledge about survivorship, metastatic breast cancer, cancer types and biology, clinical trials and research, treatment options, breast imaging, genetic testing and risk assessment, and radiotherapy; 67 percent of women initially reporting "high or extreme" anxiety became "low or no" anxiety after participation (by the way, nobody went from low to high anxiety).[102]

A breast cancer diagnosis is a distressing event. The people best equipped to dispel the distress have endured it. I have a plan. The world needs you. And the crazy thing is, you will become so blessed in the process that you will think this was all about you in the first place.

Anyone with a new breast cancer diagnosis, and everyone whose breast cancer journey feels more distant, I'm inviting you to join Breast Buddies (pinklotus.com/breastbuddies). This online venue provides a free, safe haven for women who have or have had breast cancer *all around the world* to come together for purposes of emotional and social support. Nobody cares if you were the prom queen or the class nerd. Nobody cares about your terrible teeth or your $500-a-month perfect hair. Nobody cares about your beat-up old car or your million-dollar mansion. But *everybody cares* about connecting to a community, and/or to one sister, who understands the fears you face. Breast Buddies are matched by what they choose to share, all of which is optional: cancer stage, tumor profile, treatments received, age, relationship status, children, language, religion, and more. No politics, no judgment, no fear . . . just Breast Buddies. Welcome to a sacred community of survivors—find your Breast Buddy, share a cup of coffee in person, or just post and chat online, getting answers to anything and everything, while turning strangers into friends.

DON'T GIVE CANCER A HAPPY HOME

Rogue cancer cells tumble like seeds through your bloodstream, waiting to land in fertile soil. You need to make them wait indefinitely, until they exhaust their own fuel or your host defenses identify and destroy them. How? Disable them with rough terrain that makes it impossible for them to grow. "Seed" factors that give tumors the power to grow are based in biology: malignant cells can circulate, extravasate, proliferate, and create their own blood supply (angiogenesis).[103] "Soil" factors exist wherever those cancer seeds try to take root: back in the breast, out to the liver, lung, brain, or bone.[104]

Do you recall the rat study we discussed that showed how a sugar cube–sized breast cancer sheds 3.2 million cells into your bloodstream every day?[105] Think of seed and soil like sperm and egg. Between 200 and 500 million sperm will race toward an egg, but only one is the fastest, and all the rest perish. And yet, despite beating the 1 in 500 million odds, 50 percent of those sperm will not make it past fertilization. The body requires perfect soil to create and then implant an embryo and to support that tiny life all the way through to its first gasp of air. And so it is also with the millions of shed tumor cells or potential stragglers somewhere inside you—they need perfect soil to take root, to grow, to harm you. Consider God's infinite wisdom here: the very same fertilizer that nourishes and enables you *disables* all of life's major killers: heart disease, diabetes, stroke, Alzheimer's, obesity—and yes, breast cancer.

So how do you turn that soil microenvironment into thornbushes choking seeds?

Oh, there's something so satisfying about full circles. The stars align, the puzzle pieces fit together without force, the aha moment hits . . . and you, my friend, will flip back to devour chapters 3, 4, and 5. The very same nutritional truths and healthy lifestyle behaviors that help *ward off* cancer in the first place will help *prevent* its return. Here are some evidence-based reminders about plant foods staving off breast cancer recurrence. A randomized, controlled double-blind trial of patients eating flaxseed muffins versus placebo for just five weeks prior to breast cancer surgery showed significant reductions in tumor division rates and HER2 expression, and elevated apoptosis (cell death), just from the lignans (phytoestrogens) in flaxseed.[106] Higher lignans increase endostatin—a potent inhibitor of tumor angiogenesis—in your bloodstream;[107] flaxseed drops breast cancer recurrence and death between 42 to 71 percent in both ER(+) and ER(−) patients.[108] And what about how soy kept cancer away? Soy from food sources, not supplements, reduced breast cancer recurrence by 60 percent and death by 29 percent.[109] Remember the sulforaphanes in broccoli and broccoli sprouts? They can entirely eliminate cancer *stem cells* (the "mastermind cells" from which metastases are thought to spring) from implanted breast tumors in rats.[110] Cruciferous veggies are king. In women who drank broccoli sprout juice one hour before breast reduction surgery (equivalent to a quarter-cup of sprouts), researchers found sulforaphanes inside their tissue samples; it seems those stem-cell killers know exactly where to go.[111] Over 75 percent of cancer thrivers do not get enough vitamin D, so you might need some fortified foods, supplements, and sunshine.[112] Trans fats and saturated fats (cheese, pizza, donuts, ice cream, chicken, red meat) elevate cancer recurrence by 78 percent and 41 percent, respectively.[113] Trim the fat.

DR. FUNK'S "BEAT IT, BREAST CANCER" CHECKLIST

☐ Whole food, plant-based eating that prioritizes vegetables, fruits, 100 percent whole grains, and legumes (beans, peas, lentils), whole food soy, ground flaxseed; eliminate all meat, poultry, fish, dairy, and eggs; minimize saturated fat, simple sugars, processed foods, and refined cereals.

☐ Exercise: 5 hours a week moderate effort, or 2.5 hours a week vigorous, sweaty workouts.

☐ Minimize or eliminate alcohol: 7 drinks or fewer a week, favor 4 to 8 ounces of red wine.

☐ No smoking.

☐ Stress management techniques: 20 minute daily minimum (prayer, meditation, *tai chi*, yoga, guided imagery, focused breathing).

☐ Social connectedness: 30 minute daily minimum (no computers or phones or screens when with others in person). Examples: date night, coffee with a friend, church group, tennis team, uplifting online community, bridge club.

☐ Monthly breast self-exam, annual clinical breast exam, annual mammogram, plus additional imaging (ultrasound, MRI) and clinical exams when indicated.

☐ Extra credit: Give back. Smile. Laugh.

A study compared lifestyle factors with cancer recurrence and mortality among 6,295 five-year ER(+) stage I to III breast cancer survivors.[114] Here's anticancer fertilizer for your soil: (1) Don't *gain* weight; more than 10 percent weight gain = 24 percent increased recurrence after five years; (2) maintain a healthy BMI; obesity (BMI at or over 30) = 40 percent increase; (3) minimize alcohol; daily drinks = 28 percent increase; (4) exercise; physical inactivity = 29 percent increase; (5) don't smoke; smoking = 30 percent increased recurrence after five years. You may also want to ask your doctor about taking aspirin regularly. Aspirin use and survival was analyzed in the Nurses' Health Study. Among the 4,164 women with breast cancer who used aspirin two to five days a week, there was 71 percent less death than never-users, irrespective of stage, BMI, menopause, or ER status.[115] Similarly, ibuprofen three or more days a week in 2,292 women showed 44 percent less recurrence.[116] Check with your doctor first, but take aspirin 325 mg and ibuprofen 200 mg every two to three days.

Control the controllable in your life; heaven knows there's enough outside our sphere of influence, from natural disasters to the date you got diagnosed, so don't perseverate on that stuff. No matter how long you ponder it, you cannot change it. Focus on what dwells within your grasp, and make sure each area of your life—spiritual, physical, emotional, relational—gets daily attention. Whether in the form of toxic activities, foods, thoughts, or people, toxins aren't good for your body's soil. A psychological intervention trial randomized 227 women with early breast cancer to receive twenty-six sessions of either routine psychological assessment *only* or the addition of psychologist-led interventions like progressive muscle relaxation for stress reduction and other strategies to improve mood and alter health behaviors. Eleven years later, the intervention arm showed 45 percent less recurrence and 56 percent less death than the control group.[117] If you're stressed out, get the stress *out*. Consider changing one thing about your habits or exposures that you know creates the wrong soil within or around you. Master that, and then add another.

Perhaps above all, broaden and deepen meaning in your life. Studies show meaning can be found by giving to the world through creative activities.[118] Use your innate gifts, hobbies, or vocation to give back. I've had breast cancer patients put their existing skills into action, working as full-time physical therapists, yoga instructors, psychologists, oncology aestheticians, and writers with a newfound passionate focus on breast cancer survivors. I've known women in the beauty industry who provide pre-chemo haircuts and post-chemo styling, and makeup lessons for patients. A musician patient makes meditative CDs for survivors, another makes sunglasses with pink themes, and all proceeds go to the Pink Lotus Foundation (pinklotus.com/foundation). You can also find an easy way to support your favorite charity by hosting a fun event. I've seen thrivers spearhead office golf tournaments, tennis round-robins, movie screenings, bake sales, book signings, jewelry booths, and wine tastings. Run a race. If that sounds exhausting, walk a walk . . . or just sit down with a Breast Buddy and smile and laugh. (You wanted that extra credit, didn't you?)

Acknowledgments

To Andy. My True North, my true love. Thank you for being oxygen.

To Ethan, Sebastian, and Justin. I have known no greater honor than to be your mother. How boring would life be without epic bike rides, game nights, sleeping in forts, and farts?

To Mom and Dad. Your love shines brighter than a thousand suns. Seriously, you almost blinded me with all that love.

To Jacqueline Busse, Diana Franklin, Donna Rapson, Natalie Razavi, and Fernanda Carvalho. Your constant prayers and text messages while I wrote kept me fired up.

To my patients. Thank you for asking me to come alongside one of life's darkest moments, and to walk with you until the light shines. What a privilege! You are so beautiful.

To my surgical mentors. Dr. John A. Ryan Jr., you taught me surgical excellence and clinical acumen like none other; Dr. Edward H. Phillips, you jump-started my breast career and saved me from a life spent with the esophagus.

To medical researchers all over the world. You spend years and sometimes whole careers to discover the evidence that I write in one single sentence. I am humbled by your contributions to unraveling the mysteries of life and death.

To Dr. Mike Dow. A chance encounter and one minute later, you had me writing this book. Your advice: write as if you love the reader. I did and I do.

To Chrissy and J. D. Roth. Everything happens for a reason. Grateful.

To Daisy Blackwell Hutton, Lori Cloud, Meaghan Porter, and Mark Schoenwald, my enthusiastic publishing family; to Kristina Grish, my cleaner; and to Celeste Fine and John Maas, my stellar literary agents. Let's Save Lives!

APPENDIX

Acronyms and Abbreviations

10YS	ten-year survival
15YS	fifteen-year survival
3DCRT	three-dimensional conformal radiation therapy
5YS	five-year survival
AASECT	American Association of Sexuality Educators, Counselors, and Therapists
ABUS	automated breast ultrasound
ACOG	American College of Obstetricians and Gynecologists
ACS	American Cancer Society
ADH	atypical ductal hyperplasia
AHA	American Heart Association
AI	aromatase inhibitor
AICR	American Institute for Cancer Research
ALA	*alpha*-Linolenic acid
ALCL	anaplastic large cell lymphoma
ALH	atypical lobular hyperplasia
ALND	axillary lymph node dissection
AML	acute myeloid leukemia
APBI	accelerated partial breast irradiation
ASA	acetylsalicylic acid
ASBS	American Society of Breast Surgeons

ASCO	American Society of Clinical Oncology
ATRA	all-trans retinoic acid
AWBI	accelerated whole breast irradiation
AWS	axillary web syndrome
BCI	breast cancer index
BHRT	bioidentical hormone replacement therapy
BI-RADS	Breast Imaging Reporting and Data System
BLV	bovine leukemia virus
BMD	bone mineral density
BMI	body mass index
BPA	bisphenol A
BPM	bilateral prophylactic mastectomy
BRCA-1; BRCA-2	BReast CAncer-1 and -2
BSE	breast self-exam
CAM	complementary and alternative medicine
CBC	contralateral breast cancer
CBD	cannabidiol
CBE	clinical breast exam
CCL	columnar cell lesions
CDK	cyclin-dependent kinase
CESM	contrast-enhanced spectral mammography
cfDNA	cell-free DNA
CNB	core needle biopsy
CPM	contralateral prophylactic mastectomy
CT	computed tomography
CTCs	circulating tumor cells
DCIS	ductal carcinoma *in situ*
DDT	dichlorodiphenyltrichloroethane
DES	diethylstilbestrol
DHEA	dehydroepiandrosterone
DNA	deoxyribonucleic acid
DVT	deep vein thrombosis
DXA	dual-energy X-ray absorptiometry

EDCs	endocrine disrupting compounds
EEC	European Economic Community
EGCG	epigallocatechin gallate
EMF	electromagnetic fields
EPA	Environmental Protection Agency
EPIC	European Prospective Investigation into Cancer and Nutrition
ER	estrogen receptor
ER(-)	estrogen receptor-negative
ER(+)	estrogen receptor-positive
ERD	ER-downregulator
EU	European Union
EWG	Environmental Working Group
FA	fibroadenoma
FAO	Food and Agriculture Organization of the United Nations
FCC	fibrocystic change
FDA	Food and Drug Administration
FEA	flat epithelial atypia
FISH	fluorescence *in situ* hybridization
FNA	fine needle aspiration
GINA	Genetic Information Nondiscrimination Act
GMO	genetically modified organism
HCAs	heterocyclic amines
HEPA	high efficiency particulate air
HER2	human epidermal growth factor receptor 2 oncogene
HER2(-)	HER2 negative
HER2(+)	HER2 positive
HGF	hepatocyte growth factor
HIPAA	Health Insurance Portability and Accountability Act
HR-	hormone receptor negative

HR+	hormone receptor positive
HRT	hormone replacement therapy
IAEA	International Atomic Energy Agency
IARC	International Agency for Research on Cancer
IBTR	ipsilateral breast tumor recurrence
IDC	invasive ductal carcinoma
IGF-1	insulin-like growth factor-1
IGFBP	insulin-like growth factor binding protein
IGM	idiopathic granulomatous mastitis
IHC	immunohistochemistry
IL-1	interleukin 1
IL-6	interleukin 6
IMRT	intensity-modulated radiation therapy
IORT	intraoperative radiation therapy
IVF	*in vitro* fertilization
LACE	Life After Cancer Epidemiology Study
LCIS	lobular carcinoma *in situ*
LRF	locoregional failure
MBC	metastatic breast cancer
MINDACT	microarray in node negative and 1 to 3 positive lymph node disease may avoid chemotherapy
MRI	magnetic resonance imaging
MTHFR	methylenetetrahydrofolate reductase
MUFA	monounsaturated fatty acids
NCCN	National Comprehensive Cancer Network
NCI	National Cancer Institute
NHANES	National Health and Nutrition Examination Surveys
NIH	National Institutes of Health
NIH-AARP	National Institutes of Health-American Association of Retired Persons
NK	natural killer
NRDC	Natural Resources Defense Council

NSAID	nonsteroidal anti-inflammatory drug
NSM	nipple-sparing mastectomy
NTP	National Toxicology Program
OCP	oral contraceptive pill
PAHs	polycyclic aromatic hydrocarbons
PAL	physical activity and lymphedema
PARP	poly (ADP-ribose) polymerase
PASH	pseudoangiomatous stromal hyperplasia
PBDE	polybrominated diphenyl ether
PBDI	prophylactic breast dye injection
PCB	polychlorinated biphenyl
pCR	pathologic complete response
PCRM	Physicians Committee for Responsible Medicine
PE	pulmonary embolism
PET	positron emission tomography
PGD	preimplantation genetic diagnosis
PLCIS	pleomorphic lobular carcinoma *in situ*
PR(-)	progesterone receptor-negative
PR(+)	progesterone receptor-positive
PTH	parathyroid hormone
PUFA	polyunsaturated fatty acids
PVC	polyvinyl chloride
rBGH	recombinant bovine growth hormone
rBST	recombinant bovine somatotropin
RDA	recommended daily allowance
RF	radio-frequency
RRSO	risk-reducing salpingo-oophorectomy
SAD	standard American diet
SBRT	stereotactic body radiotherapy
SEER	Surveillance, Epidemiology and End Results
SERM	selective estrogen receptor modulator
SES	socioeconomic status

SLN   sentinel lymph node
SLNB   sentinel lymph node biopsy
SNP   single-nucleotide polymorphism
STAR   Study of Tamoxifen and Raloxifene
TBBPA   tetrabromobisphenol A
TCM   traditional chinese medicine
THC   tetrahydrocannabinol
TMAO   trimethylamine *N*-oxide
TNBC   triple-negative breast cancer
TNFα   tumor necrosis factor-*alpha*
TNM   tumor size, nodes, metastases
UDH   usual ductal hyperplasia
UK   United Kingdom
US   United States
USDA   United States Department of Agriculture
UV   ultraviolet
VEGF   vascular endothelial growth factor
WBI   whole breast irradiation
WCRF   World Cancer Research Fund
WHI   Women's Health Initiative
WHO   World Health Organization

UNITS OF MEASURE

cm	centimeter(s)	mcg	microgram(s)
g	gram(g)	mg	milligram(s)
k	kilogram(s)	ml	milliliter(s)
kcal	calorie(s)	mm	millimeter(s)
IU	International Units	ng	nanogram(s)
lb	pound(s)	oz	ounce(s)
m	meter(s)		

Notes

Introduction

1. Collaborative Group on Hormonal Factors in Breast Cancer, "Familial Breast Cancer: Collaborative Reanalysis of Individual Data from 52 Epidemiological Studies Including 58,209 Women with Breast Cancer and 101,986 Women Without the Disease," *Lancet* 358, no. 9291 (2001): 1389–99.

2. J. A. Dumalaon-Canaria et al., "What Causes Breast Cancer? A Systematic Review of Causal Attributions Among Breast Cancer Survivors and How These Compare to Expert-Endorsed Risk Factors," *Cancer Causes & Control* 25, no. 7 (2014): 771–85.

3. L. M. Sánchez-Zamorano et al., "Healthy Lifestyle on the Risk of Breast Cancer," *Cancer Epidemiology and Prevention Biomarkers* 20, no. 5 (2011): 912–22.

4. D. Evans et al., "The Angelina Jolie Effect: How High Celebrity Profile Can Have a Major Impact on Provision of Cancer-Related Services," *Breast Cancer Research* 16, no. 5 (2014): 442; D. Evans et al., "Longer-Term Effects of the Angelina Jolie Effect: Increased Risk-Reducing Mastectomy Rates in BRCA Carriers and Other High-Risk Women," *Breast Cancer Research* 17, no. 1 (2015): 143; R. H. Juthe, A. Zaharchuk, and C. Wang, "Celebrity Disclosures and Information Seeking: The Case of Angelina Jolie," *Genetics in Medicine* 17, no. 7 (2014): 545–53; P. B. Lebo et al., "The Angelina Effect Revisited: Exploring a Media-Related Impact on Public Awareness," *Cancer* 121, no. 22 (2015): 3959–64; C. M. Malcolm, M. U. Javed, and D. Nguyen, "Has the Angelina Jolie Effect Led to an Increase in Risk-Reducing Mastectomy and Breast Reconstruction in Wales: A Retrospective, Single-Centre Cohort Study," *Journal of Plastic, Reconstructive & Aesthetic Surgery* 69, no. 2 (2016): 288–89; C. Staudigl et al., "Changes of Socio-demographic Data of Clients Seeking Genetic Counseling for Hereditary Breast and Ovarian Cancer Due to the 'Angelina Jolie Effect,'" *BMC Cancer* 16, no. 1 (2016): 436; J. Lee et al., "Influence of the Angelina Jolie Announcement and Insurance Reimbursement on Practice Patterns for Hereditary Breast Cancer," *Journal of Breast Cancer* 20, no. 2 (2017): 203–7.

5. P. Anand et al., "Cancer Is a Preventable Disease That Requires Major Lifestyle Changes," *Pharmaceutical Research* 25, no. 9 (2008): 2097–116; L. M. Sánchez-Zamorano et al., "Healthy Lifestyle on the Risk of Breast Cancer," *Cancer Epidemiology and Prevention Biomarkers* 20, no. 5 (2011): 912–22.

Chapter 1: Breast Care ABCs

1. C. Adem et al., "Primary Breast Sarcoma: Clinicopathologic Series from the Mayo Clinic and Review of the Literature," *British Journal of Cancer* 91, no. 2 (2004): 237–41.
2. R. P. Rapini, J. L. Bolognia, and J. L. Jorizzo, *Dermatology: 2-Volume Set* (St. Louis: Mosby, 2007).

Chapter 2: Debunking Breast Cancer Myths

1. A. S. Hamilton and T. M. Mack, "Puberty and Genetic Susceptibility to Breast Cancer in a Case-Control Study in Twins," *New England Journal of Medicine* 348, no. 23 (2003): 2313–22.
2. American Cancer Society, *Breast Cancer Facts & Figures 2017–2018* (2017), accessed December 3, 2017, https://www.cancer.org/content/dam/cancer-org/research /cancer-facts-and-statistics/breast-cancer-facts-and-figures/breast-cancer-facts-and -figures-2017-2018.pdf.
3. American Cancer Society, *Breast Cancer Facts & Figures 2017–2018* (2017), accessed December 7, 2017, https://www.cancer.org/content/dam/cancer-org/research /cancer-facts-and-statistics/breast-cancer-facts-and-figures/breast-cancer-facts-and -figures-2017-2018.pdf.
4. American Cancer Society, *Breast Cancer Facts & Figures 2017–2018* (2017), accessed December 3, 2017, https://www.cancer.org/content/dam/cancer-org/research /cancer-facts-and-statistics/breast-cancer-facts-and-figures/breast-cancer-facts-and -figures-2017-2018.pdf.
5. American Cancer Society, *Breast Cancer Facts & Figures 2017–2018* (2017), accessed December 6, 2017, https://www.cancer.org/content/dam/cancer-org/research /cancer-facts-and-statistics/breast-cancer-facts-and-figures/breast-cancer-facts-and -figures-2017-2018.pdf.
6. D. Ornish et al., "Changes in Prostate Gene Expression in Men Undergoing an Intensive Nutrition and Lifestyle Intervention," *Proceedings of the National Academy of Sciences* 105, no. 24 (2008): 8369–74.
7. K. B. Michels et al., "Coffee, Tea, and Caffeine Consumption and Breast Cancer Incidence in a Cohort of Swedish Women," *Annals of Epidemiology* 12, no. 1 (January 2002): 21–26; L. J. Vatten, K. Solvoll, and E. B. Løken, "Coffee Consumption and the Risk of Breast Cancer: A Prospective Study of 14,593 Norwegian Women," *British Journal of Cancer* 62 (1990): 267–70.
8. J. A. Baker et al., "Consumption of Coffee, but Not Black Tea, Is Associated with Decreased Risk of Premenopausal Breast Cancer," *Journal of Nutrition* 136, no. 1 (January 2006): 166–71; J. Li et al., "Coffee Consumption Modifies Risk of Estrogen-Receptor Negative Breast Cancer," *Breast Cancer Research* 13, no. 3 (2011): R49.
9. P. W. Parodi, "Dairy Product Consumption and the Risk of Breast Cancer," *Journal of the American College of Nutrition* 24, no. 6 (December 2005): 556S–68S; W. Al Sarakbi, M. Salhab, and K. Mokbel, "Dairy Products and Breast Cancer Risk: A Review of the Literature," *International Journal of Fertility and Women's Medicine* 50, no. 6 (November–December 2005): 244–49; P. G. Moorman and P. D. Terry, "Consumption of Dairy Products and the Risk of Breast Cancer: A Review of the

Literature," *American Journal of Clinical Nutrition* 80, no. 1 (2004): 5–14; M. H. Shin et al., "Intake of Dairy Products, Calcium, and Vitamin D and Risk of Breast Cancer," *Journal of the National Cancer Institute* 94, no. 17 (September 2002): 1301–11.

10. S. A. Missmer et al., "Meat and Dairy Food Consumption and Breast Cancer: A Pooled Analysis of Cohort Studies," *International Journal of Epidemiology* 31, no. 1 (February 2002): 78–85; M. D. Holmes et al., "Meat, Fish and Egg Intake and Risk of Breast Cancer," *International Journal of Cancer* 104, no. 2 (March 2003): 221–27; D. D. Alexander et al., "A Review and Meta-analysis of Red and Processed Meat Consumption and Breast Cancer," *Nutrition Research Reviews* 23, no. 2 (2010): 349–65.

11. V. Estrella et al., "Acidity Generated by the Tumor Microenvironment Drives Local Invasion," *Cancer Research* 73, no. 5 (2013): 1524–35; J. B. McGillen et al., "A General Reaction–Diffusion Model of Acidity in Cancer Invasion," *Journal of Mathematical Biology* 68, no. 5 (2014): 1199–224; K. O. Alfarouk, A. K. Muddathir, and M. E. A. Shayoub, "Tumor Acidity as Evolutionary Spite," *Cancers* 3, no. 1 (2011): 408–14; M. F. McCarty and J. Whitaker, "Manipulating Tumor Acidification as a Cancer Treatment Strategy," *Alternative Medicine Review* 15, no. 3 (2010): 264–72.

12. C. R. Cassileth, *Principles and Practice of Gastrointestinal Oncology* (Philadelphia: Lippincott Williams & Wilkins, 2008): 137.

13. S. R. Harris et al., "Clinical Practice Guidelines for the Care and Treatment of Breast Cancer: 11. Lymphedema," *Canadian Medical Association Journal* 164, no. 2 (2001): 191–99.

14. L. Chen, K. E. Malone, and C. I. Li, "Bra Wearing Not Associated with Breast Cancer Risk: A Population-Based Case-Control Study," *Cancer Epidemiology, Biomarkers & Prevention* 23, no. 10 (2014): 2181–85.

15. D. K. Mirick, S. Davis, and D. B. Thomas, "Antiperspirant Use and the Risk of Breast Cancer," *Journal of the National Cancer Institute* 94 (2002): 1578–80; P. D. Gikas, L. Mansfield, and K. Mokbel, "Do Underarm Cosmetics Cause Breast Cancer?" *International Journal of Fertility and Women's Medicine* 49 (2004): 212–14.

16. P. D. Darbre, "Aluminum, Antiperspirants and Breast Cancer," *Journal of Inorganic Biochemistry* 99, no. 9 (2005): 1912–19.

17. P. D. Darbre, F. Mannello, and C. Exley, "Aluminium and Breast Cancer: Sources of Exposure, Tissue Measurements and Mechanisms of Toxicological Actions on Breast Biology," *Journal of Inorganic Biochemistry* 128 (2013): 257–61.

18. C. C. Willhite et al., "Systematic Review of Potential Health Risks Posed by Pharmaceutical, Occupational and Consumer Exposures to Metallic and Nanoscale Aluminum, Aluminum Oxides, Aluminum Hydroxide and Its Soluble Salts," *Critical Reviews in Toxicology* 44, no. 4 (2014): 1–80.

19. P. D. Darbre et al., "Concentrations of Parabens in Human Breast Tumours," *Journal of Applied Toxicology* 24 (2004): 5–13.

20. L. Barr et al., "Measurement of Paraben Concentrations in Human Breast Tissue at Serial Locations Across the Breast from Axilla to Sternum," *Journal of Applied Toxicology* 32 (2012): 219–32.

21. D. K. Mirick, S. Davis, and D. B. Thomas, "Antiperspirant Use and the Risk of Breast Cancer," *Journal of the National Cancer Institute* 94 (2002): 1578–80.

22. S. Fakri, A. Al-Azzawi, and N. Al-Tawil, "Antiperspirant Use as a Risk Factor for Breast Cancer in Iraq," *Eastern Mediterranean Health Journal* 12, nos. 3–4 (2006): 478–82.

23. K. G. McGrath, "An Earlier Age of Breast Cancer Diagnosis Related to More Frequent Use of Antiperspirants/Deodorants and Underarm Shaving," *European Journal of Cancer Prevention* 12 (2003): 479–85.

24. "Breast Cancer Statistics," World Cancer Research Fund International, accessed June 10, 2017, http://www.wcrf.org/int/cancer-facts-figures/data-specific-cancers /breast-cancer-statistics.

25. M. Donovan et al., "Personal Care Products That Contain Estrogens or Xenoestrogens May Increase Breast Cancer Risk," *Medical Hypotheses* 68 (2007): 756–66.

26. L. Rosenberg et al., "Hair Relaxers Not Associated with Breast Cancer Risk: Evidence from the Black Women's Health Study," *Cancer Epidemiology and Prevention Biomarkers* 16, no. 5 (2007): 1035–37.

27. M. E. Herman-Giddens et al., "Secondary Sexual Characteristics and Menses in Young Girls Seen in Office Practice: A Study from the Pediatric Research in Office Settings Network," *Pediatrics* 99, no. 4 (1997): 505–12.

28. M. Donovan et al., "Personal Care Products That Contain Estrogens or Xenoestrogens May Increase Breast Cancer Risk," *Medical Hypotheses* 68, no. 4 (2007): 756–66.

29. V. R. Jacobs et al., "Mastitis Nonpuerperalis After Nipple Piercing: Time to Act," *International Journal of Fertility and Women's Medicine* 48, no. 5 (2002): 226–31; J. Martin, "Is Nipple Piercing Compatible with Breastfeeding?" *Journal of Human Lactation* 20, no. 3 (2004): 319–21.

30. N. Kluger and V. Koljonen, "Tattoos, Inks, and Cancer," *Lancet Oncology* 13, no. 4 (2012): e161–e168.

31. K. Lehner et al., "Black Tattoo Inks Are a Source of Problematic Substances such as Dibutyl Phthalate," *Contact Dermatitis* 65 (2011): 231–38.

32. M. Shermer, "Can You Hear Me Now? The Truth About Cell Phones and Cancer," *Scientific American* 303, no. 4 (2010): 98.

33. B. Leikind, "Do Cell Phones Cause Cancer?" *Skeptic* 15, no. 4 (2010): 30.

34. E. Cardis et al., "Brain Tumour Risk in Relation to Mobile Telephone Use: Results of the INTERPHONE International Case-Control Study," *International Journal of Epidemiology* 39 (2010): 675; C. Johansen et al., "Cellular Telephones and Cancer: A Nationwide Cohort Study in Denmark," *Journal of the National Cancer Institute* 93 (2001): 203; V. G. Khurana et al., "Cell Phones and Brain Tumors: A Review Including the Long-Term Epidemiologic Data," *Surgical Neurology* 70 (2009): 205; V. S. Benson et al., "Mobile Phone Use and Risk of Brain Neoplasms and Other Cancers: Prospective Study," *International Journal of Epidemiology* 42, no. 3 (2013): 792–802.

35. V. G. Khurana et al., "Cell Phones and Brain Tumors: A Review Including the Long-Term Epidemiologic Data," *Surgical Neurology* 70 (2009): 205.

36. E. R. Schoenfeld et al., "Electromagnetic Fields and Breast Cancer on Long Island: A Case-Control Study," *American Journal of Epidemiology* 158, no. 1 (2003): 47–58.

37. P. K. Verkasalo et al., "Magnetic Fields of High Voltage Power Lines and Risk of Cancer in Finnish Adults: Nationwide Cohort Study," *British Medical Journal* 313

(1996): 1047–51; S. Davis, D. K. Mirick, and R. G. Stevens, "Residential Magnetic Fields and the Risk of Breast Cancer," *American Journal of Epidemiology* 155, no. 5 (2002): 446–54.

38. R. K. Adair, "Constraints on Biological Effects of Weak Extremely-Low-Frequency Electromagnetic Fields," *Physics Review* A43 (1991): 1039–48.

39. Collaborative Group on Hormonal Factors in Breast Cancer, "Breast Cancer and Hormonal Contraceptives: Collaborative Reanalysis of Individual Data on 53,297 Women with Breast Cancer and 100,239 Women Without Breast Cancer from 54 Epidemiological Studies," *Lancet* 347, no. 9017 (1996): 1713–27.

40. Jennifer M. Gierisch et al., "Oral Contraceptive Use and Risk of Breast, Cervical, Colorectal, and Endometrial Cancers: A Systematic Review," *Cancer Epidemiology and Prevention Biomarkers* 22, no. 11 (2013): 1931–43.

41. S. A. Narod et al., "Oral Contraceptives and the Risk of Hereditary Ovarian Cancer: Hereditary Ovarian Cancer Clinical Study Group," *New England Journal of Medicine* 339, no. 7 (1998): 424–28.

42. G. Nikas et al., "Endometrial Pinopodes Indicate a Shift in the Window of Receptivity in IVF Cycles," *Human Reproduction* 14 (1999): 787–92.

43. C. Fei et al., "Fertility Drugs and Young-Onset Breast Cancer: Results from the Two Sister Study," *Journal of the National Cancer Institute* 104 (2012): 1021–27; L. G. Liat et al., "Are Infertility Treatments a Potential Risk Factor for Cancer Development? Perspective of 30 Years of Follow-Up," *Gynecological Endocrinology* 28, no. 10 (2012): 809–14; L. M. Stewart et al., "In Vitro Fertilization and Breast Cancer: Is There Cause for Concern?" *Fertility and Sterility* 98, no. 2 (2012): 334–40; A. N. Yli-Kuha et al., "Cancer Morbidity in a Cohort of 9,175 Finnish Women Treated for Infertility," *Human Reproduction* 27, no. 4 (2012): 1149–55; L. A. Brinton et al., "In Vitro Fertilization and Risk of Breast and Gynecologic Cancers: A Retrospective Cohort Study Within the Israeli Maccabi Healthcare Services," *Fertility and Sterility* 99, no. 5 (2013): 1189–96.

44. T. N. Sergentanis et al., "IVF and Breast Cancer: A Systematic Review and Meta-analysis," *Human Reproduction Update* 20, no. 1 (2013): 106–23.

45. A. Q. van den Belt-Dusebout et al., "Ovarian Stimulation for In Vitro Fertilization and Long-Term Risk of Breast Cancer," *Journal of the American Medical Association* 316, no. 3 (2016): 300–312.

46. L. M. Stewart, "In Vitro Fertilization and Breast Cancer: Is There Cause for Concern?" *Fertility and Sterility* 98, no. 2 (2012): 334–40.

47. V. Beral et al., "Breast Cancer and Abortion: Collaborative Reanalysis of Data from 53 Epidemiological Studies, including 83,000 Women with Breast Cancer from 16 Countries," *Lancet* 363, no. 9414 (2004): 1007–16; K. B. Michels et al., "Induced and Spontaneous Abortion and Incidence of Breast Cancer Among Young Women: A Prospective Cohort Study," *Archives of Internal Medicine* 167, no. 8 (2007): 814–20; G. K. Reeves et al., "Breast Cancer Risk in Relation to Abortion: Results from the EPIC Study," *International Journal of Cancer* 119, no. 7 (2006): 1741–45; J. Couzin, "Cancer Risk: Review Rules Out Abortion–Cancer Link," *Science* 299, no. 5612 (2003): 1498.

48. National Cancer Institute, "Abortion, Miscarriage, and Breast Cancer Risk:

2003 Workshop," reviewed January 2010, http://www.cancer.gov/types/breast /abortion-miscarriage-risk.

49. V. Beral et al., "Breast Cancer and Abortion: Collaborative Reanalysis of Data from 53 Epidemiological Studies, Including 83,000 Women with Breast Cancer from 16 Countries," *Lancet* 363, no. 9414 (2004): 1007–16.

50. D. M. Deapen et al., "The Relationship Between Breast Cancer and Augmentation Mammaplasty: An Epidemiologic Study," *Plastic and Reconstructive Surgery* 77, no. 3 (1986): 361–68.

51. D. M. Deapen et al., "Cancer Risk Among Los Angeles Women with Cosmetic Breast Implants," *Plastic and Reconstructive Surgery* 119, no. 7 (2007): 1987–92.

52. E. C. Noels et al., "Breast Implants and the Risk of Breast Cancer: A Meta-analysis of Cohort Studies," *Aesthetic Surgery Journal* 35, no. 1 (2015): 55–62.

53. K. Kjøller et al., "Characteristics of Women with Cosmetic Breast Implants Compared with Women with Other Types of Cosmetic Surgery and Population-Based Controls in Denmark," *Annals of Plastic Surgery* 50, no. 1 (2003): 6–12.

54. A. Stivala et al., "Breast Cancer Risk in Women Treated with Augmentation Mammoplasty," *Oncology Reports* 28, no. 1 (2012): 3–7.

55. M. McCarthy, "Rare Lymphoma Is Linked to Breast Implants, US Officials Conclude," *British Medical Journal* 356 (2017).

56. K. Lund, M. Ewertz, and G. Schou, "Breast Cancer Incidence Subsequent to Surgical Reduction of the Female Breast," *Scandinavian Journal of Plastic and Reconstructive Surgery and Hand Surgery* 21, no. 2 (1987): 209–12; M. Baasch et al., "Breast Cancer Incidence Subsequent to Surgical Reduction of the Female Breast," *British Journal of Cancer* 73, no. 9 (1996): 961; J. D. Boice et al., "Cancer Following Breast Reduction Surgery in Denmark," *Cancer Causes and Control* 8, no. 2 (1997): 253–58; J. D. Boice et al., "Breast Cancer Following Breast Reduction Surgery in Sweden," *Plastic and Reconstructive Surgery* 106, no. 5 (2000): 755–62; M. H. Brown et al., "A Cohort Study of Breast Cancer Risk in Breast Reduction Patients," *Plastic and Reconstructive Surgery* 103, no. 8 (1999): 1674–81; J. P. Fryzek et al., "A Nationwide Study of Breast Cancer Incidence Following Breast Reduction Surgery in a Large Cohort of Swedish Women," *Breast Cancer Research and Treatment* 97, no. 2 (2006): 131–34; L. A. Brinton et al., "Breast Cancer Risk in Relation to Amount of Tissue Removed During Breast Reduction Operations in Sweden," *Cancer* 91, no. 3 (2001): 478–83; L. A. Brinton et al., "Breast Enlargement and Reduction: Results from a Breast Cancer Case-Control Study," *Plastic and Reconstructive Surgery* 97, no. 2 (1996): 269–75.

57. R. E. Tarone et al., "Breast Reduction Surgery and Breast Cancer Risk: Does Reduction Mammaplasty Have a Role in Primary Prevention Strategies for Women at High Risk of Breast Cancer?" *Plastic and Reconstructive Surgery* 113, no. 9 (2004): 2104–10.

58. A. Brodiet, B. Long, and Q. Lu, "Aromatase Expression in the Human Breast," *Breast Cancer Research and Treatment* 49, no. 1 (1998): S85–91; K. Lund, M. Ewertz, and G. Schou, "Breast Cancer Incidence Subsequent to Surgical Reduction of the Female Breast," *Scandinavian Journal of Plastic Surgery and Hand Surgery* 21, no. 2 (1987): 209–12.

59. D. Trichopoulos and L. Lipworth, "Is Cancer Causation Simpler Than We Thought,

but More Intractable?" *Epidemiology* 6, no. 4 (1995): 347–49; W. Y. J. Imagawa, R. Guzman, and S. Nandi, *Control of Mammary Gland Growth and Differentiation*, 2nd ed. (New York: Raven Press, 1994); R. T. Senie et al., "Is Breast Size a Predictor of Breast Cancer Risk or the Laterality of the Tumor?" *Cancer Causes and Control* 4, no. 3 (1993): 203–8.

60. A. S. Kusano et al., "A Prospective Study of Breast Size and Premenopausal Breast Cancer Incidence," *International Journal of Cancer* 118, no. 8 (2006): 2031–34.

61. R. T. Senie et al., "Is Breast Size a Predictor of Breast Cancer Risk or the Laterality of the Tumor?" *Cancer Causes and Control* 4, no. 3 (1993): 203–8; R. N. Katariya, A. P. Forrest, and I. H. Gravelle, "Breast Volumes in Cancer of the Breast," *British Journal of Cancer* 29, no. 3 (1974): 270–73; E. Thurfjell et al., "Breast Size and Mammographic Pattern in Relation to Breast Cancer Risk," *European Journal of Cancer Prevention* 5, no. 1 (1996): 37–41; E. L. Wynder, I. J. Bross, and T. Hirayama, "A Study of the Epidemiology of Cancer of the Breast," *Cancer* 13 (1960): 559–601; H. O. Adami and A. Rimsten, "Adipose Tissue and Aetiology of Breast Cancer," *Lancet* 2, no. 8091 (1978): 677–78; T. Hirohata, A. M. Nomura, and L. N. Kolonel, "Breast Size and Cancer," *British Medical Journal* 2, no. 6087 (1977): 641; I. Soini, "Risk Factors of Breast Cancer in Finland," *International Journal of Epidemiology* 6, no. 4 (1977): 365–73; A. Tavani et al., "Breast Size and Breast Cancer Risk," *European Journal of Cancer Prevention* 5, no. 5 (1996): 337–42.

62. C. T. Pham and S. J. McPhee, "Knowledge, Attitudes, and Practices of Breast and Cervical Cancer Screening Among Vietnamese Women," *Journal of Cancer Education* 7, no. 4 (1992): 305–10.

63. R. J. Donovan et al., "Changes in Beliefs About Cancer in Western Australia, 1964–2001," *Medical Journal of Australia* 181 (2004): 23–25.

Chapter 3: Eat This

1. T. P. Butler and P. M. Gullino, "Quantitation of Cell Shedding into Efferent Blood of Mammary Adenocarcinoma," *Cancer Research* 35, no. 3 (1975): 512–16.

2. T. C. Campbell and T. M. Campbell II, *The China Study: The Most Comprehensive Study of Nutrition Ever Conducted and the Startling Implications for Diet, Weight Loss, and Long-Term Health* (Dallas: BenBella, 2004).

3. M. O. Harris et al., "Grasses and Gall Midges: Plant Defense and Insect Adaptation," *Annual Review of Entomology* 48, no. 1 (2003): 549–77.

4. A. A. Oliveira et al., "Antimicrobial Activity of Amazonian Medicinal Plants," *SpringerPlus* 2, no. 1 (2013): 371.

5. J. Sun et al., "Antioxidant and Antiproliferative Activities of Fruits," *Journal of Agricultural and Food Chemistry* 50 (2002): 7449–54; Y. F. Chu et al., "Antioxidant and Antiproliferative Activities of Vegetables," *Journal of Agricultural and Food Chemistry* 50 (2002): 6910–16; L. O. Dragsted, M. Strube, and J. C. Larsen, "Cancer-Protective Factors in Fruits and Vegetables: Biochemical and Biological Background," *Pharmacology and Toxicology* 72 (1993): 116–35; A. R. Waladkhani and M. R. Clemens, "Effect of Dietary Phytochemicals on Cancer Development," *International Journal of Molecular Medicine* 1 (1998): 747–53.

6. M. Valko et al., "Free Radicals, Metals, and Antioxidants in Oxidative Stress -Induced Cancer," *Chemico-Biological Interactions* 160, no. 1 (2006): 1–40.

7. B. Burton-Freeman et al., "Strawberry Modulates LDL Oxidation and Postprandial Lipemia in Response to High-Fat Meal in Overweight Hyperlipidemic Men and Women," *Journal of the American College of Nutrition* 29, no. 1 (2010): 46–54.

8. M. A. Martinez-Gonzalez and N. Martin-Calvo, "Mediterranean Diet and Life Expectancy: Beyond Olive Oil, Fruits, and Vegetables," *Current Opinion in Clinical Nutrition and Metabolic Care* 19, no. 6 (2016): 401–7.

9. A. Trichopoulou et al., "Cancer and Mediterranean Dietary Traditions," *Cancer Epidemiology, Biomarkers and Prevention* 9, no. 9 (2000): 869–73; W. C. Willett et al., "Mediterranean Diet Pyramid: A Cultural Model for Healthy Eating," *American Journal of Clinical Nutrition* 61, no. 6 (1995): 1402S–6S; F. Levi, F Lucchini, and C. La Vecchia, "Worldwide Patterns of Cancer Mortality," *European Journal of Cancer Prevention* 3 (1994): 109–43.

10. A. Castelló et al., "Spanish Mediterranean Diet and Other Dietary Patterns and Breast Cancer Risk: Case-Control EpiGEICAM Study," *British Journal of Cancer* 111, no. 7 (2014): 1454–62.

11. P. A. van den Brandt and M. Schulpen, "Mediterranean Diet Adherence and Risk of Postmenopausal Breast Cancer: Results of a Cohort Study and Meta-analysis," *International Journal of Cancer* 140 (2017): 2220–31.

12. G. Buckland et al., "Adherence to the Mediterranean Diet and Risk of Breast Cancer in the European Prospective Investigation into Cancer and Nutrition Cohort Study," *International Journal of Cancer* 132, no. 12 (2013): 2918–27.

13. K. Pintha, S. Yodkeeree, and P. Limtrakul, "Proanthocyanidin in Red Rice Inhibits MDA-MB-231 Breast Cancer Cell Invasion via the Expression Control of Invasive Proteins," *Biological and Pharmaceutical Bulletin* 38, no. 4 (2015): 571–81; E. A. Hudson et al., "Characterization of Potentially Chemopreventive Phenols in Extracts of Brown Rice that Inhibit the Growth of Human Breast and Colon Cancer Cells," *Cancer Epidemiology and Prevention Biomarkers* 9, no. 11 (2000): 1163–70; C. Hui et al., "Anticancer Activities of an Anthocyanin-Rich Extract from Black Rice Against Breast Cancer Cells In Vitro and In Vivo," *Nutrition and Cancer* 62, no. 8 (2010): 1128–36.

14. American Cancer Society, *Breast Cancer Facts & Figures 2017–2018* (2017), accessed December 2, 2017, https://www.cancer.org/content/dam/cancer-org/research /cancer-facts-and-statistics/breast-cancer-facts-and-figures/breast-cancer-facts-and -figures-2017–2018.pdf.

15. American Institute for Cancer Research, *Facts on Preventing Cancer: The Cancer Fighters in Your Food* brochure, accessed December 26, 2017, https://www.aicr.org /assets/docs/pdf/brochures.

16. "5 Colors of Phytonutrients," Naturally Healthy Concepts, accessed December 26, 2017, https://www.naturalhealthyconcepts.com/resources/infographics /phytonutrients; Office of Disease Prevention and Health Promotion, "Shifts Needed to Align with Healthy Eating Patterns," in *Dietary Guidelines for Americans 2015 –2020*, 8th ed., accessed December 3, 2017, https://health.gov/dietaryguidelines/2015 /guidelines/chapter-2/a-closer-look-at-current-intakes-and-recommended-shifts/.

17. C. B. Ambrosone et al., "Breast Cancer Risk in Premenopausal Women Is Inversely Associated with Consumption of Broccoli, a Source of Isothiocyanates, but Is Not Modified by GST Genotype," *Journal of Nutrition* 134, no. 5 (2004): 1134–38.

18. Y. Li et al., "Sulforaphane, a Dietary Component of Broccoli / Broccoli Sprouts, Inhibits Breast Cancer Stem Cells," *Clinical Cancer Research* 16, no. 9 (2010): 2580–90.

19. J. J. Michnovicz, H. Adlercreutz, and H. L. Bradlow, "Changes in Levels of Urinary Estrogen Metabolites after Oral Indole-3-Carbinol Treatment in Humans," *Journal of the National Cancer Institute* 89, no. 10 (1997): 718–23.

20. D. A. Boggs et al., "Fruit and Vegetable Intake in Relation to Risk of Breast Cancer in the Black Women's Health Study," *American Journal of Epidemiology* 172, no. 11 (2010): 1268–79.

21. M. Gerber, "Fibre and Breast Cancer," *European Journal of Cancer Prevention* 7, no. 2 (May 1998): S63–67; L. A. Cohen, "Dietary Fiber and Breast Cancer," *Anticancer Research* 19, no. 5A (September–October 1999): 3685–88.

22. S. Gandini et al., "Meta-analysis of Studies on Breast Cancer Risk and Diet: The Role of Fruit and Vegetable Consumption and the Intake of Associated Micronutrients," *European Journal of Cancer* 36, no. 5 (March 2000): 636–46; T. T. Fung et al., "Diet Quality Is Associated with the Risk of Estrogen Receptor-Negative Breast Cancer in Postmenopausal Women," *Journal of Nutrition* 136, no. 2 (February 2006): 466–72.

23. I. Mattisson et al., "Intakes of Plant Foods, Fibre and Fat and Risk of Breast Cancer: A Prospective Study in the Malmo Diet and Cancer Cohort," *British Journal of Cancer* 90, no. 1 (January 2004): 122–27.

24. G. R. Howe et al., "Dietary Factors and Risk of Breast Cancer: Combined Analysis of 12 Case-Control Studies," *Journal of the National Cancer Institute* 82, no. 7 (1990): 561–69.

25. A. Moshfegh, J. Goldman, and L. Cleveland, "What We Eat in America, NHANES 2001–2002: Usual Nutrient Intakes from Food Compared to Dietary Reference Intakes," *US Department of Agriculture, Agricultural Research Service* 9 (2005).

26. G. D. Stoner, L. S. Wang, and B. C. Casto, "Laboratory and Clinical Studies of Cancer Chemoprevention by Antioxidants in Berries," *Carcinogenesis* 29, no. 9 (2008): 1665–74.

27. M. H. Carlsen et al., "The Total Antioxidant Content of More than 3,100 Foods, Beverages, Spices, Herbs and Supplements Used Worldwide," *Nutrition Journal* 9, no. 1 (2010): 3.

28. C. Gerhauser, "Cancer Chemopreventive Potential of Apples, Apple Juice, and Apple Components," *Planta Medica* 74, no. 13 (2008): 1608–24.

29. S. Gallus et al., "Does an Apple a Day Keep the Oncologist Away?" *Annals of Oncology* 16, no. 11 (2005): 1841–44.

30. K. Wolfe, W. Xianzhong, and R. H. Liu, "Antioxidant Activity of Apple Peels," *Journal of Agricultural and Food Chemistry* 51, no. 3 (2003): 609–14.

31. E. Giovannucci, "Tomatoes, Tomato-Based Products, Lycopene, and Cancer: Review of the Epidemiologic Literature," *Journal of the National Cancer Institute* 91, no. 4 (1999): 317–31; G. Masala et al., "Fruit and Vegetables Consumption and Breast Cancer Risk: The EPIC Italy study," *Breast Cancer Research and Treatment* 132, no. 3 (2012): 1127–36.

32. V. Dewanto et al., "Thermal Processing Enhances the Nutritional Value of Tomatoes by Increasing Total Antioxidant Activity," *Journal of Agricultural and Food Chemistry* 50, no. 10 (2002): 3010–14.

33. B. J. Grube et al., "White Button Mushroom Phytochemicals Inhibit Aromatase Activity and Breast Cancer Cell Proliferation," *Journal of Nutrition* 131, no. 12 (2001): 3288–93.

34. M. Zhang, "Dietary Intakes of Mushrooms and Green Tea Combine to Reduce the Risk of Breast Cancer in Chinese Women," *International Journal of Cancer* 124, no. 6 (2009): 1404–8.

35. S. P. Wasser, "Medicinal Mushroom Science: History, Current Status, Future Trends, and Unsolved Problems," *International Journal of Medicinal Mushrooms* 12, no. 1 (2010).

36. S. Oommen et al., "Allicin (from Garlic) Induces Caspase-Mediated Apoptosis in Cancer Cells," *European Journal of Pharmacology* 485, no. 1 (2004): 97–103; J. Antosiewicz et al., "Role of Reactive Oxygen Intermediates in Cellular Responses to Dietary Cancer Chemopreventive Agents," *Planta Medica* 74, no. 13 (2008): 1570–79.

37. B. Challier, J. M. Perarnau, and J. F. Viel, "Garlic, Onion and Cereal Fibre as Protective Factors for Breast Cancer: A French Case-Control Study," *European Journal of Epidemiology* 14, no. 8 (1998): 737–47.

38. B. B. Aggarwal et al., "Curcumin Suppresses the Paclitaxel-Induced Nuclear Factor-κB Pathway in Breast Cancer Cells and Inhibits Lung Metastasis of Human Breast Cancer in Nude Mice," *Clinical Cancer Research* 11, no. 20 (2005): 7490–98; T. Choudhuri et al., "Curcumin Induces Apoptosis in Human Breast Cancer Cells Through p53-Dependent BAX Induction," *FEBS Letters* 512, nos. 1–3 (2002): 334–40; S. Somasundaram et al., "Dietary Curcumin Inhibits Chemotherapy-Induced Apoptosis in Models of Human Breast Cancer," *Cancer Research* 62, no. 13 (2002): 3868–75.

39. S. Percival et al., "Bioavailability of Herbs and Spices in Humans as Determined by Ex Vivo Inflammatory Suppression and DNA Strand Breaks," *Journal of the American College of Nutrition* 31, no. 4 (2012): 288–94.

40. G. Shoba et al., "Influence of Piperine on the Pharmacokinetics of Curcumin in Animals and Human Volunteers," *Planta Medica* 64, no. 4 (1998): 353–56.

41. L. Lai et al., "Piperine Suppresses Tumor Growth and Metastasis In Vitro and In Vivo in a 4T1 Murine Breast Cancer Model," *Acta Pharmacologica Sinica* 33, no. 4 (2012): 523–30.

42. J. Kim et al., "Turmeric (Curcuma Longa) Inhibits Inflammatory Nuclear Factor (NF)-κB and NF-κB-Regulated Gene Products and Induces Death Receptors Leading to Suppressed Proliferation, Induced Chemosensitization, and Suppressed Osteoclastogenesis," *Molecular Nutrition and Food Research* 56, no. 3 (2012): 454–65.

43. A. Rasyid et al., "Effect of Different Curcumin Dosages on Human Gall Bladder," *Asia Pacific Journal of Clinical Nutrition* 11, no. 4 (2002): 314–18.

44. J. Zheng et al., "Spices for Prevention and Treatment of Cancers," *Nutrients* 8, no. 8 (2016): 495; A. Iyer et al., "Potential Health Benefits of Indian Spices in the Symptoms of the Metabolic Syndrome: A Review," *Indian Journal of Biochemistry and Biophysics* 46, no. 6 (2009): 467–81; C. M Kaefer and J. A. Milner, "The Role of

Herbs and Spices in Cancer Prevention," *Journal of Nutritional Biochemistry* 19, no. 6 (2008): 347–61; K. Krishnaswamy, "Traditional Indian Spices and Their Health Significance," *Asia Pacific Journal of Clinical Nutrition* 17, no. 1 (2008): 265–8.

45. S. S. Percival et al., "Bioavailability of Herbs and Spices in Humans as Determined by Ex Vivo Inflammatory Suppression and DNA Strand Breaks," *Journal of the American College of Nutrition* 31, no. 4 (2012): 288–94; I. Paur et al., "Extract of Oregano, Coffee, Thyme, Clove, and Walnuts Inhibits NF-κB in Monocytes and in Transgenic Reporter Mice," *Cancer Prevention Research* 3, no. 5 (2010): 653–63; N. Wang et al., "Ellagic Acid, a Phenolic Compound, Exerts Anti-angiogenesis Effects via VEGFR-2 Signaling Pathway in Breast Cancer," *Breast Cancer Research and Treatment* 134, no. 3 (2012): 943–55; K. Aruna and V. M. Sivaramakrishnan, "Plant Products as Protective Agents Against Cancer," *Indian Journal of Experimental Biology* 28, no. 11 (1990): 1008–11.

46. Federal Institute for Risk Assessment, "High Daily Intakes of Cinnamon: Daily Health Risks Cannot be Ruled Out," *BfR Health Assessment*, August 18, 2006, http://www.bfr.bund.de/cm/349/high_daily_intakes_of_cinnamon_health_risk_cannot _be_ruled_out.pdf.

47. C. M. Kaefer and J. A. Milner, "Herbs and Spices in Cancer Prevention and Treatment," in *Herbal Medicine: Biomolecular and Clinical Aspects*, 2nd ed., ed. I. F. F. Benzie and S. Wachtel-Galor (Boca Raton, FL: CRC Press, 2011), accessed December 3, 2017, https://www.ncbi.nlm.nih.gov/books/NBK92774; B. B. Aggarwal et al., "Potential of Spice-Derived Phytochemicals for Cancer Prevention," *Planta Medica* 74, no. 13 (2008): 1560–69; S. Dragland et al., "Several Culinary and Medicinal Herbs Are Important Sources of Dietary Antioxidants," *Journal of Nutrition* 133, no. 5 (2003): 1286–90.

48. J. Teas et al., "Dietary Seaweed Modifies Estrogen and Phytoestrogen Metabolism in Healthy Postmenopausal Women," *Journal of Nutrition* 139, no. 5 (2009): 939–44.

49. Y. J. Yang et al., "A Case-Control Study on Seaweed Consumption and the Risk of Breast Cancer," *British Journal of Nutrition* 103, no. 9 (2010): 1345–53.

50. F. M. Steinberg et al., "Cocoa and Chocolate Flavonoids: Implications for Cardiovascular Health," *Journal of the American Dietetic Association* 103, no. 2 (2003): 215–23.

51. Z. Faridi et al., "Acute Dark Chocolate and Cocoa Ingestion and Endothelial Function: A Randomized Controlled Crossover Trial," *American Journal of Clinical Nutrition* 88, no. 1 (2008): 58–63.

52. R. S. Muthyala et al., "Equol, a Natural Estrogenic Metabolite from Soy Isoflavones: Convenient Preparation and Resolution of R-and S-equols and Their Differing Binding and Biological Activity through Estrogen Receptors Alpha and Beta," *Bioorganic & Medicinal Chemistry* 12, no. 6 (2004): 1559–67.

53. F. V. So et al., "Inhibition of Proliferation of Estrogen Receptor-Positive MCF-7 Human Breast Cancer Cells by Flavonoids in the Presence and Absence of Excess Estrogen," *Cancer Letters* 112, no. 2 (1997): 127–33; S. O. Mueller et al., "Phytoestrogens and Their Human Metabolites Show Distinct Agonistic and Antagonistic Properties on Estrogen Receptor α (ERα) and ERβ in Human Cells," *Toxicological Sciences* 80, no. 1 (2004): 14–25.

54. J. T. Kellis Jr. and L. E. Vickery, "Inhibition of Human Estrogen Synthetase (Aromatase) by Flavones," *Science* 225 (1984): 1032–35.

55. L. J. Lu et al., "Effects of Soya Consumption for One Month on Steroid Hormones in Premenopausal Women: Implications for Breast Cancer Risk Reduction," *Cancer Epidemiology and Prevention Biomarkers* 5, no. 1 (1996): 63–70.

56. S. A. Lee et al., "Adolescent and Adult Soy Food Intake and Breast Cancer Risk: Results from the Shanghai Women's Health Study," *American Journal of Clinical Nutrition* 89, no. 6 (2009): 1920–26.

57. L. A. Korde et al., "Childhood Soy Intake and Breast Cancer Risk in Asian American Women," *Cancer Epidemiology and Prevention Biomarkers* 18, no. 4 (2009): 1050–59.

58. K. P. Ko et al., "Dietary Intake and Breast Cancer Among Carriers and Noncarriers of BRCA Mutations in the Korean Hereditary Breast Cancer Study," *American Journal of Clinical Nutrition* 98, no. 6 (2013): 1493–501.

59. N. Guha et al., "Soy Isoflavones and Risk of Cancer Recurrence in a Cohort of Breast Cancer Survivors: The Life after Cancer Epidemiology Study," *Breast Cancer Research and Treatment* 118, no. 2 (2009): 395–405.

60. P. J. Magee and I. R. Rowland, "Phyto-oestrogens, Their Mechanism of Action: Current Evidence for a Role in Breast and Prostate Cancer," *British Journal of Nutrition* 91, no. 4 (2004): 513–31; L. Varinska et al., "Soy and Breast Cancer: Focus on Angiogenesis," *International Journal of Molecular Sciences* 16, no. 5 (2015): 11728–49.

61. F. F. Zhang et al., "Dietary Isoflavone Intake and All-Cause Mortality in Breast Cancer Survivors: The Breast Cancer Family Registry," *Cancer* 123, no. 11 (2017): 2070–79.

62. X. O. Shu et al., "Soy Food Intake and Breast Cancer Survival," *Journal of the American Medical Association* 302, no. 22 (2009): 2437–43.

63. S. J. Nechuta et al., "Soy Food Intake After Diagnosis of Breast Cancer and Survival: An In-Depth Analysis of Combined Evidence from Cohort Studies of US and Chinese Women," *American Journal of Clinical Nutrition* 96, no. 1 (2012): 123–32.

64. F. Chi et al., "Post-Diagnosis Soy Food Intake and Breast Cancer Survival: A Meta-analysis of Cohort Studies," *Asian Pacific Journal of Cancer Prevention* 14, no. 4 (2013): 2407–12.

65. Economic Research Service, "Recent Trends in GE Adoption," United States Department of Agriculture, last updated July 12, 2017, http://www.ers.usda.gov /data-products/adoption-of-genetically-engineered-crops-in-the-us/recent-trends-in -ge-adoption.aspx.

66. J. A. Miller et al., "Human Breast Tissue Disposition and Bioactivity of Limonene in Women with Early-Stage Breast Cancer," *Cancer Prevention Research* 6, no. 6 (2013): 577–84.

67. U. Veronesi et al., "Randomized Trial of Fenretinide to Prevent Second Breast Malignancy in Women with Early Breast Cancer," *Journal of the National Cancer Institute* 91, no. 21 (November 1999): 1847–56.

68. S. Gandini et al., "Meta-analysis of Studies on Breast Cancer Risk and Diet:

The Role of Fruit and Vegetable Consumption and the Intake of Associated Micronutrients," *European Journal of Cancer* 36, no. 5 (March 2000): 636–46.

69. S. M. Zhang et al., "Plasma Folate, Vitamin B6, Vitamin B12, Homocysteine, and Risk of Breast Cancer," *Journal of the National Cancer Institute* 95, no. 5 (March 2003): 373–80.

70. S. Gandini, "Meta-analysis of Studies on Breast Cancer Risk and Diet: The Role of Fruit and Vegetable Consumption and the Intake of Associated Micronutrients," *European Journal of Cancer* 36, no. 5 (March 2000): 636–46.

71. M. S. Donaldson, "Metabolic Vitamin B12 Status on a Mostly Raw Vegan Diet with Follow-Up Using Tablets, Nutritional Yeast, or Probiotic Supplements," *Annals of Nutrition and Metabolism* 44, no. 5–6 (2000): 229–34.

72. S. J. P. M. Eussen et al., "Oral Cyanocobalamin Supplementation in Older People with Vitamin B12 Deficiency: A Dose-Finding Trial," *Archives of Internal Medicine* 165, no. 10 (2005): 1167–72.

73. A. J. L. Cooper, "Biochemistry of Sulfur-Containing Amino Acids," *Annual Review of Biochemistry* 52 (1983): 187–222; J. D. Hayes and L. I. McLellan, "Glutathione and Glutathione-Dependent Enzymes Represent a Co-ordinately Regulated Defence Against Oxidative Stress," *Free Radical Research* 31 (1999): 273–300.

74. S. M. Zhang et al., "Plasma Folate, Vitamin B6, Vitamin B12, Homocysteine, and Risk of Breast Cancer," *Journal of the National Cancer Institute* 95, no. 5 (2003): 373–80.

75. J. K. Song and J. M. Bae, "Citrus Fruit Intake and Breast Cancer Risk: A Quantitative Systematic Review," *Journal of Breast Cancer* 16, no. 1 (2013): 72–76.

76. G. R. Howe et al., "Dietary Factors and Risk of Breast Cancer: Combined Analysis of 12 Case-Control Studies," *Journal of the National Cancer Institute* 82, no. 7 (1990): 561–69.

77. K. Robien, G. J. Cutler, and D. Lazovich, "Vitamin D Intake and Breast Cancer Risk in Postmenopausal Women: The Iowa Women's Health Study," *Cancer Causes and Control* 18, no. 7 (September 2007): 775–82.

78. C. F. Garland et al., "Vitamin D and Prevention of Breast Cancer: Pooled Analysis," *Journal of Steroid Biochemistry and Molecular Biology* 103, nos. 3–5 (March 2007): 708–11.

79. S. B. Mohr et al., "Meta-analysis of Vitamin D Sufficiency for Improving Survival of Patients with Breast Cancer," *Anticancer Research* 34, no. 3 (2014): 1163–66.

80. C. F. Garland et al., "Vitamin D and Prevention of Breast Cancer: Pooled Analysis," *Journal of Steroid Biochemistry and Molecular Biology* 103, nos. 3–5 (March 2007): 708–11.

81. C. F. Garland et al., "Vitamin D Supplement Doses and Serum 25-Hydroxyvitamin D in the Range Associated with Cancer Prevention," *Anticancer Research* 31, no. 2 (2011): 607–11.

82. E. Kesse-Guyot et al., "Dairy Products, Calcium, and the Risk of Breast Cancer: Results of the French SU.VI.MAX Prospective Study," *Annals of Nutrition and Metabolism* 51, no. 2 (2007): 139–45; M. L. McCullough et al., "Dairy, Calcium, and Vitamin D Intake and Postmenopausal Breast Cancer Risk in the Cancer Prevention Study II Nutrition Cohort," *Cancer Epidemiology, Biomarkers and Prevention* 14, no. 12 (December 2005): 2898–904.

83. P. W. Parodi, "Dairy Product Consumption and the Risk of Breast Cancer," *Journal of the American College of Nutrition* 24 (2005): 556S–68S; Y. Cui and T. E. Rohan, "Vitamin D, Calcium, and Breast Cancer Risk: A Review," *Cancer Epidemiology, Biomarkers and Prevention* 15, no. 8 (2006): 1427–37.

84. B. C. Davis and P. M. Kris-Etherton, "Achieving Optimal Essential Fatty Acid Status in Vegetarians: Current Knowledge and Practical Implications," *The American Journal of Clinical Nutrition* 78, no. 3 (2003): 640S–46S.

85. E. D. Rosen and B. M. Spiegelman, "What We Talk About When We Talk About Fat," *Cell* 156, no. 1 (2014): 20–44.

86. M. Khodarahmi and L. Azadbakht, "The Association Between Different Kinds of Fat Intake and Breast Cancer Risk in Women," *International Journal of Preventive Medicine* 5, no. 1 (2014): 6–15.

87. S. Sieri et al., "Dietary Fat Intake and Development of Specific Breast Cancer Subtypes," *Journal of the National Cancer Institute* 106, no. 5 (2014): dju068.

88. Y. Liu et al., "Adolescent Dietary Fiber, Vegetable Fat, Vegetable Protein, and Nut Intakes and Breast Cancer Risk," *Breast Cancer Research and Treatment* 145, no. 2 (2014): 461–70; G. A. Colditz, K. Bohlke, and C. S. Berkey, "Breast Cancer Risk Accumulation Starts Early: Prevention Must Also," *Breast Cancer Research and Treatment* 145, no. 3 (2014): 567–79.

89. A. L. Frazier et al., "Adolescent Diet and Risk of Breast Cancer," *Cancer Causes and Control* 15, no. 1 (February 2004): 73–82.

90. A. I. Smeds et al., "Quantification of a Broad Spectrum of Lignans in Cereals, Oilseeds, and Nuts," *Journal of Agricultural and Food Chemistry* 55, no. 4 (2007): 1337–46.

91. L. B. Kardono et al., "Cytotoxic Constituents of the Bark of Plumeria Rubra Collected in Indonesia," *Journal of Natural Products* 53 (1990): 1447–55; T. Hirano et al., "Antiproliferative Activity of Mammalian Lignan Derivatives Against the Human Breast Carcinoma Cell Line, ZR-75–1," *Cancer Investigation* 8 (1990): 592–602; M. Serraino and L. U. Thompson, "The Effect of Flaxseed Supplementation on Early Risk Markers for Mammary Carcinogenesis," *Cancer Letters* 60 (1991): 135–42; L. U. Thompson et al., "Antitumorigenic Effect of a Mammalian Lignan Precursor from Flaxseed," *Nutrition and Cancer* 26, no. 2 (1996): 159–65; C. Wang et al., "Lignans and Flavonoids Inhibit Aromatase Enzyme in Human Preadipocytes," *Journal of Steroid Biochemistry and Molecular Biology* 50, nos. 3–4 (1994): 205–12; H. Adlercreutz et al., "Dietary Phytoestrogens and Cancer: In Vitro and In Vivo Studies," *Journal of Steroid Biochemistry and Molecular Biology* 41, nos. 3–8 (1992): 331–37.

92. C. J. Fabian et al., "Reduction in Ki-67 in Benign Breast Tissue of High-Risk Premenopausal Women with the SERM Acolbifene," *Journal of Clinical Oncology* 30, no. 15 (2012): 520.

93. H. L. Newmark, "Squalene, Olive Oil, and Cancer Risk: Review and Hypothesis," *Annals of the New York Academy of Sciences* 889, no. 1 (1999): 193–203.

94. G. K. Beauchamp et al., "Phytochemistry: Ibuprofen-like Activity in Extra-Virgin Olive Oil," *Nature* 437, no. 7055 (2005): 45–46.

95. L. Bozzetto et al., "Extra-Virgin Olive Oil Reduces Glycemic Response to a

High–Glycemic Index Meal in Patients with Type 1 Diabetes: A Randomized Controlled Trial," *Diabetes Care* 39, no. 4 (2016): 518–24.

96. A. Trichopoulou et al., "Consumption of Olive Oil and Specific Food Groups in Relation to Breast Cancer Risk in Greece," *Journal of the National Cancer Institute* 87, no. 2 (1995): 110–16; J. M. Martin-Moreno et al., "Dietary Fat, Olive Oil Intake and Breast Cancer Risk," *International Journal of Cancer* 58, no. 6 (1994): 774–80; L. Lipworth et al., "Olive Oil and Human Cancer: An Assessment of the Evidence," *Preventive Medicine* 26, no. 2 (1997): 181–90.

97. E. Toledo et al., "Mediterranean Diet and Invasive Breast Cancer Risk Among Women at High Cardiovascular Risk in the PREDIMED Trial: A Randomized Clinical Trial," *Journal of the American Medical Association Internal Medicine* 14 (September 2015).

98. C. Razquin et al., "A 3 Years Follow-Up of a Mediterranean Diet Rich in Virgin Olive Oil Is Associated with High Plasma Antioxidant Capacity and Reduced Body Weight Gain," *European Journal of Clinical Nutrition* 63, no. 12 (2009): 1387–93.

99. M. Ni, *Secrets of Longevity* (San Francisco: Chronicle Books, 2006).

100. M. R. Sartippour et al., "Green Tea and Its Catechins Inhibit Breast Cancer Xenografts," *Nutrition and Cancer* 40, no. 2 (2001): 149–56; S. F. Eddy, S. E. Kane, and G. E. Sonenshein, "Trastuzumab-Resistant HER2-Driven Breast Cancer Cells Are Sensitive to Epigallocatechin-3 Gallate," *Cancer Research* 67, no. 19 (2007): 9018–23.

101. A. Büyükbalci, "Determination of In Vitro Antidiabetic Effects, Antioxidant Activities, and Phenol Contents of Some Herbal Teas," *Plant Foods for Human Nutrition* 63, no. 1 (March 2008): 27–33.

102. M. Inoue et al., "Regular Consumption of Green Tea and the Risk of Breast Cancer Recurrence: Follow-Up Study from the Hospital-Based Epidemiologic Research Program at Aichi Cancer Center (HERPACC), Japan," *Cancer Letters* 167, no. 2 (June 2001): 175–82.

103. A. H. Wu et al., "Green Tea and Risk of Breast Cancer in Asian Americans," *International Journal of Cancer* 106, no. 4 (September 2003): 574–79.

104. A. A. Ogunleye, F. Xue, and K. B. Michels, "Green Tea Consumption and Breast Cancer Risk or Recurrence: A Meta-analysis," *Breast Cancer Research and Treatment* 119, no. 2 (2010): 477–84.

105. M. Inoue et al., "Regular Consumption of Green Tea and the Risk of Breast Cancer Recurrence: Follow-Up Study from the Hospital-Based Epidemiologic Research Program at Aichi Cancer Center (HERPACC), Japan," *Cancer Letters* 167, no. 2 (June 2001): 175–82.

106. K. Nakachi et al., "Influence of Drinking Green Tea on Breast Cancer Malignancy Among Japanese Patients," *Japanese Journal of Cancer Research* 89, no. 3 (1998): 254–61.

107. S. Pianetti et al., "Green Tea Polyphenol Epigallocatechin-3 Gallate Inhibits Her-2/neu Signaling, Proliferation, and Transformed Phenotype of Breast Cancer Cells," *Cancer Research* 62, no. 3 (2002): 652–55.

108. J. Jankun et al., "Why Drinking Green Tea Could Prevent Cancer," *Nature* 387, no. 6633 (1997): 561.

109. C. Cabrera, R. Giménez, and M. C. López, "Determination of Tea Components with Antioxidant Activity," *Journal of Agricultural and Food Chemistry* 51, no. 15 (2003): 4427–35.

110. R. J. Green et al., "Common Tea Formulations Modulate In Vitro Digestive Recovery of Green Tea Catechins," *Molecular Nutrition and Food Research* 51, no. 9 (2007): 1152–62.

111. World Cancer Research Fund, "Food, Nutrition, and the Prevention of Cancer: A Global Perspective" (Washington, DC: American Institute for Cancer Research, 1997).

112. K. B. Michels et al., "Coffee, Tea, and Caffeine Consumption and Breast Cancer Incidence in a Cohort of Swedish Women," *Annals of Epidemiology* 12, no. 1 (January 2002): 21–26; A. Tavani et al., "Coffee Consumption and the Risk of Breast Cancer," *European Journal of Cancer Prevention* 7, no. 1 (February 1998): 77–82.

113. J. A. Baker et al., "Consumption of Coffee, but Not Black Tea, Is Associated with Decreased Risk of Premenopausal Breast Cancer," *Journal of Nutrition* 136, no. 1 (January 2006): 166–71; J. Li et al., "Coffee Consumption Modifies Risk of Estrogen-Receptor Negative Breast Cancer," *Breast Cancer Research* 13, no. 3 (2011): R49.

114. N. Bhoo-Pathy et al., "Coffee and Tea Consumption and Risk of Pre- and Postmenopausal Breast Cancer in the European Prospective Investigation into Cancer and Nutrition (EPIC) Cohort Study," *Breast Cancer Research* 17, no. 1 (2015): 15.

115. I. E. Milder et al., "Lignan Contents of Dutch Plant Foods: A Database Including Lariciresinol, Pinoresinol, Secoisolariciresinol, and Matairesinol," *British Journal of Nutrition* 93, no. 3 (2005): 393–402.

116. Ann. H. Rosendahl et al., "Caffeine and Caffeic Acid Inhibit Growth and Modify Estrogen Receptor and Insulin-like Growth Factor I Receptor Levels in Human Breast Cancer," *Clinical Cancer Research* 21, no. 8 (April 2015): 1877–87.

117. E. C. Lowcock et al., "High Coffee Intake, but Not Caffeine, Is Associated with Reduced Estrogen Receptor Negative and Postmenopausal Breast Cancer Risk with No Effect Modification by CYP1A2 Genotype," *Nutrition and Cancer* 65, no. 3 (2013): 398–409.

118. A. Nkondjock et al., "Coffee Consumption and Breast Cancer Risk among BRCA1 and BRCA2 Mutation Carriers," *International Journal of Cancer* 118, no. 1 (2006): 103–7.

119. L. J. Vatten, K. Solvoll, and E. B. Løken, "Coffee Consumption and the Risk of Breast Cancer: A Prospective Study of 14,593 Norwegian Women," *British Journal of Cancer* 62, no. 2 (August 1990): 267–70.

120. L. Zhu et al., "Coffee Consumption Increases Risk of Advanced Breast Cancer Among Singapore Chinese Women," *CSU Theses and Dissertations* (Fort Collins, CO: Colorado State University, 2013), 135.

121. S. C. Killer, A. K. Blannin, and A. E. Jeukendrup, "No Evidence of Dehydration with Moderate Daily Coffee Intake: A Counterbalanced Cross-Over Study in a Free-Living Population," *PloS One* 9, no. 1 (2014): e84154.

122. B. Benelam and L. Wyness, "Hydration and Health: A Review," *Nutrition Bulletin* 35, no. 1 (2010): 3–25.

123. B. M. Popkin et al., "A New Proposed Guidance System for Beverage Consumption in the United States," *American Journal of Clinical Nutrition* 83, no. 3 (2006): 529–42.

124. M. A. Saleh et al., "Chemical, Microbial, and Physical Evaluation of Commercial Bottled Waters in Greater Houston Area of Texas," *Journal of Environmental Science and Health Part A* 43, no. 4 (2008): 335–47.

125. S. Arranz, J. M. Silván, and F. Saura-Calixto, "Nonextractable Polyphenols, Usually Ignored, Are the Major Part of Dietary Polyphenols: A Study on the Spanish Diet," *Molecular Nutrition and Food Research* 54, no. 11 (November 2010): 1646–58.

126. I. Muraki et al., "Fruit Consumption and Risk of Type 2 Diabetes: Results from Three Prospective Longitudinal Cohort Studies," *British Medical Journal* 347 (2013): f5001.

127. H. Ali and J. F. Tahmassebi, "The Effects of Smoothies on Enamel Erosion: An In Situ Study," *International Journal of Paediatric Dentistry* 24, no. 3 (May 2014): 184–91.

Chapter 4: Don't Eat That

1. D. Ornish et al., "Can Lifestyle Changes Reverse Coronary Heart Disease?: The Lifestyle Heart Trial," *Lancet* 336, no. 8708 (1990): 129–33.

2. J. W. Anderson and K. Ward, "High-Carbohydrate, High-Fiber Diets for Insulin-Treated Men with Diabetes Mellitus," *American Journal of Clinical Nutrition* 32, no. 11 (1979): 2312–21.

3. D. Ornish et al., "Intensive Lifestyle Changes May Affect the Progression of Prostate Cancer," *Journal of Urology* 174, no. 3 (2005): 1065–70.

4. C. R. Daniel et al., "Trends in Meat Consumption in the USA," *Public Health Nutrition* 14, no. 4 (2011): 575–83.

5. Y. T. Szeto, T. C. Kwok, and I. F. Benzie, "Effects of a Long-Term Vegetarian Diet on Biomarkers of Antioxidant Status and Cardiovascular Disease Risk," *Nutrition* 20, no. 10 (October 2004): 863–66; V. Wijendran and K. C. Hayes, "Dietary n-6 and n-3 Fatty Acid Balance and Cardiovascular Health," *Annual Review Nutrition* 24: 597–615; J. M. Genkinger and A. Koushik, "Meat Consumption and Cancer Risk," *PLoS Medicine* 4, no. 12 (2007): e345; A. Tappel, "Heme of Consumed Red Meat Can Act as a Catalyst of Oxidative Damage and Could Initiate Colon, Breast and Prostate Cancers, Heart Disease, and Other Diseases," *Medical Hypotheses* 68, no. 3 (2007): 562–64.

6. M. Inoue-Choi et al., "Red and Processed Meat, Nitrite, and Heme Iron Intakes and Postmenopausal Breast Cancer Risk in the NIH-AARP Diet and Health Study," *International Journal of Cancer* 138, no. 7 (2016): 1609–18; V. Pala et al., "Meat, Eggs, Dairy Products, and Risk of Breast Cancer in the European Prospective Investigation into Cancer and Nutrition (EPIC) Cohort," *American Journal of Clinical Nutrition* 90, no. 3 (2009): 602–12; S. C. Larsson, L. Bergkvist, and A. Wolk, "Long-Term Meat Intake and Risk of Breast Cancer by Oestrogen and Progesterone Receptor Status in a Cohort of Swedish Women," *European Journal of Cancer* 45, no. 17 (2009): 3042–46; J. M. Genkinger et al., "Consumption of Dairy and Meat in Relation to Breast Cancer Risk in the Black Women's Health Study," *Cancer Causes and Control* 24, no. 4 (2013): 675–84.

7. E. F. Taylor et al., "Meat Consumption and Risk of Breast Cancer in the UK Women's Cohort Study," *British Journal of Cancer* 96, no. 7 (2007): 1139.

8. Y. Tantamango-Bartley et al., "Vegetarian Diets and the Incidence of Cancer in a Low-Risk Population," *Cancer Epidemiology and Prevention Biomarkers* (2012): cebp-1060.

9. S. S. Epstein, "The Chemical Jungle: Today's Beef Industry," *International Journal of Health Services* 20, no. 2 (1990): 277–80.

10. G. M. Fara et al., "Epidemic of Breast Enlargement in an Italian School," *Lancet* 314, no. 8137 (1979): 295–97.

11. Henrik Leffers et al., "Oestrogenic Potencies of Zeranol, Oestradiol, Diethylstilboestrol, Bisphenol-A and Genistein: Implications for Exposure Assessment of Potential Endocrine Disrupters," *Human Reproduction* 16, no. 5 (2001): 1037–45.

12. W. Ye et al., "In Vitro Transformation of MCF-10A Cells by Sera Harvested from Heifers Two Months Post-Zeranol Implantation," *International Journal of Oncology* 38, no. 4 (2011b): 985–92; R. Khosrokhavar et al., "Effects of Zearalenone and α-Zearalenol in Comparison with Raloxifene on T47D Cells," *Toxicology Mechanisms and Methods* 19, no. 3 (2009): 246–50.

13. E. V. Bandera et al., "Urinary Mycoestrogens, Body Size and Breast Development in New Jersey Girls," *Science of the Total Environment* 409, no. 24 (2011): 5221–27.

14. F. Massart and G. Saggese, "Oestrogenic Mycotoxin Exposures and Precocious Pubertal Development," *International Journal of Andrology* 33, no. 2 (2010): 369–76.

15. E. Linos et al., "Red Meat Consumption During Adolescence Among Premenopausal Women and Risk of Breast Cancer," *Cancer Epidemiology and Prevention Biomarkers* 17, no. 8 (2008): 2146–51.

16. M. S. Farvid et al., "Premenopausal Dietary Fat in Relation to Pre- and Post-menopausal Breast Cancer," *Breast Cancer Research and Treatment* 145, no. 1 (2014): 255.

17. J. Niu et al., "The Association Between Leptin Level and Breast Cancer: A Meta-analysis." *PloS One* 8, no. 6 (2013): e67349.

18. P. Xu et al., "Zeranol Enhances Leptin-Induced Proliferation in Primary Cultured Human Breast Cancer Epithelial Cells," *Molecular Medicine Reports* 3, no. 5 (2010): 795–800.

19. A. C. Vergnaud et al., "Meat Consumption and Prospective Weight Change in Participants of the EPIC-PANACEA Study," *American Journal of Clinical Nutrition* 92, no. 2 (2010): 398–407.

20. C. P. Velloso, "Regulation of Muscle Mass by Growth Hormone and IGF-1," *British Journal of Pharmacology* 154 (2008): 557–68, doi:10.1038/bjp.2008.153; M. Llorens-Martin, I. Torres-Aleman, and J. L. Trejo, "Mechanisms Mediating Brain Plasticity: IGF1 and Adult Hippocampal Neurogenesis," *Neuroscientist* 15 (2009): 134–48, doi:10.1177/1073858408331371.

21. S. Y. Yang et al., "Growth Factors and Their Receptors in Cancer Metastases," *Frontiers in Bioscience (Landmark Edition)* 16 (2011): 531–38.

22. M. E. Levine et al., "Low Protein Intake Is Associated with a Major Reduction in IGF-1, Cancer, and Overall Mortality in the 65 and Younger but not Older Population," *Cell Metabolism* 19, no. 3 (2014): 407–17.

23. M. Leslie, "Growth Defect Blocks Cancer and Diabetes," *Science* 331, no. 6019 (2011): 837.

24. J. Guevara-Aguirre et al., "Growth Hormone Receptor Deficiency Is Associated with

a Major Reduction in Pro-aging Signaling, Cancer, and Diabetes in Humans," *Science Translational Medicine* 16, no. 3 (February 2011): 70ra13.

25. P. F. Christopoulos, P. Msaouel, and M. Koutsilieris, "The Role of the Insulin-Like Growth Factor-1 System in Breast Cancer," *Molecular Cancer* 14, no. 1 (2015): 43; S. Sarkissyan et al., "IGF-1 Regulates Cyr61 Induced Breast Cancer Cell Proliferation and Invasion," *PloS One* 9, no. 7 (2014): e103534.

26. Hormones, the Endogenous, and Breast Cancer Collaborative Group, "Insulin-Like Growth Factor 1 (IGF1), IGF Binding Protein 3 (IGFBP3), and Breast Cancer Risk: Pooled Individual Data Analysis of 17 Prospective Studies," *Lancet Oncology* 11, no. 6 (2010): 530–42.

27. R. J. Barnard et al., "Effects of a Low-Fat, High-Fiber Diet and Exercise Program on Breast Cancer Risk Factors In Vivo and Tumor Cell Growth and Apoptosis In Vitro," *Nutrition and Cancer* 55, no. 1 (2006): 28–34.

28. R. J. Barnard et al., "A Low-Fat Diet and/or Strenuous Exercise Alters the IGF Axis In Vivo and Reduces Prostate Tumor Cell Growth In Vitro," *Prostate* 56, no. 3 (2003): 201–6.

29. N. E. Allen et al., "The Associations of Diet with Serum Insulin-Like Growth Factor 1 and Its Main Binding Proteins in 292 Women Meat-Eaters, Vegetarians, and Vegans," *Cancer Epidemiology and Prevention Biomarkers* 11, no. 11 (2002): 1441–48.

30. S. E. Steck et al., "Cooked Meat and Risk of Breast Cancer: Lifetime Versus Recent Dietary Intake," *Epidemiology* 18, no. 3 (May 2007): 373–82.

31. R. Zaidi, S. Kumar, and P. R. Rawat, "Rapid Detection and Quantification of Dietary Mutagens in Food Using Mass Spectrometry and Ultra Performance Liquid Chromatography," *Food Chemistry* 135, no. 4 (2012): 2897–903.

32. H. P. Thiebaud et al., "Airborne Mutagens Produced by Frying Beef, Pork and a Soy-based Food," *Food and Chemical Toxicology* 33, no. 10 (1995): 821–28.

33. W. Zheng et al., "Well-Done Meat Intake and the Risk of Breast Cancer," *Journal of the National Cancer Institute* 90, no. 22 (November 1998): 1724–29.

34. S. N. Lauber, S. Ali, and N. J. Gooderham, "The Cooked Food Derived Carcinogen 2-amino-1-methyl-6-phenylimidazo [4, 5-b] Pyridine Is a Potent Oestrogen: A Mechanistic Basis for Its Tissue-Specific Carcinogenicity," *Carcinogenesis* 25, no. 12 (2004): 2509–17.

35. L. S. DeBruin, P. A. Martos, and P. D. Josephy, "Detection of PhIP (2-amino-1-methyl-6-phenylimidazo [4, 5-b] Pyridine) in the Milk of Healthy Women," *Chemical Research in Toxicology* 14, no. 11 (2001): 1523–28.

36. R. D. Holland et al., "Formation of a Mutagenic Heterocyclic Aromatic Amine from Creatinine in Urine of Meat Eaters and Vegetarians," *Chemical Research in Toxicology* 18, no. 3 (2005): 579–90.

37. S. Murray et al., "Effect of Cruciferous Vegetable Consumption on Heterocyclic Aromatic Amine Metabolism in Man," *Carcinogenesis* 22, no. 9 (2001): 1413–20.

38. H. A. J. Schut and R. Yao, "Tea as a Potential Chemopreventive Agent in PhIP Carcinogenesis: Effects of Green Tea and Black Tea on PhIP-DNA Adduct Formation in Female F-344 Rats," *Nutrition and Cancer* 36, no. 1 (2000): 52–58.

39. E. F. Taylor et al., "Meat Consumption and Risk of Breast Cancer in the UK Women's Cohort Study," *British Journal of Cancer* 96, no. 7 (2007): 1139.

40. D. D. Alexander et al., "A Review and Meta-analysis of Red and Processed Meat Consumption and Breast Cancer," *Nutrition Research Reviews* 23, no. 2 (2010): 349–65.

41. V. Bouvard et al., "Carcinogenicity of Consumption of Red and Processed Meat," *Lancet Oncology* 16, no. 16 (2015): 1599.

42. M. Inoue-Choi et al., "Red and Processed Meat, Nitrite, and Heme Iron Intakes and Postmenopausal Breast Cancer Risk in the NIH-AARP Diet and Health Study," *International Journal of Cancer* 138, no. 7 (2016): 1609–18.

43. "Animal Foods," World Cancer Research Fund International, accessed October 14, 2017, http://www.wcrf.org/int/research-we-fund/cancer-prevention-recommendations/animal-foods.

44. R. Sinha et al., "Meat Intake and Mortality: A Prospective Study of over Half a Million People," *Archives of Internal Medicine* 169, no. 6 (2009): 562–71; S. Rohrmann et al., "Meat Consumption and Mortality: Results from the European Prospective Investigation into Cancer and Nutrition," *BMC Medicine* 11, no. 1 (2013): 63.

45. A. J. Cross et al., "A Prospective Study of Red and Processed Meat Intake in Relation to Cancer Risk," *PLoS Medicine* 4, no. 12 (December 2007): e325.

46. T. P. Robinson et al., "Mapping the Global Distribution of Livestock," *PloS One* 9, no. 5 (2014): e96084, accessed December 3, 2017, https://doi.org/10.1371/journal.pone.0096084.

47. USDA, *USDA Climate Change Science Plan* 4, 2010, http://www.usda.gov/oce/climate_change/science_plan2010/USDA_CCSPlan_120810.pdf.

48. P. Ross, "Cow Farts Have 'Larger Greenhouse Gas Impact' Than Previously Thought; Methane Pushes Climate Change," *International Business Times,* November 26, 2013, http://www.ibtimes.com/cow-farts-have-larger-greenhouse-gas-impact-previously-thought-methane-pushes-climate-change-1487502.

49. USDA Economic Research Service, "How Important Is Irrigation to US Agriculture?" October 12, 2016, https://www.ers.usda.gov/topics/farm-practices-management/irrigation-water-use/background/.

50. EPA, "Draft Plan to Study the Potential Impacts of Hydraulic Fracturing on Drinking Water Resources," February 2011, http://www2.epa.gov/sites/production/files/documents/HFStudyPlanDraft_SAB_020711.pdf.

51. D. Pimentel et al., "Water Resources: Agricultural and Environmental Issues," *BioScience* 54 (2004): 909, 911.

52. M. M. Mekonnen and A. Y. Hoekstra, "A Global Assessment of the Water Footprint of Farm Animal Products," *Ecosystems* 15 (2012): 401–15.

53. P. Thornton, M. Herrero, and P. Ericksen, "Livestock and Climate Change," *Livestock Exchange* 3 (November 2011).

54. S. Margulis, *Causes of Deforestation of the Brazilian Amazon* (The World Bank, 2004), http://www-wds.worldbank.org/servlet/WDSContentServer/WDSP/IB/2004/02/02/000090341_20040202130625/Rendered/PDF/277150PAPER0wbwp0no1022.pdf.

55. R. Oppenlander, "The World Hunger-Food Choice Connection: A Summary," *Comfortably Unaware* (blog), April 22, 2012, http://comfortablyunaware.com/blog

/the-world-hunger-food-choice-connection-a-summary/; United Nations Children's Fund, *Improving Child Nutrition: The Achievable Imperative for Global Progress* (New York: UNICEF, 2013).

56. "General Situation of World Fish Stocks," Food and Agricultural Organization of the United Nations, accessed December 26, 2007, http://www.fao.org/newsroom /common/ecg/1000505/en/stocks.pdf.

57. Annenberg Learner, "Unit 9: Biodiversity Decline, Section 7: Habitat Loss—Causes and Consequences," Habitable Planet multimedia course, accessed December 26, 2007, https://www.learner.org/courses/envsci/unit/text.php?unit=9&secNum=7.

58. R. Maughan, "Wedge Wolf Pack Will Be Killed Because of Its Increasing Beef Consumption," *Wildlife News,* September 28, 2012, http://www.thewildlifenews .com/2012/09/22/wedge-wolf-pack-will-be-killed-because-of-increasing-beef -consumption/.

59. D. Tilman and M. Clark, "Global Diets Link Environmental Sustainability and Human Health," *Nature* 515, no. 7528 (November 2014): 518–22.

60. H. Davoodi, S. Esmaeili, and A. M. Mortazavian, "Effects of Milk and Milk Products Consumption on Cancer: A Review," *Comprehensive Reviews in Food Science and Food Safety* 12, no. 3 (2013): 249–64.

61. P. W. Parodi, "Dairy Product Consumption and the Risk of Breast Cancer," *Journal of the American College of Nutrition* 24, no. 6 (December 2005): 556S–68S; W. Al Sarakbi, M. Salhab, and K. Mokbel, "Dairy Products and Breast Cancer Risk: A Review of the Literature," *International Journal of Fertility and Women's Medicine* 50, no. 6 (November–December 2005): 244–49; P. G. Moorman and P. D. Terry, "Consumption of Dairy Products and the Risk of Breast Cancer: A Review of the Literature," *American Journal of Clinical Nutrition* 80, no. 1 (July 2004): 5–14; M. H. Shin et al., "Intake of Dairy Products, Calcium, and Vitamin D and Risk of Breast Cancer," *Journal of the National Cancer Institute* 94, no. 17 (September 2002): 1301–11.

62. H. Davoodi, S. Esmaeili, and A. M. Mortazavian, "Effects of Milk and Milk Products Consumption on Cancer: A Review," *Comprehensive Reviews in Food Science and Food Safety* 12, no. 3 (2013): 249–64.

63. M. H. Shin et al., "Intake of Dairy Products, Calcium, and Vitamin D and Risk of Breast Cancer," *Journal of the National Cancer Institute* 94, no. 17 (2002): 1301–10.

64. C. H. Kroenke et al., "High- and Low-Fat Dairy Intake, Recurrence, and Mortality After Breast Cancer Diagnosis," *Journal of the National Cancer Institute* 105, no. 9 (2013): 616–23.

65. D. Ganmaa and A. Sato, "The Possible Role of Female Sex Hormones in Milk from Pregnant Cows in the Development of Breast, Ovarian and Corpus Uteri Cancers," *Medical Hypotheses* 65, no. 6 (2005): 1028–37.

66. D. A. Pape-Zambito, R. F. Roberts, and R. S. Kensinger, "Estrone and 17β-estradiol Concentrations in Pasteurized-Homogenized Milk and Commercial Dairy Products," *Journal of Dairy Science* 93, no. 6 (2010): 2533–40.

67. S. Stender and J. Dyerberg, "Influence of Trans Fatty Acids on Health," *Annals of Nutrition and Metabolism* 48, no. 2 (2004): 61–66.

68. A. Trichopoulou et al., "Consumption of Olive Oil and Specific Food Groups in

Relation to Breast Cancer Risk in Greece," *Journal of the National Cancer Institute* 87, no. 2 (1995): 110–16.

69. J. R. Hebert, T. G. Hurley, and Y. Ma, "The Effect of Dietary Exposures on Recurrence and Mortality in Early Stage Breast Cancer," *Breast Cancer Research and Treatment* 51, no. 1 (September 1998): 17–28; A. J. McEligot et al., "Dietary Fat, Fiber, Vegetable, and Micronutrients Are Associated with Overall Survival in Postmenopausal Women Diagnosed with Breast Cancer," *Nutrition and Cancer* 55, no. 2 (2006): 132–40.

70. D. Doell et al., "Updated Estimate of Trans Fat Intake by the US Population," *Food Additives and Contaminants: Part A* 29, no. 6 (2012): 861–74.

71. I. Laake et al., "A Prospective Study of Intake of Trans-Fatty Acids from Ruminant Fat, Partially Hydrogenated Vegetable Oils, and Marine Oils and Mortality from CVD," *British Journal of Nutrition* 108, no. 4 (2012): 743–54.

72. D. Mozaffarian et al., "Trans Fatty Acids and Cardiovascular Disease," *New England Journal of Medicine* 354, no. 15 (2006): 1601–13.

73. J. M. Beasley et al., "Post-diagnosis Dietary Factors and Survival after Invasive Breast Cancer," *Breast Cancer Research and Treatment* 128, no. 1 (2011): 229–36.

74. A. C. Thiebaut et al., "Dietary Fat and Postmenopausal Invasive Breast Cancer in the National Institutes of Health-AARP Diet and Health Study Cohort," *Journal of the National Cancer Institute* 99, no. 6 (March 2007): 451–62.

75. Y. Liu et al., "Adolescent Dietary Fiber, Vegetable Fat, Vegetable Protein, and Nut Intakes and Breast Cancer Risk," *Breast Cancer Research and Treatment* 145, no. 2 (2014): 461–70.

76. Division of Cancer Control and Population Sciences, "Top Food Sources of Saturated Fat Among US Population," National Cancer Institute, last updated April 20, 2016, https://epi.grants.cancer.gov/diet/foodsources/sat_fat/sf.html.

77. A. P. Simopoulos, "Evolutionary Aspects of Diet, the Omega-6/Omega-3 Ratio and Genetic Variation: Nutritional Implications for Chronic Diseases," *Biomedicine and Pharmacotherapy* 60, no. 9 (2006): 502–7.

78. M. Hansen et al., "Potential Public Health Impacts of the Use of Recombinant Bovine Somatotropin in Dairy Production," Consumers Union, September 1997, http://consumersunion.org/news/potential-public-health-impacts-of-the-use-of -recombinant-bovine-somatotropin-in-dairy-production-part-1/.

79. R. P. Heaney et al., "Dietary Changes Favorably Affect Bone Remodeling in Older Adults," *Journal of the American Dietetic Association* 99, no. 10 (1999): 1228–33.

80. USDA Animal and Plant Health Inspection Service, "Dairy 2007, Part IV: Reference of Dairy Cattle Health and Management Practices in the United States" *NAHMS Dairy 2007* (2007).

81. P. G. Moorman and P. D. Terry, "Consumption of Dairy Products and the Risk of Breast Cancer: A Review of the Literature," *American Journal of Clinical Nutrition* 80, no. 1 (2004): 5–14.

82. Centers for Epidemiology and Animal Health, "Bovine Leukosis Virus (BLV) on U.S. Dairy Operations," *APHIS Info Sheet* (October 2008).

83. G. C. Buehring, S. M. Philpott, and K. Y. Choi, "Humans Have Antibodies Reactive

with Bovine Leukemia Virus," *AIDS Research and Human Retroviruses* 19, no. 12 (2003): 1105–13.

84. G. C. Buehring et al., "Exposure to Bovine Leukemia Virus Is Associated with Breast Cancer: A Case-Control Study," *PLoS One* 10, no. 9 (2015): e0134304.

85. P. C. Bartlett et al., "Options for the Control of Bovine Leukemia Virus in Dairy Cattle," *Journal of the American Veterinary Medical Association* 244, no. 8 (2014): 914–22.

86. K. E. Nachman et al., "Roxarsone, Inorganic Arsenic, and Other Arsenic Species in Chicken: A US-Based Market Basket Sample," *Environmental Health Perspectives* 121, no. 7 (2013): 818.

87. R. Vogt et al., "Cancer and Non-cancer Health Effects from Food Contaminant Exposures for Children and Adults in California: A Risk Assessment," *Environmental Health* 11, no. 1 (2012): 83.

88. B. P. Jackson et al., "Arsenic, Organic Foods, and Brown Rice Syrup," *Environmental Health Perspectives* 120, no. 5 (2012): 623.

89. K. E. Nachman et al., "Arsenic Species in Poultry Feather Meal," *Science of the Total Environment* 417 (2012): 183–88.

90. R. Si et al., "Egg Consumption and Breast Cancer Risk: A Meta-analysis," *Breast Cancer* 21, no. 3 (2014): 251–61.

91. S. A. Missmer et al., "Meat and Dairy Food Consumption and Breast Cancer: A Pooled Analysis of Cohort Studies," *International Journal of Epidemiology* 31, no. 1 (February 2002): 78–85.

92. Z. Wang et al., "Gut Flora Metabolism of Phosphatidylcholine Promotes Cardiovascular Disease," *Nature* 472, no. 7341 (2011): 57–63.

93. E. L. Richman et al., "Egg, Red Meat, and Poultry Intake and Risk of Lethal Prostate Cancer in the Prostate-Specific Antigen-Era: Incidence and Survival," *Cancer Prevention Research* 4, no. 12 (December 2011): 2110–21.

94. R. D. Holland et al., "Formation of a Mutagenic Heterocyclic Aromatic Amine from Creatinine in Urine of Meat Eaters and Vegetarians," *Chemical Research in Toxicology* 18, no. 3 (2005): 579–90.

95. M. J. Rudling et al., "Content of Low Density Lipoprotein Receptors in Breast Cancer Tissue Related to Survival of Patients," *British Medical Journal (Clinical Research Edition)* 292, no. 6520 (1986): 580–82.

96. A. H. Lichtenstein et al., "Diet and Lifestyle Recommendations Revision 2006: A Scientific Statement from the American Heart Association Nutrition Committee," *Circulation* 114, no. 1 (2006): 82–96.

97. C. M. Kitahara et al., "Total Cholesterol and Cancer Risk in a Large Prospective Study in Korea," *Journal of Clinical Oncology* 29, no. 12 (2011): 1592–98.

98. E. B. Rimm et al., "Review of Moderate Alcohol Consumption and Reduced Risk of Coronary Heart Disease: Is the Effect Due to Beer, Wine, or Spirits?" *British Medical Journal* 312, no. 7033 (1996): 731–36.

99. NIAAA Publications, "Tips for Cutting Down on Drinking," National Institute on Alcohol Abuse and Alcoholism, September 2008, http://pubs.niaaa.nih.gov /publications/Tips/tips.htm.

100. R. C. Ellison et al., "Exploring the Relation of Alcohol Consumption to Risk of

Breast Cancer," *American Journal of Epidemiology* 154, no. 8 (October 2001): 740–47; S. M. Zhang et al., "Alcohol Consumption and Breast Cancer Risk in the Women's Health Study," *American Journal of Epidemiology* 165, no. 6 (March 2007): 667–76; N. Hamajima et al., "Alcohol, Tobacco and Breast Cancer: Collaborative Reanalysis of Individual Data from 53 Epidemiological Studies, including 58,515 Women with Breast Cancer and 95,067 Women Without the Disease," *British Journal of Cancer* 87, no. 11 (November 2002): 1234–45.

101. D. G. Weir, P. G. McGing, and J. M. Scott, "Folate Metabolism, the Enterohepatic Circulation and Alcohol," *Biochemical Pharmacology* 34, no. 1 (1985): 1–7; I. P. Pogribny et al., "Breaks in Genomic DNA and Within the p53 Gene Are Associated with Hypomethylation in Livers of Folate/Methyl-Deficient Rats," *Cancer Research* 55, no. 9 (May 1995): 1894–901.

102. E. Ergul et al., "Polymorphisms in the MTHFR Gene Are Associated with Breast Cancer," *Tumor Biology* 24, no. 6 (2003): 286–90.

103. J. Chen et al., "One-Carbon Metabolism, MTHFR Polymorphisms, and Risk of Breast Cancer," *Cancer Research* 65, no. 4 (2005): 1606–14; I. G. Campbell et al., "Methylenetetrahydrofolate Reductase Polymorphism and Susceptibility to Breast Cancer," *Breast Cancer Research* 4, no. 6 (2002): R14.

104. S. M. Zhang et al., "Plasma Folate, Vitamin B6, Vitamin B12, Homocysteine, and Risk of Breast Cancer," *Journal of the National Cancer Institute* 95, no. 5 (2003): 373–80; S. Zhang et al., "A Prospective Study of Folate Intake and the Risk of Breast Cancer," *Journal of the American Medical Association* 281, no. 17 (May 1999): 1632–37.

105. T. A. Sellers et al., "Interaction of Dietary Folate Intake, Alcohol, and Risk of Hormone Receptor-Defined Breast Cancer in a Prospective Study of Postmenopausal Women," *Cancer Epidemiology, Biomarkers and Prevention* 11, no. 10 (October 2002): 1104–10.

106. S. Zhang et al., "Dietary Carotenoids and Vitamins A, C, and E and Risk of Breast Cancer," *Journal of the National Cancer Institute* 91, no. 6 (1999): 547–56.

107. D. E. Nelson et al., "Alcohol-Attributable Cancer Deaths and Years of Potential Life Lost in the United States," *American Journal of Public Health* 103, no. 4 (April 2013): 641–48.

108. M. Grønbæk et al., "Type of Alcohol Consumed and Mortality from All Causes, Coronary Heart Disease, and Cancer," *Annals of Internal Medicine* 133, no. 6 (2000): 411–29.

109. C. Shufelt et al., "Red Versus White Wine as a Nutritional Aromatase Inhibitor in Premenopausal Women: A Pilot Study," *Journal of Women's Health* 21, no. 3 (2012): 281–84.

110. M. Jang et al., "Cancer Chemopreventive Activity of Resveratrol, a Natural Product Derived from Grapes," *Science* 275, no. 5297 (1997): 218–20.

111. S. Chen et al., "Suppression of Breast Cancer Cell Growth with Grape Juice," *Pharmaceutical Biology* 36, no. 1 (1998): 53–61.

112. R. Baan et al., "Carcinogenicity of Alcoholic Beverages," *Lancet Oncology* 8, no. 4 (2007): 292.

113. T. A. Hastert et al., "Adherence to WCRF/AICR Cancer Prevention

Recommendations and Risk of Postmenopausal Breast Cancer," *Cancer Epidemiology and Prevention Biomarkers* 22, no. 9 (September 2013): 1498–508.

114. S. Takayama et al., "Long-Term Feeding of Sodium Saccharin to Nonhuman Primates: Implications for Urinary Tract Cancer," *Journal of the National Cancer Institute* 90, no. 1 (1998): 19–25; O. M. Jensen and C. Kamby, "Intra-uterine Exposure to Saccharine and Risk of Bladder Cancer in Man," *International Journal of Cancer* 29, no. 5 (1982): 507–9; H. A. Risch et al., "Dietary Factors and the Incidence of Cancer of the Urinary Bladder," *American Journal of Epidemiology* 127, no. 6 (1988): 1179–91.

115. S. R. Sturgeon et al., "Associations Between Bladder Cancer Risk Factors and Tumor Stage and Grade at Diagnosis," *Epidemiology* 5, no. 2 (March 1994): 218–25.

116. M. B. Azad et al., "Nonnutritive Sweeteners and Cardiometabolic Health: A Systematic Review and Meta-analysis of Randomized Controlled Trials and Prospective Cohort Studies," *Canadian Medical Association Journal* 189, no. 28 (July 2017): e929–e939; S. E. Swithers, "Artificial Sweeteners Produce the Counterintuitive Effect of Inducing Metabolic Derangements," *Trends in Endocrinology and Metabolism* 24, no. 9 (2013): 431–41; J. A. Nettleton et al., "Diet Soda Intake and Risk of Incident Metabolic Syndrome and Type 2 Diabetes in the Multi-Ethnic Study of Atherosclerosis (MESA)," *Diabetes Care* 32, no. 4 (2009): 688–94; S. S. Schiffman and K. I. Rother, "Sucralose, a Synthetic Organochlorine Sweetener: Overview of Biological Issues," *Journal of Toxicology and Environmental Health, Part B* 16, no. 7 (2013): 399–451.

117. R. Mattes, "Effects of Aspartame and Sucrose on Hunger and Energy Intake in Humans," *Physiology and Behavior* 47, no. 6 (1990): 1037–44.

118. Q. Yang, "Gain Weight by 'Going Diet?' Artificial Sweeteners and the Neurobiology of Sugar Cravings: Neuroscience 2010," *Yale Journal of Biology and Medicine* 83, no. 2 (2010): 101.

119. Joint FAO/WHO Expert Committee on Food Additives, "Evaluation of Certain Food Additives," *World Health Organization Technical Report Series* 952 (2009): 1–208.

120. G. J. M. den Hartog et al., "Erythritol Is a Sweet Antioxidant," *Nutrition* 26, no. 4 (2010): 449–58.

121. N. M. Avena, P. Rada, and B. G. Hoebel, "Evidence for Sugar Addiction: Behavioral and Neurochemical Effects of Intermittent, Excessive Sugar Intake," *Neuroscience and Biobehavioral Reviews* 32, no. 1 (2008): 20–39.

122. D. G. Liem and C. de Graaf, "Sweet and Sour Preferences in Young Children and Adults: Role of Repeated Exposure," *Physiology and Behavior* 83, no. 3 (December 2004): 421–29.

123. S. Thongprakaisang et al., "Glyphosate Induces Human Breast Cancer Cells Growth via Estrogen Receptors," *Food and Chemical Toxicology* 59 (2013): 129–36.

124. K. E. Bradbury et al., "Organic Food Consumption and the Incidence of Cancer in a Large Prospective Study of Women in the United Kingdom," *British Journal of Cancer* 110, no. 9 (2014): 2321.

125. C. Smith-Spangler et al., "Are Organic Foods Safer or Healthier than Conventional Alternatives? A Systematic Review," *Annals of Internal Medicine* 157, no. 5 (2012): 348–66.

126. B. P. Baker et al., "Pesticide Residues in Conventional, Integrated Pest Management (IPM)-grown and Organic Foods: Insights from Three US Data Sets," *Food Additives and Contaminants* 19, no. 5 (2002): 427–46.

127. Agricultural Marketing Service, "The National List," United States Department of Agriculture, updated December 21, 2017, https://www.ams.usda.gov/rules -regulations/organic/national-list.

128. W. J. Krol et al., "Reduction of Pesticide Residues on Produce by Rinsing," *Journal of Agricultural and Food Chemistry* 48, no. 10 (2000): 4666–70.

129. Z. Y. Zhang, X. J. Liu, and X. Y. Hong, "Effects of Home Preparation on Pesticide Residues in Cabbage," *Food Control* 18, no. 12 (2007): 1484–87.

130. G. Perelló et al., "Concentrations of Polybrominated Diphenyl Ethers, Hexachlorobenzene and Polycyclic Aromatic Hydrocarbons in Various Foodstuffs Before and After Cooking," *Food and Chemical Toxicology* 47, no. 4 (2009): 709–15.

131. U. Bajwa and K. S. Sandhu, "Effect of Handling and Processing on Pesticide Residues in Food: A Review," *Journal of Food Science and Technology* 51, no. 2 (2014): 201–20.

132. P. Chandon and B. Wansink, "The Biasing Health Halos of Fast-Food Restaurant Health Claims: Lower Calorie Estimates and Higher Side-Dish Consumption Intentions," *Journal of Consumer Research* 34, no. 3 (2007): 301–14.

133. "Distinction Between Genetic Engineering and Conventional Plant Breeding Becoming Less Clear, Says New Report on GE Crops," The National Academies of Sciences, Engineering, and Medicine, May 17, 2016, http://www8.nationalacademies .org/onpinews/newsitem.aspx?RecordID=23395.

134. United States Department of Agriculture, "Pesticide Data Program Annual Summary, Calendar Year 2011," https://www.ams.usda.gov/sites/default/files /media/2011%20PDP%20Annual%20Summary.pdf; E. Reverchon et al., "Hexane Elimination from Soybean Oil by Continuous Packed Tower Processing with Supercritical CO_2," *Journal of the American Oil Chemists' Society* 77, no. 1 (2000): 9–14.

135. M. H. Carlsen et al., "The Total Antioxidant Content of More than 3100 Foods, Beverages, Spices, Herbs and Supplements Used Worldwide," *Nutrition Journal* 9, no. 1 (2010): 3.

136. Superfoodly.com, "ORAC Values: Antioxidant Values of Foods and Beverages," https://www.superfoodly.com/orac-values.

Chapter 5: Beyond Food: What You Should Do

1. G. N. Hortobagyi et al., "The Global Breast Cancer Burden: Variations in Epidemiology and Survival," *Clinical Breast Cancer* 6, no. 5 (2005): 391–401.

2. J. Ferlay et al., "Cancer Incidence and Mortality Worldwide: Sources, Methods and Major Patterns in GLOBOCAN 2012," *International Journal of Cancer* 136, no. 5 (March 2015): E359–E386.

3. K. Katanoda and D. Qiu, "Comparison of Time Trends in Female Breast Cancer Incidence (1973–1997) in East Asia, Europe, and USA, from *Cancer Incidence in Five Continents*, Vols IV–VIII," *Japanese Journal of Clinical Oncology* 37, no. 8 (August 2007): 638–39, https://doi.org/10.1093/jjco/hym122.

4. "WHO Mortality Database," World Health Organization, accessed December 27, 2017, http://www.who.int/healthinfo/mortality_data/en/.

5. R. G. Ziegler et al., "Relative Weight, Weight Change, Height, and Breast Cancer Risk in Asian-American Women," *Journal of the National Cancer Institute* 88, no. 10 (1996): 650–60.

6. L. A. Torre et al., "Global Cancer Statistics, 2012," *CA: A Cancer Journal for Clinicians* 65 (2015): 87–108.

7. R. G. Ziegler et al., "Migration Patterns and Breast Cancer Risk in Asian-American Women," *Journal of the National Cancer Institute* 85, no. 22 (1993): 1819–27.

8. S. L. Gomez et al., "Cancer Incidence Trends Among Asian American Populations in the United States, 1990–2008," *Journal of the National Cancer Institute* 105, no. 15 (2013): 1096–110.

9. Centers for Disease Control and Prevention, Division for Heart Disease and Stroke Prevention, "Women and Heart Disease Fact Sheet," accessed November 4, 2017, https://www.cdc.gov/dhdsp/data_statistics/fact_sheets/fs_women_heart .htm; American Cancer Society, *Breast Cancer Facts & Figures 2017–2018* (Atlanta: American Cancer Society, Inc., 2017), accessed November 4, 2017, https://www .cancer.org/content/dam/cancer-org/research/cancer-facts-and-statistics/breast-cancer -facts-and-figures/breast-cancer-facts-and-figures-2017-2018.pdf.

10. IARC Working Group on the Evaluation of Cancer-Preventive Agents, "Weight Control and Physical Activity," *IARC Handbook of Cancer Prevention*, vol. 6 (Lyon, France: IARC, 2002).

11. J. M. Petrelli et al., "Body Mass Index, Height, and Postmenopausal Breast Cancer Mortality in a Prospective Cohort of US Women," *Cancer Causes and Control* 13, no. 4 (May 2002): 325–32.

12. A. Afshin et al., "Health Effects of Overweight and Obesity in 195 Countries over 25 Years," *New England Journal of Medicine* 377 (2017): 13–27.

13. E. Weiderpass et al., "A Prospective Study of Body Size in Different Periods of Life and Risk of Premenopausal Breast Cancer," *Cancer Epidemiology and Prevention Biomarkers* 13, no. 7 (2004): 1121–27.

14. A. McTiernan, "Behavioral Risk Factors in Breast Cancer: Can Risk Be Modified?" *Oncologist* 8, no. 4 (2003): 326–34.

15. S. Loi et al., "Obesity and Outcomes in Premenopausal and Postmenopausal Breast Cancer," *Cancer Epidemiology, Biomarkers and Prevention* 14, no. 7 (July 2005): 1686–91.

16. E. E. Calle et al., "Overweight, Obesity, and Mortality from Cancer in a Prospectively Studied Cohort of U.S. Adults," *New England Journal of Medicine* 348 (2003): 1625–38.

17. J. M. Petrelli et al., "Body Mass Index, Height, and Postmenopausal Breast Cancer Mortality in a Prospective Cohort of US Women," *Cancer Causes and Control* 13, no. 4 (May 2002): 325–32.

18. S. A. Khan et al., "Estrogen Receptor Expression of Benign Breast Epithelium and Its Association with Breast Cancer," *Cancer Research* 54, no. 4 (1994): 993–97.

19. A. R. Carmichael, "Obesity as a Risk Factor for Development and Poor Prognosis

335

of Breast Cancer," *BJOG: An International Journal of Obstetrics and Gynaecology* 113, no. 10 (October 2006): 1160–66.

20. R. M. Cento et al., "Leptin Levels in Menopause: Effect of Estrogen Replacement Therapy," *Hormone Research in Paediatrics* 52, no. 6 (1999): 269–73.

21. A. A. J. Van Landeghem et al., "Endogenous Concentration and Subcellular Distribution of Androgens in Normal and Malignant Human Breast Tissue," *Cancer Research* 45, no. 6 (1985): 2907–12.

22. A. Kendall, E. J. Folkerd, and M. Dowsett, "Influences on Circulating Oestrogens in Postmenopausal Women: Relationship with Breast Cancer," *Journal of Steroid Biochemistry and Molecular Biology* 103, no. 2 (2007): 99–109; H. Kuhl, "Breast Cancer Risk in the WHI Study: The Problem of Obesity," *Maturitas* 51, no. 1 (May 2005): 83–97.

23. L. M. Morimoto et al., "Obesity, Body Size, and Risk of Postmenopausal Breast Cancer: The Women's Health Initiative (United States)," *Cancer Causes and Control* 13, no. 8 (October 2002): 741–51.

24. D. P. Rose, D. Komninou, and G. D. Stephenson, "Obesity, Adipocytokines, and Insulin Resistance in Breast Cancer," *Obesity Reviews* 5, no. 3 (2004): 153–65.

25. A. Tchernof et al., "Weight Loss Reduces C-Reactive Protein Levels in Obese Postmenopausal Women," *Circulation* 105, no. 5 (2002): 564–69.

26. N. V. Christou et al., "Bariatric Surgery Reduces Cancer Risk in Morbidly Obese Patients," *Surgery for Obesity and Related Diseases* 4, no. 6 (2008): 691–95.

27. M. Harvie et al., "Association of Gain and Loss of Weight Before and After Meno-pause with Risk of Postmenopausal Breast Cancer in the Iowa Women's Health Study," *Cancer Epidemiology, Biomarkers and Prevention* 14, no. 3 (March 2005): 656–61.

28. P. T. Bradshaw et al., "Postdiagnosis Change in Bodyweight and Survival after Breast Cancer Diagnosis," *Epidemiology* 23 (2012): 320–27.

29. A. McTiernan et al., "Recreational Physical Activity and the Risk of Breast Cancer in Postmenopausal Women: The Women's Health Initiative Cohort Study," *Journal of the American Medical Association* 290, no. 10 (September 2010): 1331–36.

30. A. McTiernan, "Behavioral Risk Factors in Breast Cancer: Can Risk Be Modified?" *Oncologist* 8, no. 4 (2003): 326–34.

31. L. Bernstein et al., "Physical Exercise and Reduced Risk of Breast Cancer in Young Women," *Journal of the National Cancer Institute* 86, no. 18 (1994): 1403–8.

32. J. P. Pierce et al., "Greater Survival after Breast Cancer in Physically Active Women with High Vegetable-Fruit Intake Regardless of Obesity," *Journal of Clinical Oncology* 25, no. 17 (2007): 2345–51.

33. M. L. Irwin et al., "Influence of Pre- and Postdiagnosis Physical Activity on Mortality in Breast Cancer Survivors: The Health, Eating, Activity, and Lifestyle Study," *Journal of Clinical Oncology* 26, no. 24 (2008): 3958–64.

34. A. McTiernan et al., "Relation of BMI and Physical Activity to Sex Hormones in Postmenopausal Women," *Obesity* 14, no. 9 (2006): 1662–77.

35. J. F. Meneses-Echávez et al., "The Effect of Exercise Training on Mediators of Inflammation in Breast Cancer Survivors: A Systematic Review with Meta-analysis," *Cancer Epidemiology, Biomarkers and Prevention* 25, no. 7 (2016): 1009–17.

36. C. M. Dieli-Conwright and B. Z. Orozco, "Exercise after Breast Cancer Treatment: Current Perspectives," *Breast Cancer: Targets and Therapy* 7 (2015): 353.

37. "Physical Activity and Your Heart: Recommendations for Physical Activity," National Heart, Lung, and Blood Institute, accessed July 31, 2017, https://www.nhlbi .nih.gov/health/health-topics/topics/phys/recommend.

38. J. M. Beasley et al., "Meeting the Physical Activity Guidelines and Survival after Breast Cancer: Findings from the After Breast Cancer Pooling Project," *Breast Cancer Research and Treatment* 131, no. 2 (January 2012): 637–43.

39. B. MacMahon et al., "Age at First Birth and Breast Cancer Risk," *Bulletin of the World Health Organization* 43, no. 2 (1970): 209–21.

40. B. MacMahon, "Reproduction and Cancer of the Breast," *Cancer* 71, no. 10 (1993): 3185–88.

41. P. Bruzzi et al., "Short Term Increase in Risk of Breast Cancer After Full Term Pregnancy," *British Medical Journal* 297, no. 6656 (October 1988): 1096–98.

42. B. MacMahon et al., "Age at First Birth and Breast Cancer Risk," *Bulletin of the World Health Organization* 43, no. 2 (1970): 209–21.

43. B. MacMahon et al., "Age at First Birth and Breast Cancer Risk," *Bulletin of the World Health Organization* 43, no. 2 (1970): 209–21.

44. Y. Zhou et al., "Association Between Breastfeeding and Breast Cancer Risk: Evidence from a Meta-analysis," *Breastfeeding Medicine* 10, no. 3 (2015): 175–82.

45. P. A. Newcomb, "Lactation and Breast Cancer Risk," *Journal of Mammary Gland Biology and Neoplaisa* 2, no. 3 (1997): 311–18; S. Y. Lee et al., "Effect of Lifetime Lactation on Breast Cancer Risk: A Korean Women's Cohort Study," *International Journal of Cancer* 105, no. 3 (June 2003): 390–93; J. L. Freudenheim et al., "Lactation History and Breast Cancer Risk," *American Journal of Epidemiology* 146, no. 11 (December 1997): 932–38.

46. F. Islami, et al., "Breastfeeding and Breast Cancer Risk by Receptor Status—a Systematic Review and Meta-analysis," *Annals of Oncology* 26, no. 12 (2015): 2398–407.

47. J. Kotsopoulos et al., "Breastfeeding and the Risk of Breast Cancer in BRCA1 and BRCA2 Mutation Carriers," *Breast Cancer Research* 14, no. 2 (2012): R42.

48. G. Brignone et al., "A Case-Control Study on Breast Cancer Risk Factors in a Southern European Population," *International Journal of Epidemiology* 16, no. 3 (September 1987): 356–61; E. Negri et al., "Lactation and the Risk of Breast Cancer in an Italian Population," *International Journal of Cancer* 67, no. 2 (July 1996): 161–64; S. J. London et al., "Lactation and Risk of Breast Cancer in a Cohort of US Women," *American Journal of Epidemiology* 132, no. 1 (July 1990): 17–26.

49. J. Russo et al., "17-Beta-estradiol Induces Transformation and Tumorigenesis in Human Breast Epithelial Cells," *FASEB Journal* 20, no. 10 (2006): 1622–34.

50. B. T. Zhu and A. H. Conney, "Functional Role of Estrogen Metabolism in Target Cells: Review and Perspectives," *Carcinogenesis* 19, no. 1 (1998): 1–27.

51. A. McTiernan et al., "Estrogen-Plus-Progestin Use and Mammographic Density in Postmenopausal Women: Women's Health Initiative Randomized Trial," *Journal of the National Cancer Institute* 97, no. 18 (September 2005): 1366–76.

52. J. E. Rossouw et al., "Risks and Benefits of Estrogen Plus Progestin in Healthy Postmenopausal Women: Principal Results from the Women's Health Initiative Randomized Controlled Trial," *Journal of the American Medical Association* 288, no. 3 (July 2002): 321–33.

53. Million Women Study Collaborators, "Breast Cancer and Hormone-Replacement Therapy in the Million Women Study," *Lancet* 362, no. 9382 (2003): 419–27.

54. G. Heiss et al., "Health Risks and Benefits 3 Years after Stopping Randomized Treatment with Estrogen and Progestin," *Journal of the American Medical Association* 299, no. 9 (2008): 1036–45.

55. V. Beralet al., "Breast Cancer Risk in Relation to the Interval between Menopause and Starting Hormone Therapy," *Journal of the National Cancer Institute* 103, no. 4 (2011): 296–305.

56. W. Y. Chen et al., "Unopposed Estrogen Therapy and the Risk of Invasive Breast Cancer," *Archives of Internal Medicine* 166, no. 9 (2006): 1027–32.

57. J. E. Manson et al., "Estrogen Therapy and Coronary-Artery Calcification," *New England Journal of Medicine* 356 (June 2007): 2591–602.

58. T. M. Brasky et al., "Specialty Supplements and Breast Cancer Risk in the Vitamins and Lifestyle (VITAL) Cohort," *Cancer Epidemiology, and Biomarkers and Prevention* 19, no. 7 (2010): 1696–708; C. L. Loprinzi et al., "Venlafaxine in Management of Hot Flashes in Survivors of Breast Cancer: A Randomised Controlled Trial," *Lancet* 356, no. 9247 (2000): 2059–63.

59. A. Chang et al., "The Effect of Herbal Extract (EstroG-100) on Pre-, Peri- and Post-menopausal Women: A Randomized Double-Blind, Placebo-Controlled Study," *Phytotherapy Research* 26, no. 4 (2012): 510–16.

60. J. V. Pinkerton and G. D. Constantine, "Compounded Non-FDA–Approved Menopausal Hormone Therapy Prescriptions Have Increased: Results of a Pharmacy Survey," *Menopause* 23, no. 4 (2016): 359.

61. A. Fournieret et al., "Use of Different Postmenopausal Hormone Therapies and Risk of Histology- and Hormone Receptor–Defined Invasive Breast Cancer," *Journal of Clinical Oncology* 26, no. 8 (2008): 1260–68.

62. American Cancer Society, *Cancer Facts & Figures 2017* (Atlanta: American Cancer Society, Inc., 2017), accessed January 14, 2018, https://www.cancer.org/content/dam/cancer-org/research/cancer-facts-and-statistics/annual-cancer-facts-and-figures/2017/cancer-facts-and-figures-2017.pdf.

63. American Cancer Society, *Cancer Prevention and Early Detection 2005.*

64. P. D. Terry and T. E. Rohan, "Cigarette Smoking and the Risk of Breast Cancer in Women: A Review of the Literature," *Cancer Epidemiology, Biomarkers and Prevention* 11, no. 10 (October 2002): 953–71.

65. M. D. Gammon et al., "Cigarette Smoking and Breast Cancer Risk among Young Women (United States)," *Cancer Causes and Control* 9, no. 6 (December 1998): 583–90.

66. P. Reynolds, "Smoking and Breast Cancer," *Journal of Mammary Gland Biology and Neoplasia* 18 (2013): 15–23; S. A. Glantz and K. C. Johnson, "The Surgeon General Report on Smoking and Health 50 Years Later: Breast Cancer and the Cost

of Increasing Caution," *Cancer Epidemiology, Biomarkers and Prevention* 23, no. 1 (January 2014): 37–46.

67. L. Dossus et al., "Active and Passive Cigarette Smoking and Breast Cancer Risk: Results from the EPIC Cohort," *International Journal of Cancer* 134, no. 8 (2014): 1871–88.

68. Y. Cui, A. B. Miller, and T. E. Rohan, "Cigarette Smoking and Breast Cancer Risk: Update of a Prospective Cohort Study," *Breast Cancer Research and Treatment* 100, no. 3 (December 2006): 293–99.

69. P. Reynolds et al., "Active Smoking, Household Passive Smoking, and Breast Cancer: Evidence from the California Teachers Study," *Journal of the National Cancer Institute* 96, no. 1 (2004): 29–37.

70. M. N. Passarelli et al., "Cigarette Smoking Before and After Breast Cancer Diagnosis: Mortality from Breast Cancer and Smoking-Related Diseases," *Journal of Clinical Oncology* 34, no. 12 (April 2016): 1315–22.

71. J. Russo et al., "Cancer Risk Related to Mammary Gland Structure and Development," *Microscopy Research and Technique* 52, no. 2 (2001): 204–23.

72. M. R. Bonner et al., "Breast Cancer Risk and Exposure in Early Life to Polycyclic Aromatic Hydrocarbons Using Total Suspended Particulates as a Proxy Measure," *Cancer Epidemiology, Biomarkers and Prevention* 14 (2005): 53–60.

73. R. A. Rudel et al., "Chemicals Causing Mammary Gland Tumors in Animals Signal New Directions for Epidemiology, Chemicals Testing, and Risk Assessment for Breast Cancer Prevention," *Cancer* 109, no. 12 (2007): 2635–66.

74. C. D. Land, "Radiation and Breast Cancer Risk," *Progress in Clinical Biological Research* 396 (1997): 115–24; E. Pukkala et al., "Breast Cancer in Belarus and Ukraine After the Chernobyl Accident," *International Journal of Cancer* 119 (2006): 651–58.

75. M. Morin-Doody et al., "Breast Cancer Mortality after Diagnostic Radiography: Findings from the U.S. Scoliosis Cohort Study," *Spine* 25 (2005): 2052–63.

76. N. G. Hildreth, R. E. Shore, and P. M. Dvoretsky, "The Risk of Breast Cancer After Irradiation of the Thymus in Infancy," *New England Journal of Medicine* 321, no. 19 (1989): 1281–84.

77. S. L. Hancock, M. A. Tucker, and R. T. Hoppe, "Breast Cancer After Treatment of Hodgkin's Disease," *Journal of the National Cancer Institute* 85 (1993): 25–31; A. C. Aisenberg et al., "High Risk of Breast Carcinoma After Irradiation of Young Women with Hodgkin's Disease," *Cancer* 79 (1997): 1203–10.

78. K. Deniz et al., "Breast Cancer in Women After Treatment for Hodgkin's Disease," *Lancet Oncology* 4, no. 4 (April 2003): 207–14.

79. K. C. Oeffinger et al., "Breast Cancer Surveillance Practices Among Women Previously Treated with Chest Radiation for a Childhood Cancer," *Journal of the American Medical Association* 301, no. 4 (2009): 404–14.

80. National Cancer Institute, *Cancer and the Environment: What You Need to Know, What You Can Do* (National Institutes of Health, 2003).

81. J. G. Brody and R. A. Rudel, "Environmental Pollutants and Breast Cancer," *Environmental Health Perspectives* 111, no. 8 (2003): 1007.

82. K. Wada et al., "Life Style-Related Diseases of the Digestive System: Endocrine Disruptors Stimulate Lipid Accumulation in Target Cells Related to Metabolic Syndrome," *Journal of Pharmacological Sciences* 105, no. 2 (2007): 133–37.

83. J. Gray et al., "State of the Evidence: The Connection Between Breast Cancer and the Environment," *International Journal of Occupational and Environmental Health* 15, no. 1 (2009): 43–78; National Research Council Committee, *Hormonally Active Agents in the Environment* (Washington, DC: National Academies Press, 1999).

84. "Plastics—The Facts 2013," PlasticsEurope, accessed December 10, 2017, http://www.plasticseurope.org/Document/plastics-the-facts-2013.aspx?FolID=2.

85. International Baby Food Action Network, "Brazil, China, Malaysia, and Now the US Follow the EU with Bans on BPA in Feeding Bottles and Infant Food Containers," IBFAN.org, accessed December 10, 2017, http://ibfan.org/stop-press-bpa-sept-2012.

86. A. Schecter et al., "Polybrominated Diphenyl Ether (PBDE) Levels in an Expanded Market Basket Survey of US Food and Estimated PBDE Dietary Intake by Age and Sex," *Environmental Health Perspectives* 114, no. 10 (2006): 1515.

87. M. K. Kettles et al., "Triazine Herbicide Exposure and Breast Cancer Incidence: An Ecologic Study of Kentucky Counties," *Environmental Health Perspectives* 105, no. 11 (1997): 1222; United States Environmental Protection Agency, "Pesticides Industry Sales and Usage, 2008–2012 Market Usage," EPA.gov, accessed January 2, 2018, https://www.epa.gov/sites/production/files/2017-01/documents/pesticides-industry-sales-usage-2016_0.pdf.

88. T. B. Hayes et al., "Atrazine Induces Complete Feminization and Chemical Castration in Male African Clawed Frogs (Xenopus Laevis)," *Proceedings of the National Academy of Sciences* 107, no. 10 (2010): 4612–17.

89. R. J. Biggar et al., "Digoxin Use and the Risk of Breast Cancer in Women," *Journal of Clinical Oncology* 29, no. 16 (2011): 2165–70.

90. A. L. Herbst, H. Ulfelder, and D. C. Poskanzer, "Adenocarcinoma of the Vagina: Association of Maternal Stilbestrol Therapy with Tumor Appearance in Young Women," *New England Journal of Medicine* 284 (1971): 878–81.

91. J. R. Palmer et al., "Prenatal Diethylstilbestrol Exposure and Risk of Breast Cancer," *Cancer Epidemiology, Biomarkers and Prevention* 15 (2006): 1509–14.

92. F. S. vom Saal et al., "Chapel Hill Bisphenol A Expert Panel Consensus Statement: Integration of Mechanisms, Effects in Animals and Potential to Impact Human Health at Current Levels of Exposure," *Reproductive Toxicology* 24, no. 2 (August–September 2007): 131–8.

93. C. M. Jandegian et al., "Developmental Exposure to Bisphenol A (BPA) Alters Sexual Differentiation in Painted Turtles (Chrysemys Picta)," *General and Comparative Endocrinology* 216 (2015): 77–85.

94. D. Case, "The Real Story Behind Bisphenol A," *Fast Company*, February 1, 2009, https://www.fastcompany.com/1139298/real-story-behind-bisphenol.

95. F. S. vom Saal and C. Hughes, "An Extensive New Literature Concerning Low-Dose Effects of Bisphenol A Shows the Need for a New Risk Assessment," *Environmental Health Perspectives* 113, no. 8 (2005): 926–33.

96. G. M. Gray et al., "Weight of the Evidence Evaluation of Low-Dose Reproductive

and Developmental Effects of Bisphenol A," *Human and Ecological Risk Assessment* 10, no. 5 (2004): 875–921.

97. J. Gray et al., "State of the Evidence: The Connection Between Breast Cancer and the Environment," *International Journal of Occupational and Environmental Health* 15, no. 1 (2009): 43–78.

98. P. Franklin, "Down the Drain: Plastic Water Bottles Should No Longer Be a Wasted Resource," *Waste Management World*, February 6, 2006, https://waste-management -world.com/a/down-the-drain.

99. J. R. Jambeck et al., "Plastic Waste Inputs from Land into the Ocean," *Science* 347, no. 6223 (2015): 768–71.

100. S. Spear, "Stomach Contents of Seabirds Show that Marine Plastic Pollution Is Out of Control," EcoWatch, July 9, 2012, https://www.ecowatch.com/stomach-contents -of-seabirds-show-that-marine-plastic-pollution-is-out-1881631462.html.

101. B. C. Wolverton, A. Johnson, and K. Bounds, *Interior Landscape Plants for Indoor Air Pollution Abatement: Final Report—September 1989* (Bay Saint Louis, MS: National Aeronautics and Space Administration, John C. Stennis Space Center, 1989).

102. S. J. Genuis et al., "Blood, Urine, and Sweat (BUS) Study: Monitoring and Elimination of Bioaccumulated Toxic Elements," *Archives of Environmental Contamination and Toxicology* 61, no. 2 (2011): 344–57.

103. S. C. Segerstrom and G. E. Miller, "Psychological Stress and the Human Immune System: A Meta-analytic Study of 30 Years of Inquiry," *Psychological Bulletin* 130, no. 4 (2004): 601.

104. D. S. Krantz and M. K. McCeney, "Effects of Psychological and Social Factors on Organic Disease: A Critical Assessment of Research on Coronary Heart Disease," *Annual Review of Psychology* 53 (2002): 341–69.

105. C. Hammen, "Stress and Depression," *Annual Review of Clinical Psychology* 1 (2005): 293–319.

106. R. J. Wright, M. Rodriguez, and S. Cohen, "Review of Psychosocial Stress and Asthma: An Integrated Biopsychosocial Approach," *Thorax* 53, no. 12 (1998): 1066–74.

107. M. F. Dallman et al., "Chronic Stress and Obesity: A New View of 'Comfort Food,'" *Proceedings of the National Academy of Sciences* 100, no. 20 (2003): 11696–701.

108. K. E. Wellen and G. S. Hotamisligil, "Inflammation, Stress, and Diabetes," *Journal of Clinical Investigation* 115, no. 5 (2005): 1111.

109. J. Leserman et al., "Progression to AIDS, a Clinical AIDS Condition and Mortality: Psychosocial and Physiological Predictors," *Psychological Medicine* 32, no. 6 (2002): 1059–73.

110. J. Passchier and J. F. Orlebeke, "Headaches and Stress in Schoolchildren: An Epidemiological Study," *Cephalalgia* 5, no. 3 (1985): 167–76.

111. M. A. Smith et al., "Oxidative Stress in Alzheimer's Disease," *Biochimica et Biophysica Acta (BBA)-Molecular Basis of Disease* 1502, no. 1 (2000): 139–44.

112. E. A. Mayer, "The Neurobiology of Stress and Gastrointestinal Disease," *Gut* 47, no. 6 (2000): 861–69.

113. K. W. Davidson, E. Mostofsky, and W. Whang, "Don't Worry, Be Happy: Positive

Affect and Reduced 10-Year Incident Coronary Heart Disease: The Canadian Nova Scotia Health Survey," *European Heart Journal* 31, no. 9 (2010): 1065–70.

114. E. L. Worthington and M. Scherer, "Forgiveness Is an Emotion-Focused Coping Strategy that Can Reduce Health Risks and Promote Health Resilience: Theory, Review, and Hypotheses," *Psychology & Health* 19, no. 3 (2004): 385–405; C. van Oyen Witvliet, T. E. Ludwig, and K. L. Vander Laan, "Granting Forgiveness or Harboring Grudges: Implications for Emotion, Physiology, and Health," *Psychological Science* 12, no. 2 (2001): 117–23.

115. K. A. Lawler et al., "The Unique Effects of Forgiveness on Health: An Exploration of Pathways," *Journal of Behavioral Medicine* 28, no. 2 (2005): 157–67.

116. M. E. McCullough et al., "Religious Involvement and Mortality: A Meta-analytic Review," *Health Psychology* 19, no. 3 (2000): 211.

117. Y. Jia et al., "Does Night Work Increase the Risk of Breast Cancer? A Systematic Review and Meta-analysis of Epidemiological Studies," *Cancer Epidemiology* 37 (2013): 197–206.

118. International Agency for Research on Cancer, *IARC Monographs on the Evaluation of Carcinogenic Risks to Humans, Volume 98: Painting, Firefighting, and Shiftwork* (Lyon, France: International Agency for Research on Cancer, 2007).

119. G. C. Brainard, R. Kavet, and L. I. Kheifets, "The Relationship Between Electromagnetic Field and Light Exposures to Melatonin and Breast Cancer Risk: A Review of the Relevant Literature," *Journal of Pineal Research* 26, no. 2 (1999): 65–100; R. G. Stevens et al., "Breast Cancer and Circadian Disruption from Electric Lighting in the Modern World," *CA: A Cancer Journal for Clinicians* 64 (2014): 207–18.

120. E. E. Flynn-Evans et al., "Total Visual Blindness Is Protective Against Breast Cancer," *Cancer Causes and Control* 20, no. 9 (2009): 1753–56.

121. M. Cohen, M. Lippman, and B. Chabner, "Pineal Gland and Breast Cancer," *Lancet* 2, no. 8104–5 (December 1978): 1381–82.

122. I. Kloog et al., "Light at Night Co-distributes with Incident Breast but Not Lung Cancer in the Female Population of Israel," *Chronobiology International* 25, no. 1 (2008): 65–81.

Chapter 6: Uncontrollable Risk Factors: Do You Have Them?

1. L. M. Sánchez-Zamorano et al., "Healthy Lifestyle on the Risk of Breast Cancer," *Cancer Epidemiology, Biomarkers and Prevention* 20, no. 5 (2011): 912–22.

2. L. A. Brinton et al., "Anthropometric and Hormonal Risk Factors for Male Breast Cancer: Male Breast Cancer Pooling Project Results," *Journal of the National Cancer Institute* 106, no. 3 (March 2014): djt465; K. J. Ruddy and E. P. Winer, "Male Breast Cancer: Risk Factors, Biology, Diagnosis, Treatment, and Survivorship," *Annals of Oncology* 24, no. 6 (2013): 1434–43.

3. American Cancer Society, *Breast Cancer Facts & Figures 2017–2018* (Atlanta: American Cancer Society, Inc., 2017), accessed November 4, 2017, https://www.cancer.org/content/dam/cancer-org/research/cancer-facts-and-statistics/breast-cancer-facts-and-figures/breast-cancer-facts-and-figures-2017-2018.pdf.

4. "World Health Statistics 2016: Monitoring Health for the SDGs: Annex B: Tables of Health Statistics by Country, WHO Region and Globally," World Health Organization, 2016, accessed November 4, 2017, http://www.who.int/gho/publications /world_health_statistics/2016/EN_WHS_AnnexB.pdf.

5. M. Pierce and R. Hardy, "Commentary: The Decreasing Age of Puberty—As Much a Psychosocial as Biological Problem?" *International Journal of Epidemiology* 41, no. 1 (2012): 300–302.

6. M. E. Herman-Giddens et al., "Secondary Sexual Characteristics and Menses in Young Girls Seen in Office Practice: A Study from the Pediatric Research in Office Settings Network," *Pediatrics* 99, no. 4 (1997): 505–12.

7. M. M. Grumbach, "Puberty: Ontogeny, Neuroendocrinology, Physiology, and Disorder," *Williams Textbook of Endocrinology* (Philadelphia: Saunders, 1998), 1509–625.

8. S. J. Jordan, P. M. Webb, and A. C. Green, "Height, Age at Menarche, and Risk of Epithelial Ovarian Cancer," *Cancer Epidemiology, Biomarkers and Prevention* 14 (2005): 2045–48.

9. M. B. Pierce and D. A. Leon, "Age at Menarche and Adult BMI in the Aberdeen Children of the 1950s Cohort Study," *American Journal of Clinical Nutrition* 82 (2005): 733–98.

10. M. B. Pierce, D. Kuh, and R. Hardy, "The Role of BMI Across the Life Course in the Relationship Between Age at Menarche and Diabetes, in a British Birth Cohort," *Diabetic Medicine* 29, no. 5 (May 2012): 600–603.

11. G. C. Patton and R. Viner, "Pubertal Transitions in Health," *Lancet* 369, no. 9567 (March 2007): 1130–39.

12. M. B. Pierce, D. Kuh, and R. Hardy, "Role of Lifetime Body Mass Index in the Association Between Age at Puberty and Adult Lipids: Findings from Men and Women in a British Birth Cohort," *Annals of Epidemiology* 20, no. 9 (September 2010): 676–82.

13. M. R. Palmert et al., "Is Obesity an Outcome of Gonadotropin-Releasing Hormone Agonist Administration? Analysis of Growth and Body Composition in 110 Patients with Central Precocious Puberty," *Journal of Clinical Endocrinology and Metabolism* 84, no. 12 (1999): 4480–88; F. Massart et al., "How Do Environmental Estrogen Disruptors Induce Precocious Puberty?" *Minerva Pediatrica* 58, no. 3 (2006): 247–54.

14. J. Dratva et al., "Is Age at Menopause Increasing Across Europe? Results on Age at Menopause and Determinants from Two Population-Based Studies," *Menopause* 16, no. 2 (2009): 385–94.

15. J. R. Wisbey et al., "Natural History of Breast Pain," *Lancet* 322, no. 8351 (1983): 672–74.

16. Collaborative Group on Hormonal Factors in Breast Cancer, "Menarche, Menopause, and Breast Cancer Risk: Individual Participant Meta-analysis, Including 118,964 Women with Breast Cancer from 117 Epidemiological Studies," *Lancet Oncology* 13, no. 11 (2012): 1141–51.

17. G. Copeland et al., *Cancer in North America: 2008–2012. Volume One: Combined Cancer Incidence for the United States, Canada and North America* (Springfield, IL: North American Association of Central Cancer Registries, 2015).

18. American Cancer Society, *Breast Cancer Facts & Figures 2017–2018* (Atlanta: American Cancer Society, Inc., 2017), accessed November 5, 2017, https://www .cancer.org/content/dam/cancer-org/research/cancer-facts-and-statistics/breast-cancer -facts-and-figures/breast-cancer-facts-and-figures-2017-2018.pdf.

19. L. X. Clegg et al., "Cancer Survival Among US Whites and Minorities: A SEER (Surveillance, Epidemiology and End Results) Program Population-Based Study," *Archives of Internal Medicine* 162, no. 17 (September 2002): 1985–93.

20. American Cancer Society, "Cancer Facts & Figures for African Americans, 2016–18," accessed November 4, 2017, https://www.cancer.org/content/dam/cancer-org /research/cancer-facts-and-statistics/cancer-facts-and-figures-for-african-americans /cancer-facts-and-figures-for-african-americans-2016-2018.pdf.

21. D. Huo et al., "Comparison of Breast Cancer Molecular Features and Survival by African and European Ancestry in The Cancer Genome Atlas," *JAMA Oncology*, accessed December 10, 2017, doi:10.1001/jamaoncol.2017.0595.

22. R. T. Chlebowski et al., "Ethnicity and Breast Cancer: Factors Influencing Differences in Incidence and Outcome," *Journal of the National Cancer Institute* 97, no. 6 (March 2005): 439–48; A. Naeim et al., "Do Age and Ethnicity Predict Breast Cancer Treatment Received? A Cross-Sectional Urban Population–Based Study, Breast Cancer Treatment: Age and Ethnicity," *Critical Reviews in Oncology-Hematology* 59, no. 3 (September 2006): 234–42; G. Maskarinec et al., "A Longitudinal Investigation of Mammographic Density: The Multiethnic Cohort," *Cancer Epidemiology, Biomarkers and Prevention* 15, no. 4 (April 2006): 732–39; C. P. Kaplan et al., "Breast Cancer Risk Reduction Options: Awareness, Discussion, and Use Among Women from Four Ethnic Groups," *Cancer Epidemiology, Biomarkers and Prevention* 15, no. 1 (January 2006): 162–66; L. Tillman et al., "Breast Cancer in Native American Women Treated at an Urban-Based Indian Health Referral Center 1982–2003," *American Journal of Surgery* 190, no. 6 (December 2005): 895–902; R. Nanda et al., "Genetic Testing in an Ethnically Diverse Cohort of High-Risk Women: A Comparative Analysis of BRCA1 and BRCA2 Mutations in American Families of European and African Ancestry," *Journal of the American Medical Association* 294, no. 15 (2005): 1925–33; Hunt et al., "Increasing Black:White Disparities in Breast Cancer Mortality in the 50 Largest Cities in the US," *Cancer Epidemiology* 38, no. 2 (April 2014): 118–23; S. Percac-Lima et al., "Decreasing Disparities in Breast Cancer Screening in Refugee Women Using Culturally Tailored Patient Navigation," *Journal of General Internal Medicine* 28 (2013): 1463–68.

23. J. S. Lawson, "The Link Between Socioeconomic Status and Breast Cancer—a Possible Explanation," *Scandinavian Journal of Public Health* 27, no. 3 (September 1999): 203–5.

24. S. A. Robert et al., "Socioeconomic Risk Factors for Breast Cancer: Distinguishing Individual- and Community-Level Effects," *Epidemiology* 15, no. 4 (July 2004): 442–50.

25. Centers for Disease Control and Prevention (CDC), "Breast Cancer Screening and Socioeconomic Status—35 Metropolitan Areas, 2000 and 2002," *Morbidity and Mortality Weekly Report* 54, no. 39 (October 2005): 981–85.

26. A. Downing et al., "Socioeconomic Background in Relation to Stage at Diagnosis, Treatment and Survival in Women with Breast Cancer," *British Journal of Cancer* 96, no. 5 (March 2007): 836–40; L. E. Rutqvist and A. Bern, "Socioeconomic Gradients in Clinical Stage at Presentation and Survival Among Breast Cancer Patients in the Stockholm Area 1977–1997," *International Journal of Cancer* 119, no. 6 (September 2006): 1433–39.

27. R. Shi, "Effects of Payer Status on Breast Cancer Survival: A Retrospective Study," *BMC Cancer* 15 (2015): 211.

28. L. A. Newman et al., "Impact of Breast Carcinoma on African-American Women: The Detroit Experience," *Cancer* 91, no. 9 (May 2001): 1834–43.

29. H. J. Baer et al., "Adult Height, Age at Attained Height, and Incidence of Breast Cancer in Premenopausal Women," *International Journal of Cancer* 119, no. 9 (November 2006): 2231–35.

30. J. M. Petrelli et al., "Body Mass Index, Height, and Postmenopausal Breast Cancer Mortality in a Prospective Cohort of US Women," *Cancer Causes and Control* 13, no. 4 (May 2002): 325–32.

31. R. G. Ziegler, "Anthropometry and Breast Cancer," *Journal of Nutrition* 127, no. 5 (May 1997): 924S–928S.

32. Hormones, the Endogenous, and Breast Cancer Collaborative Group, "Insulin-like Growth Factor 1 (IGF1), IGF Binding Protein 3 (IGFBP3), and Breast Cancer Risk: Pooled Individual Data Analysis of 17 Prospective Studies," *Lancet Oncology* 11, no. 6 (2010): 530–42.

33. R. Pacifici, "Cytokines, Estrogen, and Postmenopausal Osteoporosis—the Second Decade," *Endocrinology* 139, no. 6 (June 1998): 2659–61.

34. Y. Zhang et al., "Bone Mass and the Risk of Breast Cancer Among Postmenopausal Women," *New England Journal of Medicine* 336, no. 9 (February 1997): 611–17; J. A. Cauley et al., "Bone Mineral Density and Risk of Breast Cancer in Older Women: The Study of Osteoporotic Fractures; Study of Osteoporotic Fractures Research Group," *Journal of the American Medical Association* 276, no. 17 (November 1996): 1404–8.

35. I. Persson et al., "Reduced Risk of Breast and Endometrial Cancer Among Women with Hip Fractures," *Cancer Causes and Control* 5, no. 6 (November 1994): 523–28; H. Olsson and G. Hagglund, "Reduced Cancer Morbidity and Mortality in a Prospective Cohort of Women with Distal Forearm Fractures," *American Journal of Epidemiology* 136, no. 4 (August 1992): 422–27.

36. N. F. Boyd et al., "Mammographic Density: A Hormonally Responsive Risk Factor for Breast Cancer," *Journal of the British Menopause Society* 12, no. 4 (December 2006): 186–93; M. P. V. Shekhar et al., "Breast Stroma Plays a Dominant Regulatory Role in Breast Epithelial Growth and Differentiation: Implications for Tumor Development and Progression," *Cancer Research* 61, no. 4 (2001): 1320–26.

37. T. M. Kolb, J. Lichy, and J. H. Newhouse, "Comparison of the Performance of Screening Mammography, Physical Examination, and Breast US and Evaluation of Factors that Influence Them: An Analysis of 27,825 Patient Evaluations," *Radiology* 225, no. 1 (2002): 165–75.

38. N. F. Boyd et al., "Quantitative Classification of Mammographic Densities and

Breast Cancer Risk: Results from the Canadian National Breast Screening Study," *Journal of the National Cancer Institute* 87, no. 9 (May 1995): 670–75; R. M. Tamimi et al., "Endogenous Hormone Levels, Mammographic Density, and Subsequent Risk of Breast Cancer in Postmenopausal Women," *Journal of the National Cancer Institute* 99, no. 15 (August 2007): 1178–87.

39. J. A. Knight et al., "Macronutrient Intake and Change in Mammographic Density at Menopause: Results from a Randomized Trial," *Cancer Epidemiology, Biomarkers and Prevention* 8, no. 2 (February 1999): 123–28; G. A. Greendale et al., "Effects of Estrogen and Estrogen-Progestin on Mammographic Parenchymal Density: Postmenopausal Estrogen/Progestin Interventions (PEPI) Investigators," *Annals of Internal Medicine* 130, no. 4 (February 1999): 262–69.

40. G. Ursin et al., "Can Mammographic Densities Predict Effects of Tamoxifen on the Breast?" *Journal of the National Cancer Institute* 88, no. 2 (January 1996): 128–29.

41. A. McTiernan et al., "Estrogen-Plus-Progestin Use and Mammographic Density in Postmenopausal Women: Women's Health Initiative Randomized Trial," *Journal of the National Cancer Institute* 97, no. 18 (2005): 1366–76.

42. J. Cuzick et al., "Tamoxifen-Induced Reduction in Mammographic Density and Breast Cancer Risk Reduction: A Nested Case-Control Study," *Journal of the National Cancer Institute* 103, no. 9 (2011): 744–52.

43. K. A. Ely et al., "Core Biopsy of the Breast with Atypical Ductal Hyperplasia: A Probabilistic Approach to Reporting," *American Journal of Surgical Pathology* 25, no. 8 (August 2001): 1017–21.

44. "Consensus Guideline on Concordance Assessment of Image-Guided Breast Biopsies and Management of Borderline or High-Risk Lesions," The American Society of Breast Surgeons, accessed September 9, 2017, https://www.breastsurgeons.org /new_layout/about/statements/PDF_Statements/Concordance_and_High%20 RiskLesions.pdf; M. Morrow, S. J. Schnitt, and L. Norton, "Reviews: Current Management of Lesions Associated with an Increased Risk of Breast Cancer," *National Review of Clinical Oncology* 12 (2015): 227–38.

45. M. Guray and A. A. Sahin, "Benign Breast Diseases: Classification, Diagnosis, and Management," *Oncologist* 11, no. 5 (2006): 435–49; R. A. Jensen et al., "Invasive Breast Cancer Risk in Women with Sclerosing Adenosis," *Cancer* 64, no. 10 (1989): 1977–83.

46. B. Fisher et al., "Tamoxifen for Prevention of Breast Cancer: Report of the National Surgical Adjuvant Breast and Bowel Project P-1 Study," *Journal of the National Cancer Institute* 90, no. 18 (September 1998): 1371–88.

47. N. Houssami et al., "The Association of Surgical Margins and Local Recurrence in Women with Early-Stage Invasive Breast Cancer Treated with Breast-Conserving Therapy: A Meta-analysis," *Annals of Surgical Oncology* 21, no. 3 (2014): 717–30.

48. R. E. Curtis et al., *New Malignancies Among Cancer Survivors: SEER Cancer Registries, 1973–2000* (Bethesda, MD: National Cancer Institute, 2006).

49. R. E. Curtis et al., "New Malignancies Following Breast Cancer," in *New Malignancies Among Cancer Survivors: SEER Cancer Registries, 1973–2000* (Bethesda, MD: National Cancer Institute, 2006).

50. "Familial Breast Cancer: Collaborative Reanalysis of Individual Data from 52 Epidemiological Studies Including 58,209 Women with Breast Cancer and 101,986 Women Without the Disease," *Lancet* 358, no. 9291 (2001): 1389–99.

51. P. Pharoah et al., "Family History and the Risk of Breast Cancer: A Systematic Review and Meta-analysis," *International Journal of Cancer* 71, no. 5 (1997): 800–9.

52. K. A. Metcalfe et al., "Breast Cancer Risks in Women with a Family History of Breast or Ovarian Cancer Who Have Tested Negative for a BRCA1 or BRCA2 Mutation," *British Journal of Cancer* 100, no. 2 (2009): 421.

53. B. N. Peshkin, M. L. Alabek, and C. Isaacs, "BRCA 1/2 Mutations and Triple Negative Breast Cancers," *Breast Disease* 32, no. 1–2 (2011): 25–33.

54. "Prevalence and Penetrance of BRCA1 and BRCA2 Mutations in a Population-Based Series of Breast Cancer Cases: Anglian Breast Cancer Study Group," *British Journal of Cancer* 83, no. 10 (2000): 1301–8; V. A. Moyer, "Risk Assessment, Genetic Counseling, and Genetic Testing for BRCA-Related Cancer in Women: US Preventive Services Task Force Recommendation Statement," *Annals of Internal Medicine* 160, no. 4 (February 2014): 271–81.

55. N. Petrucelli, M. B. Daly, and T. Pal, "BRCA1- and BRCA2-Associated Hereditary Breast and Ovarian Cancer," in M. P. Adam et al., eds., *GeneReviews* (Seattle: University of Washington, 1993–2018).

56. S. Chen and G. Parmigiani, "Meta-analysis of BRCA1 and BRCA2 Penetrance," *Journal of Clinical Oncology* 25, no. 11 (April 2007): 1329–33.

57. B. N. Peshkin, M. L. Alabek, and C. Isaacs, "BRCA 1/2 Mutations and Triple Negative Breast Cancers," *Breast Disease* 32, nos. 1–2 (2011): 25–33.

58. K. Metcalfe et al., "Contralateral Breast Cancer in BRCA1 and BRCA2 Mutation Carriers," *Journal of Clinical Oncology* 22, no. 12 (June 2004): 2328–35.

59. S. Panchal et al., "Does Family History Predict the Age at Onset of New Breast Cancers in BRCA1 and BRCA2 Mutation-Positive Families?" *Clinical Genetics* 77, no. 3 (2010): 273–79.

60. E. Mocci et al., "Risk of Pancreatic Cancer in Breast Cancer Families from the Breast Cancer Family Registry, *Cancer Epidemiology, Biomarkers and Prevention* 22, no. 5 (May 2013): 803–11.

61. D. Easton et al., "Cancer Risks in BRCA2 Mutation Carriers," *Journal of the National Cancer Institute* 91, no. 15 (August 1999): 1310–16.

62. A. Liede, B. Y. Karlan, and S. A. Narod, "Cancer Risks for Male Carriers of Germline Mutations in BRCA1 or BRCA2: A Review of the Literature," *Journal of Clinical Oncology* 22, no. 4 (February 2004): 735–42.

63. D. Easton et al., "Cancer Risks in BRCA2 Mutation Carriers," *Journal of the National Cancer Institute* 91, no. 15 (August 1999): 1310–16.

64. L. Castéra et al., "Next-Generation Sequencing for the Diagnosis of Hereditary Breast and Ovarian Cancer Using Genomic Capture Targeting Multiple Candidate Genes," *European Journal of Human Genetics* 22, no. 11 (2014): 1305.

65. K. D. Gonzalez et al., "Beyond Li Fraumeni Syndrome: Clinical Characteristics of Families with p53 Germline Mutations," *Journal of Clinical Oncology* 27, no. 8 (2009): 1250–56.

66. P. D. Pharoah, P. Guilford, and C. Caldas, "Incidence of Gastric Cancer and Breast Cancer in CDH1 (E-cadherin) Mutation Carriers from Hereditary Diffuse Gastric Cancer Families," *Gastroenterology* 121, no. 6 (2001): 1348–53.

67. M. K. Schmidt et al., "Breast Cancer Survival and Tumor Characteristics in Premenopausal Women Carrying the CHEK2* 1100delC Germline Mutation," *Journal of Clinical Oncology* 25, no. 1 (2006): 64–69.

68. M. K. Schmidt et al., "Breast Cancer Survival and Tumor Characteristics in Premenopausal Women Carrying the CHEK2* 1100delC Germline Mutation," *Journal of Clinical Oncology* 25, no. 1 (2006): 64–69.

69. B. Zhang et al., "Genetic Variants Associated with Breast Cancer Risk: Comprehensive Research Synopsis, Meta-analysis, and Epidemiological Evidence," *Lancet Oncology* 12, no. 5 (May 2011): 477–88.

70. D. F. Easton et al., "Gene-Panel Sequencing and the Prediction of Breast Cancer Risk," *New England Journal of Medicine* 372, no. 23 (2015): 2243–57.

71. A. Broeks et al., "Identification of Women with an Increased Risk of Developing Radiation-Induced Breast Cancer: A Case Only Study," *Breast Cancer Research* 9, no. 2 (2007): R26.

72. A. Broeks et al., "Identification of Women with an Increased Risk of Developing Radiation-Induced Breast Cancer: A Case Only Study," *Breast Cancer Research* 9, no. 2 (2007): R26.

73. F. J. Couch et al., "Inherited Mutations in 17 Breast Cancer Susceptibility Genes Among a Large Triple-Negative Breast Cancer Cohort Unselected for Family History of Breast Cancer," *Journal of Clinical Oncology* 33, no. 4 (2015): 304–11.

74. National Comprehensive Cancer Network, "Genetic/Familial High-Risk Assessment: Breast and Ovarian," *NCCN Clinical Practice Guidelines in Oncology*, accessed August 19, 2017, https://www.tri-kobe.org/nccn/guideline/gynecological/english/genetic_familial.pdf.

75. C. K. Kuhl et al., "Mammography, Breast Ultrasound, and Magnetic Resonance Imaging for Surveillance of Women at High Familial Risk for Breast Cancer," *Journal of Clinical Oncology* 23, no. 33 (2005): 8469–76.

76. S. Iodice et al., "Oral Contraceptives and Breast or Ovarian Cancer Risk in BRCA 1/2 Carriers: A Meta-analysis," *European Journal of Cancer* 46, no. 12 (August 2010): 2275–84.

77. American Cancer Society, *Breast Cancer Facts & Figures 2017–2018* (Atlanta: American Cancer Society, Inc., 2017), accessed December 11, 2017, https://www.cancer.org/content/dam/cancer-org/research/cancer-facts-and-statistics/breast-cancer-facts-and-figures/breast-cancer-facts-and-figures-2017-2018.pdf.

Chapter 7: Medications and Operations to Consider

1. J. Cuzick et al., "Preventive Therapy for Breast Cancer: A Consensus Statement," *Lancet Oncology* 12, no. 5 (2011): 496–503.

2. P. E. Goss et al., "Exemestane for Breast Cancer Prevention in Postmenopausal Women," *New England Journal of Medicine* 364, no. 25 (2011): 2381–91.

3. J. Cuzick et al., "Anastrozole for Prevention of Breast Cancer in High-Risk

Postmenopausal Women (IBIS-II): An International, Double-Blind, Randomised Placebo-Controlled Trial," *Lancet* 383, no. 9922 (2014): 1041–48.

4. L. E. Rutqvist et al., "Contralateral Primary Tumors in Breast Cancer Patients in a Randomized Trial of Adjuvant Tamoxifen Therapy," *Journal of the National Cancer Institute* 83: 1299–306.

5. B. Fisher et al., "Tamoxifen for Prevention of Breast Cancer: Report of the National Surgical Adjuvant Breast and Bowel Project P-1 Study," *Journal of the National Cancer Institute* 90, no. 18 (September 1998): 1371–88.

6. J. Cuzick et al., "Tamoxifen and Breast Density in Women at Increased Risk of Breast Cancer," *Journal of the National Cancer Institute* 96, no. 8 (April 2004): 621–28.

7. M. C. King et al., "Tamoxifen and Breast Cancer Incidence Among Women with Inherited Mutations in BRCA1 and BRCA2: National Surgical Adjuvant Breast and Bowel Project (NSABP-P1) Breast Cancer Prevention Trial," *Journal of the American Medical Association* 286, no. 18 (2001): 2251–56.

8. K. A. Phillips et al., "Tamoxifen and Risk of Contralateral Breast Cancer for BRCA1 and BRCA2 Mutation Carriers," *Journal of Clinical Oncology* 31, no. 25 (2013): 3091–99.

9. N. Orr et al., "Fine-Mapping Identifies Two Additional Breast Cancer Susceptibility Loci at 9q31.2," *Human Molecular Genetics* 24, no. 10 (May 2015): 2966–84.

10. A. C. Antoniou et al., "Common Alleles at 6q25.1 and 1p11.2 Are Associated with Breast Cancer Risk for BRCA1 and BRCA2 Mutation Carriers," *Human Molecular Genetics* 20, no. 16 (2011): 3304–21.

11. V. G. Vogel et al., "Effects of Tamoxifen vs Raloxifene on the Risk of Developing Invasive Breast Cancer and Other Disease Outcomes: The NSABP Study of Tamoxifen and Raloxifene (STAR) P-2 Trial," *Journal of the American Medical Association* 295, no. 23 (June 2006): 2727–41.

12. J. Cuzick et al., "Selective Oestrogen Receptor Modulators in Prevention of Breast Cancer: An Updated Meta-analysis of Individual Participant Data," *Lancet* 381, no. 9880 (2013): 1827–34.

13. R. T. Chlebowski et al., "Oral Bisphosphonate Use and Breast Cancer Incidence in Postmenopausal Women," *Journal of Clinical Oncology* 28, no. 22 (2010): 3582–90.

14. G. Rennert, M. Pinchev, and H. S. Rennert, "Use of Bisphosphonates and Risk of Postmenopausal Breast Cancer," *Journal of Clinical Oncology* 28, no. 22 (2010): 3577–81.

15. T. J. Hall and M. Schaueblin, "A Pharmacological Assessment of the Mammalian Osteoclast Vacuolar H+-ATPase," *Bone and Mineral* 27, no. 2 (1994): 159–66.

16. M. Bodmer et al., "Long-Term Metformin Use Is Associated with Decreased Risk of Breast Cancer," *Diabetes Care* 33, no. 6 (2010): 1304–8.

17. R. Govindarajan et al., "Thiazolidinediones and the Risk of Lung, Prostate, and Colon Cancer in Patients with Diabetes," *Journal of Clinical Oncology* 25, no. 12 (2007): 1476–81.

18. F. Frasca et al., "The Role of Insulin Receptors and IGF-I Receptors in Cancer and Other Diseases," *Archives of Physiology and Biochemistry* 114, no. 1 (2008): 23–37; L. L. Lipscombe et al., "The Impact of Diabetes on Survival Following Breast Cancer," *Breast Cancer Research and Treatment* 109, no. 2 (2008): 389–95.

19. A. DeCensi et al., "Metformin and Cancer Risk in Diabetic Patients: A Systematic Review and Meta-analysis," *Cancer Prevention Research* 3, no. 11 (2010): 1451–61.

20. N. D. Barnard et al., "A Low-Fat Vegan Diet Improves Glycemic Control and Cardiovascular Risk Factors in a Randomized Clinical Trial in Individuals with Type 2 Diabetes," *Diabetes Care* 29, no. 8 (2006): 1777–83.

21. M. F. Arisi et al., "All Trans-retinoic Acid (ATRA) Induces Re-differentiation of Early Transformed Breast Epithelial Cells," *International Journal of Oncology* 44, no. 6 (2014): 1831–42.

22. U. Veronesi et al., "Fifteen-Year Results of a Randomized Phase III Trial of Fenretinide to Prevent Second Breast Cancer," *Annals of Oncology* 17, no. 7 (2006): 1065–71.

23. E. Garattini et al., "Retinoids and Breast Cancer: from Basic Studies to the Clinic and Back Again," *Cancer Treatment Reviews* 40, no. 6 (2014): 739–49.

24. R. E. Harris et al., Women's Health Initiative, "Breast Cancer and Nonsteroidal Anti-inflammatory Drugs: Prospective Results from the Women's Health Initiative," *Cancer Research* 63, no. 18 (September 2003): 6096–101.

25. L. Gallicchio et al., "Nonsteroidal Anti-inflammatory Drugs and the Risk of Developing Breast Cancer in a Population-Based Prospective Cohort Study in Washington County, MD," *International Journal of Cancer* 121, no. 1 (July 2007): 211–15; E. Rahme et al., "Association Between Frequent Use of Nonsteroidal Anti-inflammatory Drugs and Breast Cancer," *BMC Cancer* 5 (2005): 159; T. M. Brasky et al., "Non-steroidal Anti-inflammatory Drug (NSAID) Use and Breast Cancer Risk in the Western New York Exposures and Breast Cancer (WEB) Study," *Cancer Causes and Control* 21, no. 9 (2010): 1503–12.

26. K. K. Ludwig et al., "Risk Reduction and Survival Benefit of Prophylactic Surgery in BRCA Mutation Carriers, a Systematic Review," *American Journal of Surgery* 212, no. 4 (2016): 660–69.

27. L. Lostumbo et al., "Prophylactic Mastectomy for the Prevention of Breast Cancer," *Cochrane Database Systematic Reviews* 4, no. 4 (October 2004).

28. J. K. Litton et al., "Earlier Age of Onset of BRCA Mutation-Related Cancers in Subsequent Generations," *Cancer* 118, no. 2 (2012): 321–25.

29. H. B. Nichols et al., "Declining Incidence of Contralateral Breast Cancer in the United States from 1975 to 2006," *Journal of Clinical Oncology* 29, no. 12 (2011): 1564–69.

30. L. Bertelsen et al., "Effect of Systemic Adjuvant Treatment on Risk for Contralateral Breast Cancer in the Women's Environment, Cancer and Radiation Epidemiology Study," *Journal of the National Cancer Institute* 100, no. 1 (2008): 32–40.

31. Y. Chen et al., "Epidemiology of Contralateral Breast Cancer," *Cancer Epidemiology, Biomarkers and Prevention* 8 (1999): 855–61.

32. A. S. Reiner et al., "Hormone Receptor Status of a First Primary Breast Cancer Predicts Contralateral Breast Cancer Risk in the WECARE Study Population," *Breast Cancer Research* 19, no. 1 (2017): 83.

33. J. Ji and K. Hemminki, "Risk for Contralateral Breast Cancers in a Population Covered by Mammography: Effects of Family History, Age at Diagnosis and Histology," *Breast Cancer and Research Treatment* 105 (2007): 229–36.

34. K. Hemminki, J. Ji, and A. Forsti, "Risks for Familial and Contralateral Breast Cancer Interact Multiplicatively and Cause a High Risk," *Cancer Research* 67 (2007): 868–70.

35. M. K. Graeser et al., "Contralateral Breast Cancer Risk in BRCA1 and BRCA2 Mutation Carriers," *Journal of Clinical Oncology* 27 (2009): 5887–92.

36. J. A. Largent et al., "Reproductive History and Risk of Second Primary Breast Cancer: The WECARE Study," *Cancer Epidemiology, Biomarkers and Prevention* 16 (2007): 906–11.

37. J. A. Largent et al., "Reproductive History and Risk of Second Primary Breast Cancer: The WECARE Study," *Cancer Epidemiology, Biomarkers and Prevention* 16 (2007): 906–11.

38. N. Druesne-Pecollo et al., "Excess Body Weight and Second Primary Cancer Risk after Breast Cancer: A Systematic Review and Meta-analysis of Prospective Studies," *Breast Cancer Research and Treatment* 135 (2012): 647–54.

39. H. B. Nichols et al., "Declining Incidence of Contralateral Breast Cancer in the United States from 1975 to 2006," *Journal of Clinical Oncology* 29, no. 12 (2011): 1564–69.

40. L. Lostumbo, N. E. Carbine, and J. Wallace, "Prophylactic Mastectomy for the Prevention of Breast Cancer," *Cochrane Database Systematic Reviews* (November 2010).

41. T. Musiello, E. Bornhammar, and C. Saunders, "Breast Surgeons' Perceptions and Attitudes Towards Contralateral Prophylactic Mastectomy," *ANZ Journal of Surgery* 83, nos. 7–8 (2013): 527–32.

42. C. E. Pesce et al., "Changing Surgical Trends in Young Patients with Early Stage Breast Cancer, 2003 to 2010: A Report from the National Cancer Data Base," *Journal of the American College of Surgeons* 219, no. 1 (2014): 19–28.

43. K. L. Kummerow et al., "Nationwide Trends in Mastectomy for Early-Stage Breast Cancer," *JAMA Surgery* 150 (2015): 9–16.

44. A. K. Arrington et al., "Patient and Surgeon Characteristics Associated with Increased Use of Contralateral Prophylactic Mastectomy in Patients with Breast Cancer," *Annals of Surgical Oncology* 16, no. 10 (2009): 2697–704.

45. U. Güth et al., "Increasing Rates of Contralateral Prophylactic Mastectomy—A Trend Made in USA?" *European Journal of Surgical Oncology* 38, no. 4 (2012): 296–301.

46. J. Gahm, M. Wickman, and Y. Brandberg, "Bilateral Prophylactic Mastectomy in Women with Inherited Risk of Breast Cancer—Prevalence of Pain and Discomfort, Impact on Sexuality, Quality of Life and Feelings of Regret Two Years After Surgery," *Breast* 19, no. 6 (2010): 462–69.

47. M. H. Frost et al., "Contralateral Prophylactic Mastectomy: Long-Term Consistency of Satisfaction and Adverse Effects and the Significance of Informed Decision-Making, Quality of Life, and Personality Traits," *Annals of Surgical Oncology* 18, no. 11 (2011): 3110.

48. S. M. Domchek et al., "Association of Risk-Reducing Surgery in BRCA1 or BRCA2 Mutation Carriers with Cancer Risk and Mortality," *Journal of the American Medical Association* 304, no. 9 (2010): 967–75.

49. C. Iavazzo, I. D. Gkegkes, and N. Vrachnis, "Primary Peritoneal Cancer in BRCA Carriers After Prophylactic Bilateral Salpingo-oophorectomy," *Journal of the Turkish German Gynecological Association* 17, no. 2 (2016): 73.

50. National Comprehensive Cancer Network, "Genetic/Familial High-Risk Assessment: Breast and Ovarian," *NCCN Clinical Practice Guidelines in Oncology*, accessed August 25, 2017, https://www.tri-kobe.org/nccn/guideline/gynecological /english/genetic_familial.pdf.

51. T. R. Rebbeck et al., "Effect of Short-Term Hormone Replacement Therapy on Breast Cancer Risk Reduction After Bilateral Prophylactic Oophorectomy in BRCA1 and BRCA2 Mutation Carriers: The PROSE Study Group," *Journal of Clinical Oncology* 23, no. 31 (2005): 7804–10.

52. K. Armstrong et al., "Hormone Replacement Therapy and Life Expectancy After Prophylactic Oophorectomy in Women with BRCA 1/2 Mutations: A Decision Analysis," *Journal of Clinical Oncology* 22, no. 6 (2004): 1045–54.

Chapter 8: Breast Cancer Screening and Detection

1. J. P. Kösters and P. C. Gøtzsche, "Regular Self-Examination or Clinical Examination for Early Detection of Breast Cancer," *Cochrane Database of Systematic Reviews* 2 (2003).

2. T. Roeke et al., "The Additional Cancer Yield of Clinical Breast Examination in Screening of Women at Hereditary Increased Risk of Breast Cancer: A Systematic Review," *Breast Cancer Research and Treatment* 147, no. 1 (2014): 15–23.

3. F. D. Schwab et al., "Self-Detection and Clinical Breast Examination: Comparison of the Two 'Classical' Physical Examination Methods for the Diagnosis of Breast Cancer," *Breast* 24, no. 1 (2015): 90–92.

4. B. L. Sprague et al., "National Performance Benchmarks for Modern Diagnostic Digital Mammography: Update from the Breast Cancer Surveillance Consortium," *Radiology* 283, no. 1 (2017): 59–69.

5. S. Sayed et al., "Training Health Workers in Clinical Breast Examination for Early Detection of Breast Cancer in Low- and Middle-Income Countries," *Cochrane Database Systematic Reviews* 1 (2017).

6. B. C. R. Devi, T. S. Tang, and M. Corbex, "Reducing by Half the Percentage of Late-Stage Presentation for Breast and Cervix Cancer over 4 Years: A Pilot Study of Clinical Downstaging in Sarawak, Malaysia," *Annals of Oncology* 18, no. 7 (2007): 1172–76.

7. M. G. Marmot et al., "The Benefits and Harms of Breast Cancer Screening—An Independent Review: A Report Jointly Commissioned by Cancer Research UK and the Department of Health (England) October 2012," *British Journal of Cancer* 108, no. 11 (2013): 2205.

8. K. L. Kummerow et al., "Nationwide Trends in Mastectomy for Early-Stage Breast Cancer," *JAMA Surgery* 150 (2015): 9–16; S. T. Hawley et al., "Social and Clinical Determinants of Contralateral Prophylactic Mastectomy," *JAMA Surgery* 149 (2014): 582–89.

9. C. P. McPherson, K. K. Swenson, and M. W. Lee, "The Effects of Mammographic Detection and Comorbidity on the Survival of Older Women with Breast Cancer," *Journal of the American Geriatrics Society* 50, no. 6 (2002): 1061–68.

10. M. M. Eberl et al., "BI-RADS Classification for Management of Abnormal Mammograms," *Journal of the American Board of Family Medicine* 19, no. 2 (2006): 161–64.

11. P. A. Carney et al., "Individual and Combined Effects of Age, Breast Density, and Hormone Replacement Therapy Use on the Accuracy of Screening Mammography," *Annals of Internal Medicine* 138 (2003): 168–75.

12. B. L. Sprague et al., "National Performance Benchmarks for Modern Diagnostic Digital Mammography: Update from the Breast Cancer Surveillance Consortium," *Radiology* 283, no. 1 (2017): 59–69.

13. S. H. Taplin et al., "Reason for Late-Stage Breast Cancer: Absence of Screening or Detection, or Breakdown in Follow-Up?" *Journal of the National Cancer Institute* 96, no. 20 (October 2004): 1518–27.

14. L. Tabar et al., "Mammography Service Screening and Mortality in Breast Cancer Patients: 20-Year Follow-Up Before and After Introduction of Screening," *Lancet* 361, no. 9367 (2003): 1405–10.

15. D. R. Youlden et al., "Incidence and Mortality of Female Breast Cancer in the Asia-Pacific Region," *Cancer Biology and Medicine* 11 (2014): 101–15.

16. R. A. Smith et al., "The Randomized Trials of Breast Cancer Screening: What Have We Learned?" *Radiologic Clinics of North America* 42, no. 5 (2004): 793–806; M. Broeders et al., "The Impact of Mammographic Screening on Breast Cancer Mortality in Europe: A Review of Observational Studies," *Journal of Medical Screening* 19, no. 1 (2012): 14–25; Preventive Services Task Force, "Screening for Breast Cancer: Recommendations and Rationale," *Annals of Internal Medicine* 137 (2002): 344–46; D. A. Berry, "Benefits and Risks of Screening Mammography for Women in Their Forties: A Statistical Appraisal," *Journal of the National Cancer Institute* 90 (1998): 1431–39.

17. E. D. Pisano et al., "Digital Mammographic Imaging Screening Trial (DMIST) Investigators Group: Diagnostic Performance of Digital Versus Film Mammography for Breast-Cancer Screening," *New England Journal of Medicine* 353, no. 17 (October 2005): 1773–83.

18. S. Ciatto et al., "Integration of 3D Digital Mammography with Tomosynthesis for Population Breast-Cancer Screening (STORM): A Prospective Comparison Study," *Lancet Oncology* 14 (2013): 583–89.

19. A. S. Tagliafico et al., "Diagnostic Performance of Contrast-Enhanced Spectral Mammography: Systematic Review and Meta-analysis," *Breast* 28 (2016): 13–19.

20. E. M. Fallenberg et al., "Contrast-Enhanced Spectral Mammography Versus MRI: Initial Results in the Detection of Breast Cancer and Assessment of Tumour Size," *European Radiology* 24, no. 1 (2014): 256–64.

21. P. A. Carney et al., "Factors Associated with Imaging and Procedural Events Used to Detect Breast Cancer After Screening Mammography," *American Journal of Roentgenology* 188, no. 2 (2007): 385–92.

22. J. G. Elmore et al., "Ten-Year Risk of False Positive Screening Mammograms and Clinical Breast Examinations," *New England Journal of Medicine* 338, no. 16 (April 1998): 1089–96.

23. S. Törnberg et al., "A Pooled Analysis of Interval Cancer Rates in Six European Countries," *European Journal of Cancer Prevention* 19, no. 2 (2010): 87–93.

24. P. A. Carney et al., "Individual and Combined Effects of Age, Breast Density, and

Hormone Replacement Therapy Use on the Accuracy of Screening Mammography," *Annals of Internal Medicine* 138, no. 3 (2003): 168–75; T. M. Kolb, J. Lichy, and J. H. Newhouse, "Comparison of the Performance of Screening Mammography, Physical Examination, and Breast US and Evaluation of Factors That Influence Them: An Analysis of 27,825 Patient Evaluations," *Radiology* 225, no. 1 (2002): 165–75.

25. S. S. K. Tang and G. P. H. Gui, "A Review of the Oncologic and Surgical Management of Breast Cancer in the Augmented Breast: Diagnostic, Surgical and Surveillance Challenges," *Annals of Surgical Oncology* 18, no. 8 (2011): 2173–81.

26. M. J. Yaffe and J. G. Mainprize, "Risk of Radiation-Induced Breast Cancer from Mammographic Screening 1," *Radiology* 258, no. 1 (2011): 98–105.

27. L. M. Warren, D. R. Dance, and K. C. Young, "Radiation Risk of Breast Screening in England with Digital Mammography," *British Journal of Radiology* 89 (November 2016): 1067; D. L. Miglioretti et al., "Radiation-Induced Breast Cancer Incidence and Mortality from Digital Mammography Screening: A Modeling Study," *Annals of Internal Medicine* 164, no. 4 (2016): 205–14.

28. "Patient Safety: Radiation Dose in X-Ray and CT Exams," RadiologyInfo.org, updated February 8, 2017, https://www.radiologyinfo.org/en/info.cfm?pg=safety-xray.

29. "Patient Safety: Radiation Dose in X-Ray and CT Exams," RadiologyInfo.org, updated February 8, 2017, https://www.radiologyinfo.org/en/info.cfm?pg=safety-xray.

30. C. H. C. Drossaert, H. Boer, and E. R. Seydel, "Monitoring Women's Experiences During Three Rounds of Breast Cancer Screening: Results from a Longitudinal Study," *Journal of Medical Screening* 9, no. 4 (2002): 168–75.

31. US Preventive Services Task Force, "Screening for Breast Cancer: US Preventive Services Task Force Recommendation Statement," *Annals of Internal Medicine* 151, no. 10 (2009): 716.

32. L. M. Schwartz et al., "US Women's Attitudes to False Positive Mammography Results and Detection of Ductal Carcinoma In Situ: Cross Sectional Survey," *British Medical Journal* 320, no. 7250 (2000): 1635–40.

33. E. K. Arleo et al., "Comparison of Recommendations for Screening Mammography Using CISNET Models," *Cancer* 123, no. 19 (October 2017): 3673–80.

34. A. S. Tagliafico et al., "Adjunct Screening with Tomosynthesis or Ultrasound in Women with Mammography-Negative Dense Breasts: Interim Report of a Prospective Comparative Trial," *Journal of Clinical Oncology* 34, no. 16 (2016): 1882–88.

35. F. Sardanelli et al., "Multicenter Surveillance of Women at High Genetic Breast Cancer Risk Using Mammography, Ultrasonography, and Contrast-Enhanced Magnetic Resonance Imaging (the High Breast Cancer Risk Italian 1 Study): Final Results," *Investigative Radiology* 46, no. 2 (2011): 94–105.

36. M. E. Brennan et al., "Magnetic Resonance Imaging Screening of the Contralateral Breast in Women with Newly Diagnosed Breast Cancer: Systematic Review and Meta-analysis of Incremental Cancer Detection and Impact on Surgical Management," *Journal of Clinical Oncology* 27, no. 33 (2009): 5640–49.

37. M. Kriege et al., "Efficacy of MRI and Mammography for Breast-Cancer Screening

in Women with a Familial or Genetic Predisposition," *New England Journal of Medicine* 351, no. 5 (2004): 427–37.

38. C. D. Lehman, "Clinical Indications: What Is the Evidence?" *European Journal of Radiology* 81 (2012): S82–S84.

39. N. Houssami, R. Turner, and M. Morrow, "Preoperative Magnetic Resonance Imaging in Breast Cancer: Meta-analysis of Surgical Outcomes," *Annals of Surgery* 257, no. 2 (2013): 249–55.

40. M. Morrow, J. Waters, and E. Morris, "MRI for Breast Cancer Screening, Diagnosis, and Treatment," *Lancet* 378, no. 9805 (2011): 1804–11.

41. National Comprehensive Cancer Network, "Guidelines for Breast Cancer Screening and Diagnosis," http://www.NCCN.org.

42. C. C. Riedl et al., "Triple-Modality Screening Trial for Familial Breast Cancer Underlines the Importance of Magnetic Resonance Imaging and Questions the Role of Mammography and Ultrasound Regardless of Patient Mutation Status, Age, and Breast Density," *Journal of Clinical Oncology* 33, no. 10 (2015): 1128–35.

43. E. M. Fallenberg et al., "Contrast-Enhanced Spectral Mammography versus MRI: Initial Results in the Detection of Breast Cancer and Assessment of Tumour Size," *European Radiology* 24, no. 1 (2014): 256–64.

44. US Food and Drug Administration, "FDA Drug Safety Communication: FDA Evaluating the Risk of Brain Deposits with Repeated Use of Gadolinium-Based Contrast Agents for Magnetic Resonance Imaging (MRI)," FDA.gov, accessed August 27, 2017, http://www.fda.gov/Drugs/DrugSafety/ucm455386.htm.

45. J. Hermans, "The Value of Aspiration Cytologic Examination of the Breast: A Statistical Review of the Medical Literature," *Cancer* 69, no. 8 (April 1992): 2104–10; F. O'Malley et al., "Clinical Correlates of False-Negative Fine Needle Aspirations of the Breast in a Consecutive Series of 1,005 Patients," *Surgery, Gynecology and Obstetrics* 176, no. 4 (April 1993): 360–64; N. J. Wollenberg et al., "Fine Needle Aspiration Cytology of the Breast: A Review of 321 Cases with Statistical Evaluation," *Acta Cytologica* 29 (1985): 425–29.

46. P. Crystal et al., "Accuracy of Sonographically Guided 14-Gauge Core-Needle Biopsy: Results of 715 Consecutive Breast Biopsies with at Least Two-Year Follow-Up of Benign Lesions," *Journal of Clinical Ultrasound* 33, no. 2 (February 2005): 47–52; M. Memarsadeghi et al., "Value of 14-Gauge Ultrasound-Guided Large-Core Needle Biopsy of Breast Lesions: Own Results in Comparison with the Literature," *RoFo* 175, no. 3 (March 2003): 374–80; J. M. Schoonjans and R. F. Brem, "Fourteen-Gauge Ultrasonographically Guided Large-Core Needle Biopsy of Breast Masses," *Journal of Ultrasound in Medicine* 20, no. 9 (September 2001): 967–72; D. N. Smith et al., "The Utility of Ultrasonographically Guided Large-Core Needle Biopsy: Results from 500 Consecutive Breast Biopsies," *Journal of Ultrasound in Medicine* 20, no. 1 (January 2001): 43–49.

47. C. F. Loughran and C. R. Keeling, "Seeding of Tumour Cells Following Breast Biopsy: A Literature Review," *British Journal of Radiology* 84, no. 1006 (2011): 869–74.

48. L. E. Hoorntje et al., "Tumour Cell Displacement after 14G Breast Biopsy," *European Journal of Surgical Oncology* 30, no. 5 (June 2004): 520–25.

49. C. Peters-Engl et al., "The Impact of Preoperative Breast Biopsy on the Risk of Sentinel Lymph Node Metastases: Analysis of 2502 Cases from the Austrian Sentinel Node Biopsy Study Group," *British Journal of Cancer* 91, no. 10 (October 2004): 1782–86.

50. N. M. Diaz, J. R. Mayes, and V. Vrcel, "Breast Epithelial Cells in Dermal Angiolymphatic Spaces: A Manifestation of Benign Mechanical Transport," *Human Pathology* 36 (2005): 310–13; I. J. Bleiweiss, C. S. Nagi, and S. Jaffer, "Axillary Sentinel Lymph Nodes Can Be Falsely Positive Due to Iatrogenic Displacement and Transport of Benign Epithelial Cells in Patients with Breast Carcinoma," *Journal of Clinical Oncology* 24, no. 13 (2006): 2013–18.

51. T. P. Butler and P. M. Gullino, "Quantitation of Cell Shedding into Efferent Blood of Mammary Adenocarcinoma," *Cancer Research* 35, no. 3 (1975): 512–16.

52. M. Silverstein, "Where's the Outrage?" *Journal of the American College of Surgeons* 208, no. 1 (January 2009): 78–79.

53. L. G. Gutwein et al., "Utilization of Minimally Invasive Breast Biopsy for the Evaluation of Suspicious Breast Lesions," *American Journal of Surgery* 202, no. 2 (2011): 127–32.

54. W. Bruening, K. Schoelles, and J. Treadwell, "Comparative Effectiveness of Core-Needle Biopsies and Open Surgical Biopsy for the Diagnosis of Breast Lesions" (Rockville, MD: Agency for Healthcare Research and Quality, 2009).

55. W. Bruening, K. Schoelles, and J. Treadwell, "Comparative Effectiveness of Core-Needle Biopsies and Open Surgical Biopsy for the Diagnosis of Breast Lesions" (Rockville, MD: Agency for Healthcare Research and Quality, 2009).

56. C. Conry, "Evaluation of a Breast Complaint: Is It Cancer?" *American Family Physician* 49 (1994): 445–50, 453–54.

57. G. Fariselli et al., "Localized Mastalgia as Presenting Symptom in Breast Cancer," *European Journal of Surgical Oncology* 14 (1988): 213–15; F. Lumachi et al., "Breast Complaints and Risk of Breast Cancer: Population-Based Study of 2,879 Self-Selected Women and Long-Term Follow-Up," *Biomedicine and Pharmacotherapy* 56 (2002): 88–92; National Breast Cancer Centre, "The Investigation of a New Breast Symptom: A Guide for General Practitioners," Cancer Australia, last updated October 23 2017, https://canceraustralia.gov.au/publications-and-resources/cancer-australia -publications/investigation-new-breast-symptom-guide-general-practitioners.

58. M. M. Koo et al., "Typical and Atypical Presenting Symptoms of Breast Cancer and Their Associations with Diagnostic Intervals: Evidence from a National Audit of Cancer Diagnosis," *Cancer Epidemiology* 48 (May 2017): 140–46.

59. J. N. Clegg-Lamptey et al., "Breast Cancer Risk in Patients with Breast Pain in Accra, Ghana," *East African Medical Journal* 84, no. 5 (May 2007): 215–18.

60. B. A. Ayoade, A. O. Tade, and B. A. Salami, "Clinical Features and Pattern of Presentation of Breast Diseases in Surgical Outpatient Clinic of a Suburban Tertiary Hospital in South-West Nigeria," *Nigerian Journal of Surgery : Official Publication of the Nigerian Surgical Research Society* 18, no. 1 (2012): 13–16.

61. D. N. Ader and M. W. Browne, "Prevalence and Impact of Cyclic Mastalgia in a United States Clinic-Based Sample," *American Journal of Obstetrics and Gynecology* 177, no. 1 (1997): 126–32.

62. M. B. Barton, J. G. Elmore, and S. W. Fletcher, "Breast Symptoms Among Women Enrolled in a Health Maintenance Organization: Frequency, Evaluation, and Outcome," *Annals of Internal Medicine* 130, no. 8 (1999): 651–57.

63. E. L. Davies et al., "The Long-Term Course of Mastalgia," *Journal of the Royal Society of Medicine* 91, no. 9 (1998): 462–64.

64. R. L. Smith, S. Pruthi, and L. A. Fitzpatrick, "Evaluation and Management of Breast Pain," *Mayo Clinic Proceedings* 79, no. 3. (2004): 353–72.

65. "Klimberg Versus Etiology and Management of Breast Pain," in *Diseases of the Breast*, J. R. Harris et al., eds., (Philadelphia: Lippincott-Raven, 1996), 99–106.

66. N. L. Pashby et al., "A Clinical Trial of Evening Primrose Oil in Mastalgia [abstract]," *British Journal of Surgery* 68 (1981): 801; P. E. Preece et al., "Evening Primrose Oil (Efamol) for Mastalgia," *Clinical Uses of Essential Fatty Acids*, D. F. Horrobin, ed., (Montreal, Quebec: Eden Press, 1982), 147–54; D. F. Horrobin, "The Role of Essential Fatty Acids and Prostaglandins in the Premenstrual Syndrome," *Journal of Reproductive Medicine* 28, no. 7 (1983): 465–68; C. A. Gateley et al., "Plasma Fatty Acid Profiles in Benign Breast Disorders," *British Journal of Surgery* 79 (1992): 407–9.

67. S. Pruthi et al., "Vitamin E and Evening Primrose Oil for Management of Cyclical Mastalgia: A Randomized Pilot Study," *Alternative Medicine Review* 15, no. 1 (2010): 59.

68. E. G. Loch, H. Selle, and N. Boblitz, "Treatment of Premenstrual Syndrome with a Phytopharmaceutical Formulation Containing Vitex Agnus Castus," *Journal of Women's Health and Gender-Based Medicine* 9, no. 3 (2000): 315–20.

69. A. Cassidy, S. Bingham, and K. D. Setchell, "Biological Effects of a Diet of Soy Protein Rich in Isoflavones on the Menstrual Cycle of Premenopausal Women," *American Journal of Clinical Nutrition* 60 (1994): 333–40.

70. C. Nagata et al., "Decreased Serum Estradiol Concentration Associated with High Dietary Intake of Soy Products in Premenopausal Japanese Women," *Nutrition and Cancer* 29, no. 3 (1997): 228–33.

71. N. F. Boyd et al., "Effect of a Low-Fat High-Carbohydrate Diet on Symptoms of Cyclical Mastopathy," *Lancet* 2, no. 8603 (1988): 128–32; P. J. Goodwin et al., "Elevated High-Density Lipoprotein Cholesterol and Dietary Fat Intake in Women with Cyclic Mastopathy," *American Journal of Obstetrics and Gynecology* 179, no. 2 (1998): 430–37.

72. N. F. Boyd et al., "Canadian Diet and Breast Cancer Prevention Study Group: Effects at Two Years of a Low-Fat, High-Carbohydrate Diet on Radiologic Features of the Breast: Results from a Randomized Trial," *Journal of the National Cancer Institute* 89, no. 7 (1997): 488–96.

73. J. P. Minton et al., "Clinical and Biochemical Studies on Methylxanthine-Related Fibrocystic Breast Disease," *Surgery* 90 (1981): 299–304; B. Bullough, M. Hindey-Alexander, H. Fetou, "Methylxanthines and Fibrocystic Breast Disease: A Study of Correlations," *Nurse Practitioner* 15 (1990): 36; J. P. Minton and H. Abou-Issa, "Nonendocrine Theories of Etiology of Benign Breast Disease," *World Journal of Surgery* 1989; 13: 680–84.

74. L. M. Dickerson, P. J. Mazyck, and M. H. Hunter, "Premenstrual Syndrome," *American Family Physician* 67, no. 8 (2003): 1743–52; P. W. Budoff, "The Use of

Prostaglandin Inhibitors for the Premenstrual Syndrome," *The Journal of Reproductive Medicine* 28, no. 7 (1983): 469–78.

75. H. Fox et al., "Are Patients with Mastalgia Anxious, and Does Relaxation Therapy Help?" *Breast* 6, no. 3 (1997): 138–42; L. Thicke et al., "Acupuncture for Treatment of Noncyclic Breast Pain: A Pilot Study," *American Journal of Chinese Medicine* 39, no. 6 (2011): 1117–29; S. Colegrave, C. Holcombe, P. Salmon, "Psychological Characteristics of Women Presenting with Breast Pain," *Journal of Psychosomatic Research* 50, no. 6 (2001): 303–7; A. A. Wren et al., "Yoga for Persistent Pain: New Findings and Directions for an Ancient Practice," *Pain* 152, no. 3 (2011): 477; F. Zeidan et al., "Mindfulness Meditation–Related Pain Relief: Evidence for Unique Brain Mechanisms in the Regulation of Pain," *Neuroscience Letters* 520, no. 2 (2012): 165–73.

76. M. C. Wilson and R. A. Sellwood, "Therapeutic Value of a Supporting Brassiere in Mastodynia," *BMJ* 2, no. 6027 (1976): 90; B. R. Mason, K. A. Page, and K. Fallon, "An Analysis of Movement and Discomfort of the Female Breast During Exercise and the Effects of Breast Support in Three Cases," *Journal of Science and Medicine in Sport* 2, no. 2 (1999): 134–44.

77. M. D. Sullivan, J. A. Turner, and J. Romano, "Chronic Pain in Primary Care: Identification and Management of Psychosocial Factors," *Journal of Family Practice* 32, no. 2 (1991): 193–99.

78. A. D. Irving and S. L. Morrison, "Effectiveness of Topical Non-steroidal Anti-inflammatory Drugs in the Management of Breast Pain," *Journal of the Royal College of Surgeons of Edinburgh* 43, no. 3 (1998): 158–59; G. Gabbrielli et al., "Nimesulide in the Treatment of Mastalgia," *Drugs* 46, suppl. 1 (1993): 137–39.

79. L. E. Hughes et al., *Benign Disorders and Diseases of the Breast* (London: WB Saunders, 2000).

80. A. N. Hussain, C. Policarpio, and M. T. Vincent, "Evaluating Nipple Discharge," *Obstetrical and Gynecological Survey* 61, no. 4 (April 2006): 278–83.

81. H. Gülay et al., "Management of Nipple Discharge," *Journal of the American College of Surgeons* 178, no. 5 (1994): 471–74.

82. J. E. Devitt, "Management of Nipple Discharge by Clinical Findings," *American Journal of Surgery* 149, no. 6 (1985): 789–92.

83. V. J. Harris and V. P. Jackson, "Indications for Breast Imaging in Women Under Age 35 Years," *Radiology* 172 (1989): 445–48; M. Morrow, S. Wong, and L. Venta, "The Evaluation of Breast Masses in Women Younger than Forty Years of Age," *Surgery* 124 (1998): 634–40.

84. F. M. Hall et al., "Nonpalpable Breast Lesions: Recommendations for Biopsy Based on Suspicion of Carcinoma at Mammography," *Radiology* 167 (1988): 353–58; P. Crone et al., "The Predictive Value of Three Diagnostic Procedures in the Evaluation of Palpable Breast Tumours," *Ovid Healthstar Annales Chirurgiae et Gynaecologiae* 73, no. 5 (1984): 273–76.

85. S. V. Hilton et al., "Real-Time Breast Sonography: Application in 300 Consecutive Patients," *American Journal of Roentgenology* 147, no. 3 (September 1986): 479–86.

86. W. A. Berg et al., "Cystic Breast Masses and the ACRIN 6666 Experience," *Radiologic Clinics of North America* 48, no. 5 (2010): 931–87.

87. R. J. Brenner et al., "Spontaneous Regression of Interval Benign Cysts of the Breast," *Radiology* 193, no. 2 (1994): 365–68.

88. C. P. Daly et al., "Complicated Breast Cysts on Sonography: Is Aspiration Necessary to Exclude Malignancy?" *Academic Radiology* 15, no. 5 (2008): 610–17; Y. W. Chang et al., "Sonographic Differentiation of Benign and Malignant Cystic Lesions of the Breast," *Journal of Ultrasound in Medicine* 26, no. 1 (2007): 47–53; W. Berg, C. Campassi, and O. Ioffe, "Cystic Lesions of the Breast: Sonographic-Pathologic Correlation," *Radiology* 227, no. 1 (2003): 183–91.

89. R. J. Santen and R. Mansel, "Benign Breast Disorders," *New England Journal of Medicine* 353 (2005): 275.

90. A. D. DiVasta, C. Weldon, and B. I. Labow, "The Breast: Examination and Lesions," in *Goldstein's Pediatric and Adolescent Gynecology*, 6th ed., ed. L. Emans and M. R. Laufer (Philadelphia: Lippincott Williams and Wilkins, 2012), 405.

91. Y. Jayasinghe and P. S. Simmons, "Fibroadenomas in Adolescence," *Current Opinion in Obstetrics and Gynecology* 21, no. 5 (October 2009): 402.

92. J. A. Harvey et al., "Short-Term Follow-Up of Palpable Breast Lesions with Benign Imaging Features: Evaluation of 375 Lesions in 320 Women," *American Journal of Roentgenology* 193, no. 6 (December 2009): 1723.

93. D. M. Dent and P. J. Cant, "Fibroadenoma," *World Journal of Surgery* 13, no. 6 (November–December 1989): 706–10.

94. L. Deschênes et al., "Beware of Breast Fibroadenomas in Middle-Aged Women," *Canadian Journal of Surgery* 28, no. 4 (July 1985): 372–74; K. Guzanowski-Konakry, E. G. Harrison Jr., and W. S. Payne, "Lobular Carcinoma Arising in Fibroadenoma of the Breast," *Cancer* 35, no. 2 (February 1975): 450–56.

95. P. J. Littrup et al., "Cryotherapy for Breast Fibroadenomas," *Radiology* 234, no. 1 (January 2005): 63–72; C. S. Kaufman et al., "Office-Based Ultrasound-Guided Cryoablation of Breast Fibroadenomas," *American Journal of Surgery* 184, no. 5 (November 2002): 394–400; I. Grady, H. Gorsuch, and S. Wilburn-Bailey, "Long-Term Outcome of Benign Fibroadenomas Treated by Ultrasound-Guided Percutaneous Excision," *Breast Journal* 14 (2008): 275–78.

96. C. S. Kaufman et al., "Office-Based Cryoablation of Breast Fibroadenomas: 12-Month Follow-Up," *Journal of the American College of Surgeons* 198, no. 6 (2004): 914–23.

97. O. Kenneth Macdonald et al., "Malignant Phyllodes Tumor of the Female Breast," *Cancer* 107, no. 9 (2006): 2127–33.

98. F. A. Tavassoli and P. Devilee, eds., *Pathology and Genetics of Tumours of the Breast and Female Genital Organs* (Lyon, France: International Agency for Research on Cancer, 2003).

99. M. F. Dillon et al., "Needle Core Biopsy in the Diagnosis of Phyllodes Neoplasm," *Surgery* 140, no. 5 (2006): 779–84; A. H. Lee, "Recent Developments in the Histological Diagnosis of Spindle Cell Carcinoma, Fibromatosis and Phyllodes Tumour of the Breast," *Histopathology* 52, no. 1 (January 2008): 45–57; A. H. Lee et al., "Histological Features Useful in the Distinction of Phyllodes Tumour and Fibroadenoma on Needle Core Biopsy of the Breast," *Histopathology* 51, no. 3 (September 2007): 336.

100. R. J. Barth Jr. et al., "A Prospective, Multi-institutional Study of Adjuvant Radiotherapy After Resection of Malignant Phyllodes Tumors," *Annals of Surgical Oncology* 16, no. 8 (August 2009): 2288–94; M. L. Telli et al., "Phyllodes Tumors of the Breast: Natural History, Diagnosis, and Treatment," *Journal of the National Comprehensive Cancer Network* 5, no. 3 (March 2007): 324–30.

101. M. S. Lenhard et al., "Phyllodes Tumour of the Breast: Clinical Follow-Up of 33 Cases of This Rare Disease," *European Journal of Obstetrics & Gynecology and Reproductive Biology* 138, no. 2 (2008): 217–21.

102. J. Hoon Yu et al., "Breast Diseases During Pregnancy and Lactation," *Obstetrics & Gynecology Science* 56, no. 3 (2013): 143–59.

103. M. S. Soo et al., "Tubular Adenomas of the Breast Imaging Findings with Histologic Correlation," *American Journal of Roentgenology* 174, no. 3 (2000): 757–61; M. Guray and A. A. Sahin, "Benign Breast Diseases: Classification, Diagnosis, and Management," *Oncologist* 11, no. 5 (May 2006): 435–49.

104. W. L. Donegan, "Common Benign Conditions of the Breast," in *Cancer of the Breast*, 5th ed., W. L. Donegan and J. S. Spratt (St. Louis: Saunders, 2002): 67–110; A. D. Montemarano, P. Sau, and W. D. James, "Superficial Papillary Adenomatosis of the Nipple: A Case Report and Review of the Literature," *Journal of the American Academy of Dermatology* 33 (1995): 871–75.

105. S. Jaffer, I. J. Bleiweiss, and C. Nagi, "Incidental Intraductal Papillomas (< 2 mm) of the Breast Diagnosed on Needle Core Biopsy Do Not Need to Be Excised," *Breast Journal* 19, no. 2 (2013): 130–33.

106. M. K. Sydnor et al., "Underestimation of the Presence of Breast Carcinoma in Papillary Lesions Initially Diagnosed at Core-Needle Biopsy," *Radiology* 242, no. 1 (2007): 58–62.

107. M. S. Soo, P. J. Kornguth, and B. S. Hertzberg, "Fat Necrosis in the Breast: Sonographic Features," *Radiology* 206, no. 1 (January 1998): 261–69.

108. C. de Blacam et al., "Evaluation of Clinical Outcomes and Aesthetic Results after Autologous Fat Grafting for Contour Deformities of the Reconstructed Breast," *Plastic and Reconstructive Surgery* 128, no. 5 (2011): 411e–18e.

109. B. Erguvan-Dogan and W. T. Yang, "Direct Injection of Paraffin into the Breast: Mammographic, Sonographic, and MRI Features of Early Complications," *American Journal of Roentgenology* 186, no. 3 (March 2006): 888–94.

110. S. Majedah, I. Alhabshi, and S. Salim, "Granulomatous Reaction Secondary to Intramammary Silicone Injection," *BMJ Case Reports 2013* (February 2013).

111. R. Lewin et al., "Risk Factors for Complications After Breast Reduction Surgery," *Journal of Plastic Surgery and Hand Surgery* 48, no. 1 (2014): 10–14.

112. I. J. Wagner, W. M. Tong, and E. G. Halvorson, "A Classification System for Fat Necrosis in Autologous Breast Reconstruction," *Annals of Plastic Surgery* 70, no. 5 (2013): 553–56.

113. F. Meric et al., "Long-Term Complications Associated with Breast-Conservation Surgery and Radiotherapy," *Annals of Surgical Oncology* 9, no. 6 (July 2002): 543–49; M. D. Piroth et al., "Fat Necrosis and Parenchymal Scarring after Breast-Conserving Surgery and Radiotherapy with an Intraoperative Electron or Fractionated, Percutaneous Boost: A Retrospective Comparison," *Breast Cancer* 21, no. 4 (2004): 409–14.

114. L. H. Amir et al., "Incidence of Breast Abscess in Lactating Women: Report from an Australian Cohort," *BJOG: An International Journal of Obstetrics and Gynaecology* 111, no. 12 (2004): 1378–81.

115. A. Bharat et al., "Predictors of Primary Breast Abscesses and Recurrence," *World Journal of Surgery* 33, no. 12 (December 2009): 2582–86.

116. J. D. Berna-Serna and M. Madrigal, "Percutaneous Management of Breast Abscesses. An Experience of 39 Cases," *Ultrasound in Medicine and Biology* 30, no. 1 (January 2004): 1–6.

117. J. P. Wilson et al., "Idiopathic Granulomatous Mastitis: In Search of a Therapeutic Paradigm," *American Journal of Surgery* 73 (2007): 798–802.

118. W. S. Symmers, "Silicone Mastitis in 'Topless' Waitresses and Some Other Varieties of Foreign-Body Mastitis," *British Medical Journal* 3, no. 5609 (1968): 19–22.

119. M. E. Bouton et al., "Management of Idiopathic Granulomatous Mastitis with Observation," *American Journal of Surgery* 210 (2015): 258.

120. S. Imoto et al., "Idiopathic Granulomatous Mastitis: Case Report and Review of the Literature," *Japanese Journal of Clinical Oncology* 27, no. 4 (August 1997): 274–77; A. Krause, B. Gerber, and E. Rhode, "Puerperal and Non-puerperal Mastitis," *Zentralblatt für Gynäkologie* 116, no. 8 (1994): 488–91; S. Akbulut et al., "Is Methotrexate an Acceptable Treatment in the Management of Idiopathic Granulomatous Mastitis?" *Archives of Gynecology and Obstetrics* 284, no. 5 (2011): 1189–95.

121. K. P. Hunfeld and R. Bassler, "Lymphocytic Mastitis and Fibrosis of the Breast in Long-Standing Insulin-Dependent Diabetics," *General and Diagnostic Pathology* 143, no. 1 (July 1997): 49–58.

122. W. W. Logan and N. Y. Hoffman, "Diabetic Fibrous Breast Disease," *Radiology* 172, no. 3 (1989): 667–70.

123. G. M. K. Tse et al., "Hamartoma of the Breast: A Clinicopathological Review," *Journal of Clinical Pathology* 55, no. 12 (2002): 951–54.

124. G. M. Tse et al., "Ductal Carcinoma in Situ Arising in Mammary Hamartomas," *Journal of Clinical Pathology* 55 (2002): 541–42; M. Herbert et al., "Breast Hamartomas: Clinicopathological and Immunohistochemical Studies of 24 Cases," *Histopathology* 41 (2002): 30–34.

125. R. Salvador et al., "Pseudo-angiomatous Stromal Hyperplasia Presenting as a Breast Mass: Imaging Findings in Three Patients," *Breast* 13, no. 5 (2004): 431–35.

126. C. L. Mercado et al., "Pseudoangiomatous Stromal Hyperplasia of the Breast: Sonographic Features with Histopathologic Correlation," *Breast Journal* 10, no. 5 (2004): 427–32; S. D. Raj et al., "Pseudoangiomatous Stromal Hyperplasia of the Breast: Multimodality Review with Pathologic Correlation," *Current Problems in Diagnostic Radiology* 46, no. 2 (2017): 130–35.

127. L. Celliers, D. D. Wong, and A. Bourke, "Pseudoangiomatous Stromal Hyperplasia: A Study of the Mammographic and Sonographic Features," *Clinical Radiology* 65, no. 2 (2010): 145–49.

128. G. C. Hargaden et al., "Analysis of the Mammographic and Sonographic Features of Pseudoangiomatous Stromal Hyperplasia," *American Journal of Roentgenology* 191, no. 2 (2008): 359–63.

129. A. C. Degnim et al., "Pseudoangiomatous Stromal Hyperplasia and Breast Cancer Risk," *Annals of Surgical Oncology* 17, no. 12 (2010): 3269–77.

130. E. E. Lower, H. H. Hawkins, and R. P. Baughman, "Breast Disease in Sarcoidosis," *Sarcoidosis, Vasculitis, and Diffuse Lung Diseases: Official Journal of World Association of Sarcoidosis and Other Granulomatous Disorders* 18, no. 3 (2001): 301–6.

131. P. P. Rosen, *Breast Pathology, 3rd Edition* (Philadelphia: Lippincott Williams & Wilkins, 2009).

Chapter 9: Cancer Happens: A Newly Diagnosed Starter Kit

1. C. I. Li, D. J. Uribe, and J. R. Daling, "Clinical Characteristics of Different Histologic Types of Breast Cancer," *British Journal of Cancer* 93, no. 9 (2005): 1046–52.

2. A. Bane, "Ductal Carcinoma *In Situ:* What the Pathologist Needs to Know and Why," *International Journal of Breast Cancer* 2013 (2013).

3. M. E. Sanders et al., "Continued Observation of the Natural History of Low-Grade Ductal Carcinoma In Situ Reaffirms Proclivity for Local Recurrence Even After More than 30 Years of Follow Up," *Modern Pathology: An Official Journal of the United States and Canadian Academy of Pathology, Inc.* 28, no. 5 (May 2015): 662–69.

4. S. A. Lari and H. M. Kuerer, "Biological Markers in DCIS and Risk of Breast Recurrence: A Systematic Review," *Journal of Cancer* 2 (2011): 232–61.

5. National Comprehensive Cancer Network, "NCCN Clinical Practice Guidelines in Oncology: Breast Cancer," http://www.nccn.org/professionals/physician_gls/pdf/breast.pdf.

6. B. C. Pestalozzi et al., "Distinct Clinical and Prognostic Features of Infiltrating Lobular Carcinoma of the Breast: Combined Results of 15 International Breast Cancer Study Group Clinical Trials," *Journal of Clinical Oncology* 26, no. 18 (2008): 3006–14.

7. N. Wasif et al., "Invasive Lobular vs. Ductal Breast Cancer: A Stage-Matched Comparison of Outcomes," *Annals of Surgical Oncology* 17, no. 7 (2010): 1862–69; J. G. Molland et al., "Infiltrating Lobular Carcinoma—A Comparison of Diagnosis, Management and Outcome with Infiltrating Duct Carcinoma," *Breast* 13, no. 5 (2004): 389–96.

8. I. Jatoi et al., "Breast Cancer Adjuvant Therapy: Time to Consider Its Time-Dependent Effects," *Journal of Clinical Oncology* 29, no. 17 (2011): 2301–4.

9. K. Wu et al., "Meta-analysis on the Association Between Pathologic Complete Response and Triple-Negative Breast Cancer After Neoadjuvant Chemotherapy," *World Journal of Surgical Oncology* 12, no. 1 (2014): 95.

10. C. Liedtke et al., "Response to Neoadjuvant Therapy and Long-Term Survival in Patients with Triple-Negative Breast Cancer," *Journal of Clinical Oncology* 26, no. 8 (2008): 1275–81.

11. P. Cortazar et al., "Pathological Complete Response and Long-Term Clinical Benefit in Breast Cancer: The CTNeoBC Pooled Analysis," *Lancet* 384, no. 9938 (2014): 164–72.

12. C. E. DeSantis et al., "Breast Cancer Statistics, 2015: Convergence of Incidence Rates Between Black and White Women," *CA: A Cancer Journal for Clinicians* 66, no. 1 (2016): 31–42; B. A. Kohler et al., "Annual Report to the Nation on the

Status of Cancer, 1975–2011: Featuring Incidence of Breast Cancer Subtypes by Race/Ethnicity, Poverty, and State," *Journal of the National Cancer Institute* 107, no. 6 (2015): djv048; R. M. Amimi et al., "Traditional Breast Cancer Risk Factors in Relation to Molecular Subtypes of Breast Cancer," *Breast Cancer Research and Treatment* 131 (2012): 159–67.

13. K. C. Aalders et al., "Characterisation of Multifocal Breast Cancer Using the 70-Gene Signature in Clinical Low-Risk Patients Enrolled in the EORTC 10041/ BIG 03–04 MINDACT Trial," *European Journal of Cancer* 79 (2017): 98–105; J. A. Sparano et al., "Prospective Validation of a 21-Gene Expression Assay in Breast Cancer," *New England Journal of Medicine* 373, no. 21 (2015): 2005–14.

14. J. Iqbal et al., "Differences in Breast Cancer Stage at Diagnosis and Cancer-Specific Survival by Race and Ethnicity in the United States," *Journal of the American Medical Association* 313, no. 2 (2015): 165–73; "Breast Cancer Survival Rates," American Cancer Society, last revised December 20, 2017, http://www.cancer.org/cancer /breastcancer/detailedguide/breast-cancer-survival-by-stage.

15. American Cancer Society, *Global Cancer Facts & Figures*, 3rd ed. (Atlanta: American Cancer Society, 2015), accessed September 23, 2017, https://www.cancer.org/content /dam/cancer-org/research/cancer-facts-and-statistics/global-cancer-facts-and-figures /global-cancer-facts-and-figures-3rd-edition.pdf.

16. A. M. Soto et al., "Does Breast Cancer Start in the Womb?" *Basic and Clinical Pharmacology and Toxicology* 102, no. 2 (2008): 125–33.

17. P. G. M. Peer et al., "Age-Dependent Growth Rate of Primary Breast Cancer," *Cancer* 71 (1993): 3547–51.

18. U. Del Monte, "Does the Cell Number 109 Still Really Fit One Gram of Tumor Tissue?" *Cell Cycle* 8, no. 3 (2009): 505–6.

19. H. G. Welch and W. C. Black, "Using Autopsy Series to Estimate the Disease 'Reservoir' for Ductal Carcinoma In Situ of the Breast: How Much More Breast Cancer Can We Find?" *Annals of Internal Medicine* 127, no. 11 (1997): 1023–28.

20. P. H. Zahl, P. C. Gøtzsche, and J. Mæhlen, "Natural History of Breast Cancers Detected in the Swedish Mammography Screening Programme: A Cohort Study," *Lancet Oncology* 12, no. 12 (2011): 1118–24.

21. K. D. Miller et al., "Cancer Treatment and Survivorship Statistics," *CA: A Cancer Journal for Clinicians* 66 (2016): 271–89.

22. N. Howlader et al., *SEER Cancer Statistics Review, 1975–2012* (Bethesda, MD: National Cancer Institute, 2015), http://seer.cancer.gov/csr/1975_2012.

23. D. A. Berry et al., "Effect of Screening and Adjuvant Therapy on Mortality from Breast Cancer," *New England Journal of Medicine* 353 (2005): 1784–92.

24. F. Cardoso et al., "70-Gene Signature as an Aid to Treatment Decisions in Early-Stage Breast Cancer," *New England Journal of Medicine* 375, no. 8 (2016): 717–29.

25. R. J. Simes and A. S. Coates, "Patient Preferences for Adjuvant Chemotherapy of Early Breast Cancer: How Much Benefit Is Needed?" *JNCI Monographs* 2001, no. 30 (2001): 146–52.

26. "Dose-Dense Chemotherapy Improves Outcomes in Breast Cancer," Medscape, accessed December 9, 2017, https://www.medscape.com/viewarticle/889697?nlid=119488_2202.

27. E. L. Mayer, "Early and Late Long-Term Effects of Adjuvant Chemotherapy," in *American Society of Clinical Oncology Educational Book 2013* (Houston, TX: ASCO University, 2013), 9–14, https://meetinglibrary.asco.org/record/78715/edbook.

28. I. F. Tannock et al., "Cognitive Impairment Associated with Chemotherapy for Cancer: Report of a Workshop," *Journal of Clinical Oncology* 22, no. 11 (2004): 2233–39.

29. V. Fuchs-Tarlovsky, "Role of Antioxidants in Cancer Therapy," *Nutrition* 29, no. 1 (2013): 15–21.

30. M. G. Marmot et al., "The Benefits and Harms of Breast Cancer Screening: An Independent Review: A Report Jointly Commissioned by Cancer Research UK and the Department of Health (England), October 2012," *British Journal of Cancer* 108, no. 11 (2013): 2205–40.

31. J. A. van der Hage et al, "Preoperative Chemotherapy in Primary Operable Breast Cancer: Results from the European Organization for Research and Treatment of Cancer Trial," *Journal of Clinical Oncology* 19, no. 22 (2001): 4224–37.

32. A. F. Schott and D. F. Hayes, "Defining the Benefits of Neoadjuvant Chemotherapy for Breast Cancer," *Journal of Clinical Oncology* 30, no. 15 (May 2012): 1747–49.

33. M. Chavez-MacGregor et al., "Delayed Initiation of Adjuvant Chemotherapy Among Patients with Breast Cancer," *JAMA Oncology* 2, no. 3 (2016): 322–29.

34. B. Fisher et al., "Eight-Year Results of a Randomized Clinical Trial Comparing Total Mastectomy and Lumpectomy with or Without Irradiation in the Treatment of Breast Cancer," *New England Journal of Medicine* 320 (1989): 822–28; D. Sarrazin et al., "Conservative Treatment Versus Mastectomy in Breast Cancer Tumors with Macroscopic Diameter of 20 Millimeters or Less: The Experience of the Institut Gustave-Roussy," *Cancer* 53 (1984): 1209–13; U. Veronesi et al., "Breast Conservation Is the Treatment of Choice in Small Breast Cancer: Long-Term Results of a Randomized Trial," *European Journal of Cancer* 26 (1990): 668–70; J. A. van Dongen et al., "Randomized Clinical Trial to Assess the Value of Breast-Conserving Therapy in Stage I and II Breast Cancer, EORTC 10801 Trial," *Journal of the National Cancer Institute Monograms* 11 (1992): 8–15; M. Blichert-Toft et al., "Danish Randomized Trial Comparing Breast Conservation Therapy with Mastectomy: Six Years of Life-Table Analysis. Danish Breast Cancer Cooperative Group," *Journal of the National Cancer Institute Monograms* 11 (1992): 19–25; K. Straus et al., "Results of the National Cancer Institute Early Breast Cancer Trial," *Journal of the National Cancer Institute Monograms* 27 (1992): 11–32.

35. Early Breast Cancer Trialists' Collaborative Group, "Effects of Radiotherapy and of Differences in the Extent of Surgery for Early Breast Cancer on Local Recurrence and 15-Year Survival: An Overview of the Randomised Trials," *Lancet* 366, no. 9503 (2006): 2087–2106.

36. B. Fisher et al., "Twenty-Year Follow-Up of a Randomized Trial Comparing Total Mastectomy, Lumpectomy, and Lumpectomy Plus Irradiation for the Treatment of Invasive Breast Cancer," *New England Journal of Medicine* 347, no. 16 (2002): 1233–41; J. A. van Dongen et al., "Long-Term Results of a Randomized Trial Comparing Breast-Conserving Therapy with Mastectomy: European Organization for Research and Treatment of Cancer Trial," *Journal of the National Cancer Institute*

92 (2000): 1143–50; J. A. Jacobson et al., "Ten-Year Results of a Comparison of Conservation with Mastectomy in the Treatment of Stage I and II Breast Cancer," *New England Journal of Medicine* 332 (1995): 907–11; A. D. Morris et al., "Breast-Conserving Therapy vs Mastectomy in Early-Stage Breast Cancer: A Meta-analysis of 10-Year Survival," *Cancer Journal from Scientific American* 3 (1997): 6–12; M. M. Poggi et al., "Eighteen-Year Results in the Treatment of Early Breast Carcinoma with Mastectomy Versus Breast Conservation Therapy," *Cancer* 98, no. 4 (2003): 697–702.

37. A. P. Kiess et al., "Adjuvant Trastuzumab Reduces Locoregional Recurrence in Women Who Receive Breast-Conservation Therapy for Lymph Node-Negative, Human Epidermal Growth Factor Receptor 2-Positive Breast Cancer," *Cancer* 118, no. 8 (2012): 1982–88.

38. P. L. Nguyen et al., "Breast Cancer Subtype Approximated by Estrogen Receptor, Progesterone Receptor, and HER-2 Is Associated with Local and Distant Recurrence After Breast-Conserving Therapy," *Journal of Clinical Oncology* 26, no. 14 (2008): 2373–78.

39. J. Canavan et al., "Local Recurrence in Women with Stage I Breast Cancer: Declining Rates over Time in a Large, Population-Based Cohort," *International Journal of Radiation Oncology * Biology * Physics* 88, no. 1 (2014): 80–86.

40. N. Houssami et al., "The Association of Surgical Margins and Local Recurrence in Women with Early-Stage Invasive Breast Cancer Treated with Breast-Conserving Therapy: A Meta-analysis," *Annals of Surgical Oncology* 21, no. 3 (2014): 717–30.

41. G. M. Freedman and B. L. Fowble, "Local Recurrence After Mastectomy or Breast-Conserving Surgery and Radiation," *Oncology-Huntington* 14, no. 11 (2000): 1561–80.

42. N. Houssami et al., "Meta-analysis of the Impact of Surgical Margins on Local Recurrence in Women with Early-Stage Invasive Breast Cancer Treated with Breast-Conserving Therapy," *European Journal of Cancer* 46, no. 18 (2010): 3219–32; O. Gentilini et al., "Conservative Surgery in Patients with Multifocal/Multicentric Breast Cancer," *Breast Cancer Research and Treatment* 113, no. 3 (2009): 577–83; G. M. Freedman and B. L. Fowble, "Local Recurrence After Mastectomy or Breast-Conserving Surgery and Radiation," *Oncology-Huntington* 14, no. 11 (2000): 1561–80; A. C. Voogd et al., "Differences in Risk Factors for Local and Distant Recurrence After Breast-Conserving Therapy or Mastectomy for Stage I and II Breast Cancer: Pooled Results of Two Large European Randomized Trials," *Journal of Clinical Oncology* 19, no. 6 (2001): 1688–97; I. L. Wapnir et al., "Prognosis after Ipsilateral Breast Tumor Recurrence and Locoregional Recurrences in Five National Surgical Adjuvant Breast and Bowel Project Node-Positive Adjuvant Breast Cancer Trials," *Journal of Clinical Oncology* 24, no. 13 (2006): 2028–37.

43. I. L. Wapnir, et al., "Long-Term Outcomes of Invasive Ipsilateral Breast Tumor Recurrences After Lumpectomy in NSABP B-17 and B-24 Randomized Clinical Trials for DCIS," *Journal of the National Cancer Institute* 103, no. 6 (2011): 478–88.

44. L. Kelley, M. Silverstein, and L. Guerra, "Analyzing the Risk of Recurrence After Mastectomy for DCIS: A New Use for the USC/Van Nuys Prognostic Index," *Annals of Surgical Oncology* 18, no. 2 (2011): 459–62.

45. M. S. Moran et al., "Society of Surgical Oncology–American Society for Radiation Oncology Consensus Guideline on Margins for Breast-Conserving Surgery with

Whole-Breast Irradiation in Stages I and II Invasive Breast Cancer," *International Journal of Radiation Oncology * Biology * Physics* 88, no. 3 (2014): 553–64.

46. G.M. Freedman and B. L. Fowble, "Local Recurrence After Mastectomy or Breast-Conserving Surgery and Radiation," *Oncology (Williston Park)* 14, no. 11 (November 2000): 1561–81; M. Colleoni et al., "Annual Hazard Rates of Recurrence for Breast Cancer During 24 Years of Follow-Up: Results from the International Breast Cancer Study Group Trials I to V," *Journal of Clinical Oncology* 34, no. 9 (2016): 927–35.

47. B. Gerber, M. Freund, and T. Reimer, "Recurrent Breast Cancer: Treatment Strategies for Maintaining and Prolonging Good Quality of Life," *Deutsches Arzteblatt International* 107, no. 6 (2010): 85–91; Nick Mulcahy, "The Mystery of a Common Breast Cancer Statistic," *Medscape*, August 18, 2015, https://www.medscape.com/viewarticle/849644#vp_1.

48. K. L. Kummerow et al., "Nationwide Trends in Mastectomy for Early-Stage Breast Cancer," *JAMA Surgery* 150, no. 1 (2015): 9–16.

49. C. S. Fisher et al., "Fear of Recurrence and Perceived Survival Benefit Are Primary Motivators for Choosing Mastectomy over Breast-Conservation Therapy Regardless of Age," *Annals of Surgical Oncology* 19, no. 10 (2012): 3246–50.

50. M. A. Warmuth et al., "Complications of Axillary Lymph Node Dissection for Carcinoma of the Breast: A Report Based on a Patient Survey," *Cancer* 83 (1998): 1362–68; D. Ivens et al., "Assessment of Morbidity from Complete Axillary Dissection," *British Journal of Cancer* 66, no. 1 (1992): 136–38; E. K. Yeoh et al., "Primary Breast Cancer: Complications of Axillary Management," *Acta Radiologica Oncology* 25, no. 2 (1986): 105–8.

51. A. Lucci et al., "Surgical Complications Associated with Sentinel Lymph Node Dissection (SLND) Plus Axillary Lymph Node Dissection Compared with SLND Alone in the American College of Surgeons Oncology Group Trial," *Journal of Clinical Oncology* 25 (2007): 3657.

52. L. G. Wilke et al., "Surgical Complications Associated with Sentinel Lymph Node Biopsy: Results from a Prospective International Cooperative Group Trial," *Annals of Surgical Oncology* 13, no. 4 (2006): 491–500; R. E. Mansel et al., "Randomized Multicenter Trial of Sentinel Node Biopsy Versus Standard Axillary Treatment in Operable Breast Cancer: The ALMANAC Trial," *Journal of the National Cancer Institute* 98, no. 9 (May 2006): 599–609.

53. A. E. Giuliano et al., "Axillary Dissection vs No Axillary Dissection in Women with Invasive Breast Cancer and Sentinel Node Metastasis: A Randomized Clinical Trial," *Journal of the American Medical Association* 305 (2011): 569–75.

54. T. W. F. Yen et al., "Predictors of Invasive Breast Cancer in Patients with an Initial Diagnosis of Ductal Carcinoma In Situ: A Guide to Selective Use of Sentinel Lymph Node Biopsy in Management of Ductal Carcinoma In Situ," *Journal of the American College of Surgeons* 200, no. 4 (2005): 516–26.

55. I. A. Czyszczon, L. Roland, and S. Sahoo, "Routine Prophylactic Sentinel Lymph Node Biopsy Is Not Indicated in Women Undergoing Prophylactic Mastectomy," *Journal of Surgical Oncology* 105, no. 7 (June 2012): 650–54; S. M. Nasser, S. G. Smith, and A. B. Chagpar, "The Role of Sentinel Node Biopsy in Women

Undergoing Prophylactic Mastectomy," *Journal of Surgical Research* 164, no. 2 (2010): 188–92.

56. L. De La Cruz et al., "Overall Survival, Disease-Free Survival, Local Recurrence, and Nipple–Areolar Recurrence in the Setting of Nipple-Sparing Mastectomy: A Meta-analysis and Systematic Review," *Annals of Surgical Oncology* 22, no. 10 (2015): 3241–49.

57. K. Jonsson et al., "Tissue Oxygen Measurements in Delayed Skin Flaps: A Reconsideration of the Mechanisms of the Delay Phenomena," *Plastic and Reconstructive Surgery* 82 (1988): 328–35.

58. B. Palmieri et al., "Delayed Nipple-Sparing Modified Subcutaneous Mastectomy: Rationale and Technique," *Breast Journal* 11, no. 3 (2005): 173–78.

59. S. Ghali et al., "Vascular Delay Revisited," *Plastic and Reconstructive Surgery* 119 (2007): 1735–44.

60. J. A. Jensen et al., "Surgical Delay of the Nipple–Areolar Complex: A Powerful Technique to Maximize Nipple Viability Following Nipple-Sparing Mastectomy," *Annals of Surgical Oncology* 19, no. 10 (2012): 3171–76.

61. S. L. Spear et al., "Breast Reconstruction Using a Staged Nipple-Sparing Mastectomy Following Mastopexy or Reduction," *Plastic and Reconstructive Surgery* 129, no. 3 (2012): 572–81.

62. R. M. Leach, P. J. Rees, and P. Wilmshurst, "ABC of Oxygen: Hyperbaric Oxygen Therapy," *British Medical Journal* 317, no. 7166 (1998): 1140.

63. C. R. Albornoz et al., "A Paradigm Shift in U.S. Breast Reconstruction: Increasing Implant Rates," *Plastic and Reconstructive Surgery* 131, no. 1 (2013): 15–23.

64. A. K. Alderman et al., "Racial and Ethnic Disparities in the Use of Postmastectomy Breast Reconstruction: Results from a Population-Based Study," *Journal of Clinical Oncology* 27, no. 32 (2009): 5325–30; L. Kruper et al., "Disparities in Reconstruction Rates After Mastectomy: Patterns of Care and Factors Associated with the Use of Breast Reconstruction in Southern California," *Annals of Surgical Oncology* 18, no. 8 (2011): 2158–65.

65. M. Morrow et al., "Access to Breast Reconstruction After Mastectomy and Patient Perspectives on Reconstruction Decision Making," *JAMA Surgery* 149, no. 10 (2014): 1015–21.

66. R. J. Bleicher et al., "Time to Surgery and Breast Cancer Survival in the United States," *JAMA Oncology* 2, no. 3 (2016): 330–39.

67. D. J. MacKay and A. L. Miller, "Nutritional Support for Wound Healing," *Alternative Medicine Review* 8, no. 4 (2003): 359–78.

68. P. H. Huang et al., "Emodin and Aloe-emodin Suppress Breast Cancer Cell Proliferation Through ERα Inhibition," *Evidence-Based Complementary and Alternative Medicine* (2013); L. Zhang and I. R. Tizard, "Activation of a Mouse Macrophage Cell Line by Acemannan: The Major Carbohydrate Fraction from Aloe Vera Gel," *Immunopharmacology* 35, no. 2 (1996): 119–28.

69. B. Sweeney et al., "Evidence-Based Systematic Review of Dandelion (Taraxacum Officinale) by Natural Standard Research Collaboration," *Journal of Herbal Pharmacotherapy* 5, no. 1 (2005): 79–93.

70. P. M. Kidd, "Phosphatidyl Choline as an Aid to Liver Function," *Nutrition Science News* 1 (1996): 54.

71. H. Greenlee et al., "Clinical Applications of Silybum Marianum in Oncology," *Integrative Cancer Therapies* 6, no. 2 (2007): 158–65.

72. D. J. MacKay and A. L. Miller, "Nutritional Support for Wound Healing," *Alternative Medicine Review* 8, no. 4 (2003): 359–78.

73. N. Chaiyakunapruk et al., "The Efficacy of Ginger for the Prevention of Postoperative Nausea and Vomiting: A Meta-analysis," *American Journal of Obstetrics and Gynecology* 194 (2006): 95–99.

74. S. Prapaitrakool, A. Itharat, and L. Morinda, "Citrifolia for Prevention of Postoperative Nausea and Vomiting," *Journal of the Medical Association of Thailand* 93, no. 7 (2010): S204–9.

75. J. Webster and S. Osborne, "Preoperative Bathing or Showering with Skin Antiseptics to Prevent Surgical Site Infection," *Cochrane Database of Systematic Reviews* 2 (2007).

76. S. M. Hatfield and M. Sitkovsky, "Oxygenation to Improve Cancer Vaccines, Adoptive Cell Transfer and Blockade of Immunological Negative Regulators," *Oncoimmunology* 4, no. 12 (2015): e1052934.

77. M. L. Margolis et al., "Racial Differences Pertaining to a Belief About Lung Cancer Surgery: Results of a Multicenter Survey," *Annals of Internal Medicine* 139, no. 7 (2003): 558–63.

78. A. James, C. M. Daley, and K. A. Greiner, "'Cutting' on Cancer: Attitudes About Cancer Spread and Surgery Among Primary Care Patients in the USA," *Social Science and Medicine* 73, no. 11 (2011): 1669–73.

79. H. V. Ratajczak, R. B. Sothern, and W. J. M. Hrushesky, "Estrous Influence on Surgical Cure of a Mouse Breast Cancer," *Journal of Experimental Medicine* 168 (1988): 73–83.

80. R. A. Badwe et al., "Timing of Surgery During Menstrual Cycle and Survival of Premenopausal Women with Operable Breast Cancer," *Lancet* 337 (1991): 1261–64; R. Sainsbury et al., "Timing of Surgery for Breast Cancer and Menstrual Cycle," *Lancet* 338 (1991): 391–92.

81. U. Veronesi et al., "Effect of Menstrual Phase on Surgical Treatment of Breast Cancer," *Lancet* 343 (1994): 1544–46; R. A. Badwe, I. Mittra, and R. Havaldar, "Timing of Surgery During the Menstrual Cycle and Prognosis of Breast Cancer," *Journal of Biosciences* 25, no. 1 (2000): 113–20; I. S. Fentiman, "Timing of Surgery for Breast Cancer," *International Journal of Clinical Practice* 56, no. 3 (2002): 188–90; D. Coradini et al., "Fluctuation of Intratumor Biological Variables as a Function of Menstrual Timing of Surgery for Breast Cancer in Premenopausal Patients," *Annals of Oncology* 14, no. 6 (2003): 962–64; Z. Saad et al., "Timing of Surgery Influences Survival in Receptor-Negative as Well as Receptor-Positive Breast Cancer," *European Journal of Cancer* 30A, no. 9 (1994): 1348–52; R. T. Senie et al., "Timing of Breast Cancer Excision During the Menstrual Cycle Influences Duration of Disease-Free Survival," *Annals of Internal Medicine* 115, no. 5 (1991): 337–42.

82. A. Goldhirsch et al., "Timing Breast Cancer Surgery," *Lancet* 338 (1991): 691–92;

B. Nathan et al., "Timing of Surgery for Breast Cancer in Relation to the Menstrual Cycle and Survival of Premenopausal Women," *British Journal of Surgery* 80 (1993): 43; P. Pujol et al., "A Prospective Prognostic Study of the Hormonal Milieu at the Time of Surgery in Premenopausal Breast Carcinoma," *Cancer* 91, no. 10 (2001): 1854–61; Y. Nomura et al., "Lack of Correlation Between Timing of Surgery in Relation to the Menstrual Cycle and Prognosis of Premenopausal Patients with Early Breast Cancer," *European Journal of Cancer* 35, no. 9 (1999): 1326–30; Y. Takeda et al., "Does the Timing of Surgery for Breast Cancer in Relation to the Menstrual Cycle or Geomagnetic Activity Affect Prognoses of Premenopausal Patients?" *Biomedicine and Pharmacotherapy* 57, no. 1 (2003): 96s–103s; A. Mangia et al., "Timing of Breast Cancer Surgery Within the Menstrual Cycle: Tumor Proliferative Activity, Receptor Status and Short-Term Clinical Outcome," *Journal of Experimental and Clinical Cancer Research* 17, no. 3 (1998): 317–23; G. Mondini et al., "Timing of Surgery Related to Menstrual Cycle and Prognosis of Premenopausal Women with Breast Cancer," *Anticancer Research* 17, no. 1B (1997): 787–90; K. Holli, J. Isola, and M. Hakama, "Prognostic Effect of Timing of Operation in Relation to Menstrual Phase of Breast Cancer Patient—Fact or Fallacy," *British Journal of Cancer* 71, no. 1 (1995): 124–27; N. Kroman et al., "Timing of Surgery in Relation to Menstrual Cycle Does Not Predict the Prognosis in Primary Breast Cancer," *European Journal of Surgical Oncology* 20, no. 4 (1994): 430–35; M. F. Gnant et al., "Breast Cancer and Timing of Surgery During Menstrual Cycle: A 5-Year Analysis of 385 Premenopausal Women," *International Journal of Cancer* 52, no. 4 (1992): 707–12.

83. W. L. McGuire, "The Optimal Timing of Mastectomy: Low Tide or High Tide," *Annals of Internal Medicine* 115 (1991): 401–3.

84. H. Thorpe et al., "Timing of Breast Cancer Surgery in Relation to Menstrual Cycle Phase: No Effect on 3-Year Prognosis: The ITS Study," *British Journal of Cancer* 98, no. 1 (2008): 39–44; C. S. Grant et al., "Menstrual Cycle and Surgical Treatment of Breast Cancer: Findings from the NCCTG N9431 Study," *Journal of Clinical Oncology* 27, no. 22 (2009): 3620–26; P. Pujol et al., "A Prospective Prognostic Study of the Hormonal Milieu at the Time of Surgery in Premenopausal Breast Carcinoma," *Cancer* 91 (2001): 1854–61.

85. B. Fisher et al., "Reanalysis and Results After 12 Years of Follow-Up in a Randomized Clinical Trial Comparing Total Mastectomy with Lumpectomy with or Without Irradiation in the Treatment of Breast Cancer," *New England Journal of Medicine* 333 (1995): 1456–61.

86. R. Holland et al., "Histologic Multifocality of Tis, T1–2 Breast Carcinomas: Implications for Clinical Trials of Breast-Conserving Surgery," *Cancer* 56 (1985): 979–90.

87. M. Clarke et al., "Effects of Radiotherapy and of Differences in the Extent of Surgery for Early Breast Cancer on Local Recurrence and 15-Year Survival: An Overview of the Randomised Trials," *Lancet* 366 (2005): 2087–106.

88. J. Hastings et al., "Risk Factors for Locoregional Recurrence After Mastectomy in Stage T1 N0 Breast Cancer," *American Journal of Clinical Oncology* 37, no. 5 (2014): 486–91.

89. A. McBride et al., "Locoregional Recurrence Risk for Patients with T1, 2 Breast Cancer with 1–3 Positive Lymph Nodes Treated with Mastectomy and Systemic Treatment," *International Journal of Radiation Oncology * Biology * Physics* 89, no. 2 (2014): 392–98.

90. G. Jacobson, et al., "Randomized Trial of Pentoxifylline and Vitamin E vs Standard Follow-Up After Breast Irradiation to Prevent Breast Fibrosis, Evaluated by Tissue Compliance Meter," *International Journal of Radiation Oncology* Biology* Physics* 85, no. 3 (2013): 604–8; T. B. Chiao and A. J. Lee, "Role of Pentoxifylline and Vitamin E in Attenuation of Radiation-Induced Fibrosis," *Annals of Pharmacotherapy* 39, no. 3 (2005): 516–22.

91. T. J. Whelan et al., "Long-Term Results of Hypofractionated Radiation Therapy for Breast Cancer," *New England Journal of Medicine* 362, no. 6 (2010): 513–20.

92. T. D. Smile et al., "Accelerated Partial-Breast Irradiation: An Emerging Standard of Care," *Applied Radiation Oncology*, http://appliedradiationoncology.com/articles /accelerated-partial-breast-irradiation-an-emerging-standard-of-care.

93. U. Veronesi et al., "Radiotherapy After Breast-Conserving Surgery in Small Breast Carcinoma: Long-Term Results of a Randomized Trial," *Annals of Oncology* 12 (2001): 997–1003.

94. F. Sedlmayer, F. Zehentmayr, and G. Fastner, "Partial Breast Re-irradiation for Local Recurrence of Breast Carcinoma: Benefit and Long Term Side Effects," *Breast* 22, no. 2 (August 2013): S141–46.

95. J. S. Vaidya et al., "Targeted Intraoperative Radiotherapy (TARGIT): An Innovative Approach to Partial-Breast Irradiation," *Seminars in Radiation Oncology* 15, no. 2 (April 2005): 84–91; U. Veronesi et al., "Intraoperative Radiotherapy Versus External Beam Radiotherapy for Early Breast Cancer (ELIOT): A Randomised Controlled Equivalence Trial," *Lancet Oncology* 14, no. 13 (December 2013): 1269–77.

96. C. Shah, J. Wobb, and A. Khan, "Intraoperative Radiation Therapy in Breast Cancer: Still Not Ready for Prime Time," *Annals of Surgical Oncology* 23, no. 6 (2016): 1796–98.

97. American Cancer Society, *Global Cancer Facts & Figures*, 3rd ed. (Atlanta, GA: American Cancer Society, 2015), https://www.cancer.org/content/dam/cancer-org /research/cancer-facts-and-statistics/global-cancer-facts-and-figures/global-cancer -facts-and-figures-3rd-edition.pdf.

98. M. Clarke et al., "Effects of Radiotherapy and of Differences in the Extent of Surgery for Early Breast Cancer on Local Recurrence and 15-Year Survival: An Overview of the Randomised Trials," *Lancet* 366, no. 9503 (December 2005): 2087–106.

99. E. Styring et al., "Radiation-Associated Angiosarcoma After Breast Cancer: Improved Survival by Excision of All Irradiated Skin and Soft Tissue of the Thoracic Wall? A Report of Six Patients," *Acta Oncologica* 54, no. 7 (2015): 1078–80.

100. T. Grantzau and J. Overgaard, "Risk of Second Non-Breast Cancer Among Patients Treated with and Without Postoperative Radiotherapy for Primary Breast Cancer: A Systematic Review and Meta-analysis of Population-Based Studies Including 522,739 Patients," *Radiotherapy and Oncology* 121, no. 3 (2016): 402–13.

101. C. Shah et al., "Brachytherapy-Based Partial Breast Irradiation Is Associated with Low Rates of Complications and Excellent Cosmesis," *Brachytherapy* 12, no. 4 (2013): 278–84.

102. National Comprehensive Cancer Network (NCCN), "NCCN Clinical Practice Guidelines in Oncology: Breast Cancer," https://www.nccn.org/professionals /physician_gls/default.aspx.

103. I. H. Kunkler et al., "Breast-Conserving Surgery with or Without Irradiation in Women Aged 65 Years or Older with Early Breast Cancer (PRIME II): A Randomised Controlled Trial," *Lancet Oncology* 16, no. 3 (2015): 266–73.

104. B. McCormick et al., "RTOG 9804: A Prospective Randomized Trial for Good-Risk Ductal Carcinoma In Situ Comparing Radiotherapy with Observation," *Journal of Clinical Oncology* 33, no. 7 (March 2015): 709–15.

105. M. Donker et al., "Breast-Conserving Treatment with or Without Radiotherapy in Ductal Carcinoma In Situ: 15-Year Recurrence Rates and Outcome After a Recurrence, from the EORTC 10853 Randomized Phase III Trial," *Journal of Clinical Oncology* 31, no. 32 (2013): 4054–59.

106. L. J. Solin et al., "A Multi-Gene Expression Assay to Predict Local Recurrence Risk for Ductal Carcinoma In Situ of the Breast," *Journal of the National Cancer Institute* 105, no. 10 (May 2013): 701–10.

107. C. E. DeSantis et al., "Breast Cancer Statistics, 2015: Convergence of Incidence Rates Between Black and White Women," *CA: A Cancer Journal for Clinicians* 66, no. 1 (2016): 31–42.

108. J. F. R. Robertson et al., "Fulvestrant 500 mg Versus Anastrozole 1 mg for Hormone Receptor-Positive Advanced Breast Cancer (FALCON): An International, Randomised, Double-Blind, Phase 3 Trial," *Lancet* 388, no. 10063 (2016): 2997–3005.

109. Early Breast Cancer Trialists' Collaborative Group, "Relevance of Breast Cancer Hormone Receptors and Other Factors to the Efficacy of Adjuvant Tamoxifen: Patient-Level Meta-analysis of Randomised Trials," *Lancet* 378, no. 9793 (2011): 771–84.

110. A. Howell et al., "Results of the ATAC (Arimidex, Tamoxifen, Alone or in Combination) Trial after Completion of 5 Years' Adjuvant Treatment for Breast Cancer," *Lancet* 365, no. 9453 (2005): 60–62.

111. O. Pagani, M. M. Regan, and P. A. Francis, "TEXT and SOFT Investigators; International Breast Cancer Study Group. Exemestane with Ovarian Suppression in Premenopausal Breast Cancer," *New England Journal of Medicine* 371 (2014): 1358–59.

112. C. Davies et al., "Adjuvant Tamoxifen: Longer Against Shorter (ATLAS) Collaborative Group. Long-Term Effects of Continuing Adjuvant Tamoxifen to 10 Years Versus Stopping at 5 Years After Diagnosis of Oestrogen Receptor-Positive Breast Cancer: ATLAS, a Randomised Trial," *Lancet* 381 (2013): 805–16.

113. P. E. Goss et al., "A Randomized Trial of Letrozole in Postmenopausal Women After Five Years of Tamoxifen Therapy for Early-Stage Breast Cancer," *New England Journal of Medicine* 349 (2003): 1793–802.

114. D. C. Allred et al., "Adjuvant Tamoxifen Reduces Subsequent Breast Cancer in

Women with Estrogen Receptor-Positive Ductal Carcinoma In Situ: A Study Based on NSABP Protocol B-24," *Journal of Clinical Oncology* 30, no. 12 (April 2012): 1268–73.

115. L. Fallowfield et al., "Quality of Life of Postmenopausal Women in the Arimidex, Tamoxifen, Alone or in Combination (ATAC) Adjuvant Breast Cancer Trial," *Journal of Clinical Oncology* 22, no. 21 (November 2004): 4261–71.

116. D. Slamon et al., "Adjuvant Trastuzumab in HER2-Positive Breast Cancer," *New England Journal of Medicine* 365 (2011): 1273–83.

117. H. S. Rugo et al., "Heritage: A Phase III Safety and Efficacy Trial of the Proposed Trastuzumab Biosimilar Myl-1401O Versus Herceptin," *Journal of Clinical Oncology* 34, no. 18, LBA503.

118. R. S. Finn et al., "The Cyclin-Dependent Kinase 4/6 Inhibitor Palbociclib in Combination with Letrozole Versus Letrozole Alone as First-Line Treatment of Oestrogen Receptor-Positive, HER2-Negative, Advanced Breast Cancer (PALOMA-1 /TRIO-18): A Randomised Phase 2 Study," *Lancet Oncology* 16, no. 1 (2015): 25–35; "Ribociclib Effective in Younger Breast Cancer Patients Too," Medscape, December 8, 2017, https://www.medscape.com/viewarticle/889777?nlid=119488_2202.

119. B. Warth et al., "Metabolomics Reveals That Dietary Xenoestrogens Alter Cellular Metabolism Induced by Palbociclib/Letrozole Combination Cancer Therapy," *Cell Chemical Biology* (January 2018), accessed January 30, 2018, https://doi.org/10.1016 /j.chembiol.2017.12.010.

120. H. L. McArthur and D. B. Page, "Immunotherapy for the Treatment of Breast Cancer: Checkpoint Blockade, Cancer Vaccines, and Future Directions in Combination Immunotherapy," *Clinical Advances in Hematology and Oncology* 14, no. 11 (2016): 922–33.

121. E. M. Walker et al., "Acupuncture Versus Venlafaxine for the Management of Vasomotor Symptoms in Patients with Hormone Receptor-Positive Breast Cancer: A Randomized Controlled Trial," *Journal of Clinical Oncology* 28, no. 4 (2009): 634–40.

122. T. Gansler et al., "A Population-Based Study of Prevalence of Complementary Methods Use by Cancer Survivors," *Cancer* 113, no. 5 (2008): 1048–57.

123. M. A. Richardson et al., "Complementary/Alternative Medicine Use in a Comprehensive Cancer Center and the Implications for Oncology," *Journal of Clinical Oncology* 18, no. 13 (2000): 2505–14.

124. H. S. Boon, F. Olatunde, and S. M. Zick, "Trends in Complementary/Alternative Medicine Use by Breast Cancer Survivors: Comparing Survey Data from 1998 and 2005," *BMC Women's Health* 7, no. 1 (2007): 4.

125. A. Molassiotis et al., "Use of Complementary and Alternative Medicine in Cancer Patients: A European Survey," *Annals of Oncology* 16, no. 4 (2005): 655–63.

Chapter 10: Now What? Life After Diagnosis and Treatment

1. J. L. Khatcheressian et al., "Breast Cancer Follow-Up and Management After Primary Treatment: American Society of Clinical Oncology Clinical Practice Guideline Update," *Journal of Clinical Oncology* 31, no. 7 (2012): 961–65.

2. The GIVIO Investigators, "Impact of Follow-Up Testing on Survival and Health-Related Quality of Life in Breast Cancer Patients. A Multicenter Randomized

Controlled Trial," *Journal of the American Medical Association* 271, no. 20 (May 1994): 1587–92; S. De Placido et al., "Imaging Tests in Staging and Surveillance of Non-metastatic Breast Cancer: Changes in Routine Clinical Practice and Cost Implications," *British Journal of Cancer* 116, no. 6 (2017): 821.

3. A. Lucci et al., "Circulating Tumour Cells in Non-metastatic Breast Cancer: A Prospective Study," *Lancet Oncology* 13, no. 7 (July 2012): 688–95.

4. S. J. Dawson et al., "Analysis of Circulating Tumor DNA to Monitor Metastatic Breast Cancer," *New England Journal of Medicine* 368, no. 13 (2013): 1199–209.

5. E. Grunfeld et al., "Population-Based Longitudinal Study of Follow-Up Care for Breast Cancer Survivors," *Journal of Oncology Practice* 6, no. 4 (July 2010): 174–81.

6. LIVESTRONG, *How Cancer Has Affected Post-treatment Survivors: A LIVESTRONG Report*, https://d1un1nybq8gi3x.cloudfront.net/sites/default/files/what-we-do/reports/LSSurvivorSurveyReport.pdf.

7. Z. Koak and J. Overgaard, "Risk Factors of Arm Lymphedema in Breast Cancer Patients," *Acta Oncologica* 39 (2000): 389–92.

8. P. W. Whitworth and A. Cooper, "Reducing Chronic Breast Cancer-Related Lymphedema Utilizing a Program of Prospective Surveillance with Bioimpedance Spectroscopy," *Breast Journal* 24, no. 1 (2017): 1–4, https://doi.org/10.1111/tbj.12939; A. Soran, et al., "The Iimportance of Detection of Subclinical Lymphedema for the Prevention of Breast Cancer-Related Clinical Lymphedema After Axillary Lymph Node Dissection: A Prospective Observational Study," *Lymphatic Research and Biology* 12, no. 4 (2014): 289–94; A. Laidley and B. Anglin, "The Impact of L-Dex Measurements in Assessing Breast Cancer-Related Lymphedema as Part of Routine Clinical Practice," *Frontiers in Oncology* 6 (2016); M. T. Lacomba et al., "Effectiveness of Early Physiotherapy to Prevent Lymphoedema After Surgery for Breast Cancer: Randomised, Single Blinded, Clinical Trial," *BMJ* 340 (2010): b5396.

9. T. DiSipio et al., "Incidence of Unilateral Arm Lymphoedema After Breast Cancer: A Systematic Review and Meta-analysis," *Lancet Oncology* 14, no. 6 (2013): 500–15.

10. M. T. Lacomba et al., "Effectiveness of Early Physiotherapy to Prevent Lymphoedema After Surgery for Breast Cancer: Randomised, Single Blinded, Clinical Trial," *British Medical Journal* 340 (January 2010): b5396.

11. International Society of Lymphology, "The Diagnosis and Treatment of Peripheral Lymphedema. 2009 Concensus Document of the International Society of Lymphology," *Lymphology* 42, no. 2 (2009): 51–60.

12. R. Ito and H. Suami, "Overview of Lymph Node Transfer for Lymphedema Treatment," *Plastic and Reconstructive Surgery* 134, no. 3 (2014): 548–56.

13. S. L. Showalter et al., "Lifestyle Risk Factors Associated with Arm Swelling Among Women with Breast Cancer," *Annals of Surgical Oncology* 20, no. 3 (March 2013): 842–49.

14. C. M. Ferguson et al., "Impact of Ipsilateral Blood Draws, Injections, Blood Pressure Measurements, and Air Travel on the Risk of Lymphedema for Patients Treated for Breast Cancer," *Journal of Clinical Oncology* 34, no. 7 (2015): 691–98.

15. S. Dhesy-Thind et al., "Use of Adjuvant Bisphosphonates and Other Bone-Modifying Agents in Breast Cancer," *Journal of Clinical Oncology* 35, no. 18 (June 2017): 2062–81.

16. K. D. Crew, "Prevalence of Joint Symptoms in Postmenopausal Women Taking Aromatase Inhibitors for Early-Stage Breast Cancer," *Journal of Clinical Oncology* 25, no. 25 (September 2007): 3877–83.

17. M. Seretny et al., "Incidence, Prevalence, and Predictors of Chemotherapy-Induced Peripheral Neuropathy: A Systematic Review and Meta-analysis," *PAIN* 155, no. 12 (2014): 2461–70.

18. D. Irvine et al., "The Prevalence and Correlates of Fatigue in Patients Receiving Treatment with Chemotherapy and Radiotherapy," *Cancer Nursing* 17, no. 5 (October 1994): 367–78.

19. J. E. Bower et al., "Fatigue in Breast Cancer Survivors: Occurrence, Correlates, and Impact on Quality of Life," *Journal of Clinical Oncology* 18, no. 4 (February 2000): 743–53.

20. D. S. Dizon, "Quality of Life After Breast Cancer: Survivorship and Sexuality," *Breast Journal* 15, no. 5 (September–October 2009): 500–504.

21. J. E. Dew, B. G. Wren, and J. A. Eden, "A Cohort Study of Topical Vaginal Estrogen Therapy in Women Previously Treated for Breast Cancer," *Climacteric* 6, no. 1 (March 2003): 45–52.

22. A. Kendall et al., "Caution: Vaginal Estradiol Appears to Be Contraindicated in Postmenopausal Women on Adjuvant Aromatase Inhibitors," *Annals of Oncology* 17, no. 4 (April 2006): 584–87.

23. A. Chang et al., "The Effect of Herbal Extract (EstroG-100) on Pre-, Peri- and Post-Menopausal Women: A Randomized Double-Blind, Placebo-Controlled Study," *Phytotherapy Research* 26, no. 4 (2012): 510–16.

24. V. D. E. Simone and O. Pagani, "Pregnancy After Breast Cancer: Hope After the Storm," *Minerva Ginecologica* 69, no. 6 (December 2017): 597–607.

25. H. A. Azim et al., "Safety of Pregnancy Following Breast Cancer Diagnosis: A Meta-analysis of 14 Studies," *European Journal of Cancer* 47, no. 1 (2011): 74–83.

26. P. Fani, "Breastfeeding and Breast Cancer," *Health Science Journal* 6, no. 4 (October–December 2012): 610.

27. O. G. Palesh et al., "A Longitudinal Study of Depression, Pain, and Stress as Predictors of Sleep Disturbance Among Women with Metastatic Breast Cancer," *Biological Psychology* 75, no. 1 (April 2007): 37–44.

28. F. N. Bokhari et al., "Pilot Study of a Survey to Identify the Prevalence of and Risk Factors for Chronic Neuropathic Pain Following Breast Cancer Surgery," *Oncology Nursing Forum* 39, no. 2 (March 2012): E141–49.

29. M. C. Lauridsen, P. Christiansen, and I. B. Hessov, "The Effect of Physiotherapy on Shoulder Function in Patients Surgically Treated for Breast Cancer: A Randomized Study," *Acta Oncologica* 44, no. 5 (2005): 449–57.

30. M. T. Lacomba et al., "Axillary Web Syndrome After Axillary Dissection in Breast Cancer: A Prospective Study," *Breast Cancer Research and Treatment* 117, no. 3 (2009): 625–30.

31. K. M. Mustian et al., "A 4-Week Home-Based Aerobic and Resistance Exercise Program During Radiation Therapy: A Pilot Randomized Clinical Trial," *Journal of Supportive Oncology* 7, no. 5 (September–October 2009): 158–67; I.

Cantarero-Villanueva et al., "Effectiveness of Water Physical Therapy on Pain, Pressure Pain Sensitivity, and Myofascial Trigger Points in Breast Cancer Survivors: A Randomized, Controlled Clinical Trial," *Pain Medicine* 13, no. 11 (November 2012): 1509–19.

32. P. F. Pradat et al., "Radiation-Induced Neuropathies: Collateral Damage of Improved Cancer Prognosis," *Revue Neurologique* 168 (2012): 939–50.

33. C. P. Watson and R. J. Evans, "The Postmastectomy Pain Syndrome and Topical Capsaicin: A Randomized Trial," *Pain* 51, no. 3 (December 1992): 375–79.

34. H. S. Smith and S. X. Wu, "Persistent Pain After Breast Cancer Treatment," *Annals of Palliative Medicine* 1, no. 3 (2013): 182–94.

35. T. S. Alster and E. L. Tanzi, "Hypertrophic Scars and Keloids," *American Journal of Clinical Dermatology* 4, no. 4 (2003): 235–43.

36. M. G. Khouri et al., "Cancer Therapy–Induced Cardiac Toxicity in Early Breast Cancer," *Circulation* 126, no. 23 (2012): 2749–63.

37. I. F. Tannock et al., "Cognitive Impairment Associated with Chemotherapy for Cancer: Report of a Workshop," *Journal of Clinical Oncology* 22, no. 11 (2004): 2233–39.

38. M. Ramalho et al., "Cognitive Impairment in the First Year After Breast Cancer Diagnosis: A Prospective Cohort Study," *Breast* 32 (2017): 173–78.

39. D. H. Silverman et al. "Abnormal Regional Brain Metabolism in Breast Cancer Survivors After Adjuvant Chemotherapy Is Associated with Cognitive Changes," *Proceedings of the American Society of Clinical Oncology* 22 (2003).

40. S. B. Schagen et al., "Change in Cognitive Function After Chemotherapy: A Prospective Longitudinal Study in Breast Cancer Patients," *Journal of the National Cancer Institute* 98, no. 23 (2006): 1742–45.

41. X. Chen et al., "Decision-Making Impairments in Breast Cancer Patients Treated with Tamoxifen," *Hormones and Behavior* 66, no. 2 (2014): 449–56.

42. T. A. Ahles and A. J. Saykin, "Candidate Mechanisms for Chemotherapy-Induced Cognitive Changes," *Nature Reviews: Cancer* 7, no. 3 (March 2007): 192–201.

43. R. J. Ferguson et al., "Cognitive-Behavioral Management of Chemotherapy-Related Cognitive Change," *Psycho-Oncology* 16, no. 8 (2007): 772–77.

44. Early Breast Cancer Trialists' Collaborative Group, "Tamoxifen for Early Breast Cancer: An Overview of the Randomised Trials," *Lancet* 351, no. 9114 (May 1998): 1451–67.

45. M. Schaapveld et al., "Risk of New Primary Nonbreast Cancers After Breast Cancer Treatment: A Dutch Population-Based Study," *Journal of Clinical Oncology* 26, no. 8 (March 2008): 1239–46.

46. E. Diamandidou et al., "Treatment-Related Leukemia in Breast Cancer Patients Treated with Fluorouracil-doxorubicin-cyclophosphamide Combination Adjuvant Chemotherapy: The University of Texas M.D. Anderson Cancer Center Experience," *Journal of Clinical Oncology* 14, no. 10 (October 1996): 2722–30.

47. T. Grantzau and J. Overgaard, "Risk of Second Non-breast Cancer Among Patients Treated with and Without Postoperative Radiotherapy for Primary Breast Cancer: A Systematic Review and Meta-analysis of Population-Based Studies Including 522,739 Patients," *Radiotherapy and Oncology* 121, no. 3 (2016): 402–13.

48. H. G. Björneklett et al., "A Randomised Controlled Trial of Support Group Intervention After Breast Cancer Treatment: Results on Anxiety and Depression," *Acta Oncologica* 51, no. 2 (February 2012): 198–207; H. G. Björneklett et al., "Long-Term Follow-Up of a Randomized Study of Support Group Intervention in Women with Primary Breast Cancer," *Journal of Psychosomatic Research* 74, no. 4 (April 2013): 346–53.

49. R. Jagsi et al., "Patient-Reported Quality of Life and Satisfaction with Cosmetic Outcomes After Breast Conservation and Mastectomy with and Without Reconstruction: Results of a Survey of Breast Cancer Survivors," *Annals of Surgery* 261, no. 6 (2015): 1198.

50. M. E. Mast, "Survivors of Breast Cancer: Illness Uncertainty, Positive Reappraisal, and Emotional Distress," *Oncology Nursing Forum* 25, no. 3 (April 1998): 555–62.

51. R. R. Bouknight, C. J. Bradley, and Z. Luo, "Correlates of Return to Work for Breast Cancer Survivors," *Journal of Clinical Oncology* 24, no. 3 (2006): 345–53.

52. J. H. Lee et al., "US Screening for Detection of Nonpalpable Locoregional Recurrence After Mastectomy," *European Journal of Radiology* 82, no. 3 (2013): 485–89; Early Breast Cancer Trialists' Collaborative Group, "Effects of Radiotherapy and of Differences in the Extent of Surgery for Early Breast Cancer on Local Recurrence and 15-Year Survival: An Overview of the Randomised Trials," *Lancet* 366, no. 9503 (2006): 2087–2106.

53. I. L. Wapnir et al., "Prognosis After Ipsilateral Breast Tumor Recurrence and Locoregional Recurrences in Five National Surgical Adjuvant Breast and Bowel Project Node-Positive Adjuvant Breast Cancer Trials," *Journal of Clinical Oncology* 24, no. 13 (May 2006): 2028–37.

54. S. J. Anderson et al., "Prognosis After Ipsilateral Breast Tumor Recurrence and Locoregional Recurrences in Patients Treated by Breast-Conserving Therapy in Five National Surgical Adjuvant Breast and Bowel Project Protocols of Node-Negative Breast Cancer," *Journal of Clinical Oncology* 27, no. 15 (2009): 2466–73.

55. M. Trombetta et al., "Breast Conservation Surgery and Interstitial Brachytherapy in the Management of Locally Recurrent Carcinoma of the Breast: The Allegheny General Hospital Experience," *Brachytherapy* 7, no. 1 (January–March 2008): 29–36; T. E. Alpert et al., "Ipsilateral Breast Tumor Recurrence After Breast Conservation Therapy: Outcomes of Salvage Mastectomy vs. Salvage Breast-Conserving Surgery and Prognostic Factors for Salvage Breast Preservation," *International Journal of Radiation Oncology * Biology * Physics* 63 (2005): 845–51.

56. J. O'Shaughnessy, "Extending Survival with Chemotherapy in Metastatic Breast Cancer," *Oncologist* 10, no. 3 (2005): 20–29; S. Saadatmand et al., "Influence of Tumour Stage at Breast Cancer Detection on Survival in Modern Times: Population-Based Study in 173,797 Patients" *BMJ* 351 (2015): h4901; B. Gerber, M. Freund, and T. Reimer, "Recurrent Breast Cancer: Treatment Strategies for Maintaining and Prolonging Good Quality of Life," *Deutsches Arzteblatt International* 107, no. 6 (2010): 85–91; Nick Mulcahy, "The Mystery of a Common Breast Cancer Statistic," *Medscape*, August 18, 2015, https://www.medscape.com/viewarticle/849644#vp_1.

57. A. B. Mariotto et al., "Estimation of the Number of Women Living with Metastatic

Breast Cancer in the United States," *Cancer Epidemiology and Prevention Biomarkers* 26, no. 6 (2017): 809–15.

58. Early Breast Cancer Trialists' Collaborative Group, "Effects of Chemotherapy and Hormonal Therapy for Early Breast Cancer on Recurrence and 15-Year Survival: An Overview of the Randomised Trials," *Lancet* 365, no. 9472 (2005): 1687–17.

59. F. J. Esteva et al., "Molecular Prognostic Factors for Breast Cancer Metastasis and Survival," *Seminars in Radiation Oncology* 12, no. 4 (Philadelphia: W. B. Saunders, 2002).

60. L. Natarajan et al., "Time-Varying Effects of Prognostic Factors Associated with Disease-Free Survival in Breast Cancer," *American Journal of Epidemiology* 169, no. 12 (2009): 1463–70.

61. W. F. Anderson, I. Jatoi, and S. S. Devesa, "Distinct Breast Cancer Incidence and Prognostic Patterns in the NCI's SEER Program: Suggesting a Possible Link Between Etiology and Outcome," *Breast Cancer Research and Treatment* 90, no. 2 (2005): 127–37.

62. C. Fan et al., "Concordance Among Gene-Expression–Based Predictors for Breast Cancer," *New England Journal of Medicine* 355, no. 6 (2006): 560–69.

63. S. Paik et al., "A Multigene Assay to Predict Recurrence of Tamoxifen-Treated, Node-Negative Breast Cancer," *New England Journal of Medicine* 351, no. 27 (2004): 2817–26.

64. C. Desmedt et al., "Strong Time Dependence of the 76-Gene Prognostic Signature for Node-Negative Breast Cancer Patients in the TRANSBIG Multicenter Independent Validation Series," *Clinical Cancer Research* 13, no. 11 (June 2007): 3207–14.

65. S. Friberg and S. Mattson, "On the Growth Rates of Human Malignant Tumors: Implications for Medical Decision Making," *Journal of Surgical Oncology* 65, no. 4 (1997): 284–97.

66. M. Colleoni et al., "Annual Hazard Rates of Recurrence for Breast Cancer During 24 Years of Follow-Up: Results from the International Breast Cancer Study Group Trials I to V," *Journal of Clinical Oncology* 34, no. 9 (2016): 927–35.

67. S. H. Giordano et al., "Is Breast Cancer Survival Improving?" *Cancer* 100, no. 1 (2004): 44–52.

68. S. K. Chia et al., "The Impact of New Chemotherapeutic and Hormone Agents on Survival in a Population-Based Cohort of Women with Metastatic Breast Cancer," *Cancer* 110, no. 5 (2007): 973–79.

69. H. Kennecke et al., "Metastatic Behavior of Breast Cancer Subtypes," *Journal of Clinical Oncology* 28, no. 20 (July 2010): 3271–77.

70. G. N. Hortobagyi, "Can We Cure Limited Metastatic Breast Cancer?" *Journal of Clinical Oncology* 20, no. 3 (February 2002): 620–23.

71. E. O. Hanrahan et al., "Combined-Modality Treatment for Isolated Recurrences of Breast Carcinoma," *Cancer* 104, no. 6 (2005): 1158–71.

72. M. T. Milano et al., "Oligometastases Treated with Stereotactic Body Radiotherapy: Long-Term Follow-Up of Prospective Study," *International Journal of Radiation Oncology * Biology * Physics* 83, no. 3 (2012): 878–86.

73. M. Gerlinger et al., "Intratumor Heterogeneity and Branched Evolution Revealed by Multiregion Sequencing," *New England Journal of Medicine* 366, no. 10 (2012): 883–92.

74. L. A. Diaz Jr. and A. Bardelli, "Liquid Biopsies: Genotyping Circulating Tumor DNA," *Journal of Clinical Oncology* 32, no. 6 (2014): 579–86.

75. J. Giese-Davis et al., "Decrease in Depression Symptoms Is Associated with Longer Survival in Patients with Metastatic Breast Cancer: A Secondary Analysis," *Journal of Clinical Oncology* 29, no. 4 (2010): 413–20.

76. C. S. Cleeland et al., "Pain Outcomes in Patients with Advanced Breast Cancer and Bone Metastases," *Cancer* 119, no. 4 (2013): 832–38.

77. O. Pagani et al., "International Guidelines for Management of Metastatic Breast Cancer: Can Metastatic Breast Cancer Be Cured?" *Journal of the National Cancer Institute* 102, no. 7 (2010): 456–63.

78. O. Pagani et al., "International Guidelines for Management of Metastatic Breast Cancer: Can Metastatic Breast Cancer Be Cured?" *Journal of the National Cancer Institute* 102, no. 7 (2010): 456–63.

79. L. Ross, "The Spiritual Dimension: Its Importance to Patients' Health, Well-Being and Quality of Life and Its Implications for Nursing Practice," *International Journal of Nursing Studies* 32, no. 5 (October 1995): 457–68.

80. L. E. Ross et al., "Prayer and Self-Reported Health Among Cancer Survivors in the United States, National Health Interview Survey, 2002," *Journal of Alternative and Complementary Medicine* 14, no. 8 (2008): 931–38.

81. W. Breitbart, "Balancing Life and Death: Hope and Despair," *Palliative and Supportive Care* 3, no. 1 (2005): 57–58.

82. G. T. Reker, E. J. Peacock, and P. T. Wong, "Meaning and Purpose in Life and Well-Being: A Life-Span Perspective," *Journal of Gerontology* 42, no. 1 (January 1987): 44–49.

83. S. E. Sephton et al., "Spiritual Expression and Immune Status in Women with Metastatic Breast Cancer: An Exploratory Study," *Breast Journal* 7, no. 5 (2001): 345–53.

84. S. C. Thompson and J. Pitts, "Factors Relating to a Person's Ability to Find Meaning After a Diagnosis of Cancer," *Journal of Psychosocial Oncology* 11, no. 3 (1993): 1–21.

85. M. Preau, A. D. Bouhnik, and A. G. Le Coroller Soriano, "Two Years After Cancer Diagnosis, What Is the Relationship Between Health-Related Quality of Life, Coping Strategies and Spirituality?" *Psychology, Health and Medicine* 18 (2013): 375–86.

86. B. Skinn, "The Relationship of Belief in Control and Purpose in Life to Adult Lung Cancer Patients' Information to Use Unproven Cancer Therapies," *Canadian Oncology Nursing Journal* 4 (1994): 66–71; E. J. Taylor, "Factors Associated with Meaning in Life Among Women with Recurrent Cancer," *Oncology Nursing Forum* 9 (1993): 1399–405.

87. T. L. Gall and M. W. Cornblat, "Breast Cancer Survivors Give Voice: A Qualitative Analysis of Spiritual Factors in Long-Term Adjustment," *Psycho-Oncology* 11, no. 6 (November–December 2002): 524–35.

88. H. S. L. Jim et al., "Religion, Spirituality, and Physical Health in Cancer Patients: A Meta-analysis," *Cancer* 121, no. 21 (2015): 3760–68.

89. L. H. Powell, L. Shahabi, and C. E. Thoresen, "Religion and Spirituality: Linkages to Physical Health," *American Psychologist* 58 (2003): 36–52.

90. N. Bolger et al., "Close Relationships and Adjustment to a Life Crisis: The Case of Breast Cancer," *Journal of Personality and Social Psychology* 70, no. 2 (1996): 283–94.

91. N. Pistrang and C. Barker, "The Partner Relationship in Psychological Response to Breast Cancer," *Social Science and Medicine* 40, no. 6 (1995): 789–97.

92. S. M. Bigatti et al., "Breast Cancer in a Wife: How Husbands Cope and How Well It Works," *Cancer Nursing* 34, no. 3 (May–June 2011): 193–201; C. D. Wagner, S. M. Bigatti, and A. M. Storniolo, "Quality of Life of Husbands of Women with Breast Cancer," *Psycho-Oncology* 15, no. 2 (2006): 109–20.

93. E. H. Zahlis and F. M. Lewis, "Coming to Grips with Breast Cancer: The Spouse's Experience with His Wife's First Six Months," *Journal of Psychosocial Oncology* 28, no. 1 (2010): 79–97.

94. M. Dorval et al., "Marital Stability After Breast Cancer," *Journal of the National Cancer Institute* 91, no. 1 (1999): 54–59.

95. F. M. Lewis, M. A. Hammond, and N. F. Woods, "The Family's Functioning with Newly Diagnosed Breast Cancer in the Mother: The Development of an Explanatory Model," *Journal of Behavioral Medicine* 16, no. 4 (1993): 351–70.

96. T. Weiss, "Correlates of Posttraumatic Growth in Husbands of Breast Cancer Survivors," *Psycho-Oncology* 13, no. 4 (2004): 260–68.

97. R. R. Lichtman, S. E. Taylor, and J. V. Wood, "Social Support and Marital Adjustment After Breast Cancer," *Journal of Psychosocial Oncology* 5, no. 3 (1988): 47–74.

98. S. Hughes et al., "Social Support Predicts Inflammation, Pain, and Depressive Symptoms: Longitudinal Relationships Among Breast Cancer Survivors," *Psychoneuroendocrinology* 42 (April 2014): 38–44.

99. E. Durá-Ferrandis et al., "Personality, Coping, and Social Support as Predictors of Long-Term Quality-of-Life Trajectories in Older Breast Cancer Survivors: CALGB Protocol 369901 (Alliance)," *Psycho-Oncology* 26, no. 11 (November 2017): 1914–21.

100. C. H. Kroenke et al., "Social Networks, Social Support, and Burden in Relationships, and Mortality After Breast Cancer Diagnosis in the Life After Breast Cancer Epidemiology (LACE) Study," *Breast Cancer Research and Treatment* 137, no. 1 (2013): 261–71.

101. D. M. Crookes et al., "Social Networks and Social Support for Healthy Eating Among Latina Breast Cancer Survivors: Implications for Social and Behavioral Interventions," *Journal of Cancer Survivorship* 10, no. 2 (2016): 291–301.

102. D. J. Attai et al., "Twitter Social Media Is an Effective Tool for Breast Cancer Patient Education and Support: Patient-Reported Outcomes by Survey," *Journal of Medical Internet Research* 17, no. 7 (July 2015): e188.

103. L. Norton and J. Massagué, "Is Cancer a Disease of Self-Seeding?" *Nature Medicine* 12, no. 8 (August 2006): 875–78.

104. S. Paget, "The Distribution of Secondary Growths in Cancer of the Breast," *Cancer and Metastasis Reviews* 8, no. 2 (1989): 98–101.

105. T. P. Butler and P. M. Gullino, "Quantitation of Cell Shedding into Efferent Blood of Mammary Adenocarcinoma," *Cancer Research* 35, no. 3 (1975): 512–16.

106. L. U. Thompson et al., "Dietary Flaxseed Alters Tumor Biological Markers in Postmenopausal Breast Cancer," *Clinical Cancer Research* 11, no. 10 (May 2005): 3828–35.

107. U. W. Nilsson Åberg et al., "Tamoxifen and Flaxseed Alter Angiogenesis Regulators in Normal Human Breast Tissue In Vivo," *PLoS One* 6, no. 9 (2011): e25720.

108. K. Buck et al., "Serum Enterolactone and Prognosis of Postmenopausal Breast Cancer," *Journal of Clinical Oncology* 29, no. 28 (2011): 3730–38; S. E. McCann et al., "Dietary Lignan Intakes in Relation to Survival Among Women with Breast Cancer: The Western New York Exposures and Breast Cancer (WEB) Study," *Breast Cancer Research and Treatment* 122, no. 1 (2010): 229–35; P. Guglielmini, A. Rubagotti, and F. Boccardo, "Serum Enterolactone Levels and Mortality Outcome in Women with Early Breast Cancer: A Retrospective Cohort Study," *Breast Cancer Research and Treatment* 132, no. 2 (2012): 661–68.

109. N. Guha et al., "Soy Isoflavones and Risk of Cancer Recurrence in a Cohort of Breast Cancer Survivors: The Life After Cancer Epidemiology Study," *Breast Cancer Research and Treatment* 118, no. 2 (2009): 395–405; X. O. Shu et al., "Soy Food Intake and Breast Cancer Survival," *Journal of the American Medical Association* 302, no. 22 (December 2009): 2437–43.

110. Y. Li et al., "Sulforaphane, a Dietary Component of Broccoli / Broccoli Sprouts, Inhibits Breast Cancer Stem Cells," *Clinical Cancer Research* 16, no. 9 (2010): 2580–90.

111. B. S. Cornblatt et al., "Preclinical and Clinical Evaluation of Sulforaphane for Chemoprevention in the Breast," *Carcinogenesis* 28, no. 7 (2007): 1485–90.

112. M. L. Neuhouser et al., "Vitamin D Insufficiency in a Multiethnic Cohort of Breast Cancer Survivors," *American Journal of Clinical Nutrition* 88, no. 1 (2008): 133–39.

113. J. M. Beasley et al., "Post-diagnosis Dietary Factors and Survival After Invasive Breast Cancer," *Breast Cancer Research and Treatment* 128, no. 1 (2011): 229–36.

114. S. Nechuta et al., "A Pooled Analysis of Post-diagnosis Lifestyle Factors in Association with Late Estrogen-Receptor–Positive Breast Cancer Prognosis," *International Journal of Cancer* 138, no. 9 (2016): 2088–97.

115. M. D. Holmes et al., "Aspirin Intake and Survival After Breast Cancer," *Journal of Clinical Oncology* 28, no. 9 (2010): 1467–72.

116. M. L. Kwan et al., "NSAIDs and Breast Cancer Recurrence in a Prospective Cohort Study," *Cancer Causes and Control* 18, no. 6 (August 2007): 613–20.

117. B. L. Andersen et al., "Psychologic Intervention Improves Survival for Breast Cancer Patients," *Cancer* 113, no. 12 (2008): 3450–58.

118. V. E. Frankl, *The Will to Meaning: Foundations and Applications of Logotherapy* (New York: Meridian Books, 1988).

Index

Note that *f* refers to a figure; *t*, a table.

About the Author

Dr. Kristi Funk, board-certified breast cancer surgeon and cofounder of the Pink Lotus Breast Center, is an expert in minimally invasive diagnostic and treatment methods for all types of breast disease. She has helped thousands of women through breast treatment, including well-known celebrities such as Angelina Jolie and Sheryl Crow, who have turned to her for her surgical expertise.

After graduating with distinction from Stanford University in 1991, Dr. Funk received her medical degree from the UC Davis School of Medicine. Following her surgical residency at Virginia Mason Medical Center in Seattle, Washington, she completed a surgical breast fellowship at Cedars-Sinai Medical Center in Los Angeles, where she then excelled as a surgeon and breast center director for seven years. In 2009, Dr. Funk, alongside her entrepreneurial husband, Andy Funk, opened the Pink Lotus Breast Center in Beverly Hills. The Pink Lotus Breast Center fuses state-of-the-art screening, genetic testing, diagnosis, and treatment with preventive strategies and holistic, compassionate care.

Dr. Funk is also the founding ambassador of the Pink Lotus Foundation, whose mission is to provide low-income, uninsured, and underinsured women free access to breast cancer screening and care.

When not appearing as a breast expert and TV personality in hundreds of television segments, documentaries, news articles, and stories, Dr. Funk enjoys Half Ironman triathlon races, vegan cooking, and card games. She resides with Andy and their three sons in Santa Monica, a peaceful suburb of Los Angeles.